THE FIRST YEAR

Heart Disease

THE FIRST YEAR

Heart Disease

An Essential Guide for the Newly Diagnosed

Lawrence D. Chilnick

Da Capo
LIFE
LONG

A Member of the Perseus Books Group

Designed by BackStory Design
Set in 10.75 point Fairfield Light by BackStory Design

Cataloging-in-Publication data for this book is available from the Library of Congress.

First Da Capo Press edition 2008
ISBN-10:1-60094-029-3
ISBN-13: 978-1-60094-029-3

Published by Da Capo Press
A Member of the Perseus Books Group
www.dacapopress.com

Note: The information in this book is true and complete to the best of our knowledge. This book is intended only as an informative guide for those wishing to know more about health issues. In no way is this book intended to replace, countermand, or conflict with the advice given to you by your own physician. The ultimate decision concerning care should be made between you and your doctor. We strongly recommend you follow his or her advice. Information in this book is general and is offered with no guarantees on the part of the authors of Da Capo Press. The authors and publisher disclaim all liability in connection with the use of this book. The names and identifying details of people associated with events described in this book have been changed. Any similarity to actual persons is coincidental.

Da Capo Press books are available at special discounts for bulk purchases in the United States by corporations, institutions, and other organizations. For more information, please contact the Special Markets Department at the Perseus Books Group, 2300 Chestnut Street, Suite 200, Philadelphia, PA 19103, or call (800) 255-1514, or e-mail special.markets@perseusbooks.com.

1 2 3 4 5 6 7 8 9

To my children, Susanna and Jeremy

For your love, support, and caring
during these hard years

Remember, your health future is now.

I'm so proud of you.

Acknowledgments

Many, many people are responsible for my return to health over more than a decade. Each of them helped guide me back from the abyss of negative health behavior, taught me how to change it, and supported me at virtually every stage of my progress. It is difficult to thank one more than the other.

Over the past decade, I have had the enormous good fortune to be treated by some of the best doctors in the country, all of whom have cared for me and, in some cases, have become my friends and important sources for this book. These doctors are great advocates for change in all their patients and have worked tirelessly to improve our country's health.

Curt Rimmerman, M.D., of the Cleveland Clinic, my cardiologist and my advisor on this book, has turned my health around with his "challenges." He is one of the great doctors at the world-renowned Clinic's Heart and Cardiovascular Institute. They are lucky to have him, and I am fortunate to have found him. He has always responded quickly to questions and pointed me in the right direction. I cannot thank him enough.

Another great doctor who has influenced me tirelessly, supported and cared about me, prodded me to eat well, exercise, and "stick with the program" is Lorraine K. Doyle, M.D., an orthopedic surgeon extraordinaire.

Harold M. Solomon, M.D., in Boston has been my own and my family's physician for decades. He is a consummate clinician who communicates the message of wellness to his patients. Through the decades, he has been the person I call first. He never fails to support and to amaze me with just the right advice.

At a time when I was not sure I would survive, Robert Hanich, M.D., my cardiologist, along with Ron Caldwell, M.D., and Jeffrey Russell, M.D., in Asheville, NC, did not let up on me until I became more compliant. They inspired me to begin changing and to have hope.

Three New Jersey physicians literally saved my life early in my battle with cardiovascular disease. I will be forever grateful to my internist, Amy Rosenberg, M.D., my cardiologist, Michael Lux, M.D., and my bypass surgeon, John M. Brown, III, M.D. A very special thanks goes to Assef Ali, M.D., my former internist here in Vermilion, OH, who helped turn things around for me through his gentle manner and skills. I miss him. Thank you also to Rochelle Rosen, M.D., for her insights and advice on how to navigate an ER when your life is at stake. Also, thanks to my stress-busting guru, Andrew Slaby, M.D.

Anyone who is recovering from heart disease must have a personal support team who will always be there simply because they love you. I have been lucky to have such a group in my life. Not all of them are related by blood, but they are certainly related by the kind of "family" love and caring that is rare. A very special thanks, despite everything, for years of help way beyond the call of duty is owed to Janet Chilnick, who was by my side and with me through the years after my heart attack and during my recovery from surgery. She was selfless and is a truly good person. Others among my unofficial support group who were there for me when I first became ill include Dianne Macpherson, my sister Judy Chilnick, my other "sister", Moya Shoemaker, Sue Chorost, Susan Campbell, and Dr. Louis Petrillo. Thanks, also, to Julie Heim and Kevin Mooney at the Cleveland Clinic.

No book comes to life through the efforts of a single person. This one is no different. First and foremost, my deepest thanks go to the brilliant Patricia Fernberg, whose editorial skills, thoughtful suggestions, intelligence, knowledge, humor, and encouragement constantly saved the day and helped shape the text. Joe Kanaz, both a friend and a colleague, created the illustrations for the book. Just one look will tell you how special, talented, and smart he is. Steve Travaras, also a great friend, contributed the author photo. Thank you very much, Rae Ann Houghton: Your skills, dedication, and hard work brought this book to the finish line smoothly and on time. Others who have been essential are Martin Kanovsky, M.D., a Washington, DC, cardiologist who is both brilliant and funny, and Michael Crawford, the supervisor of the cardio-rehabilitation program at the Cleveland Clinic, whose insights and help were right on target.

During the writing of this book, I joined the Vermilion Weight Watchers group and fell under the spell of three marvelous people who also influenced my recovery more than they know. Becky Pragg, Denise Carreon, and Rachel Donley prodded me, made me laugh, and put me on the right weight-loss/back-to-health track, which is now a permanent part of my life. They never let me give up on myself. Thank you, ladies, for all those Thursday-night weigh-ins and meetings!

I am especially grateful to Katie McHugh, my editor at Da Capo; a number of sources at Barnes-Jewish Hospital in St. Louis; my friend and teacher Bert Stern; Linda Richards at OTR; the staff at the American Heart Association; the March of Dimes; and multiple EP lab directors from New England to California who talked to me about the more controversial issues in cardiac catheterization today. Their willingness to give me data helped shape some of the important recommendations in this book.

In the great tradition of publishing—saving the ones who have really believed in you longest for the last, but not least—my undying gratitude goes to my mentor, the legendary Toni Burbank; my brother-in-arms, Michael Carlisle; and, especially, my patient, sympathetic, and always optimistic agent, Colleen O'Shea. Colleen, you supported, trusted, and stood up for me, but thank you most for your friendship.

One last thanks goes to Mr. Sneakers, who never left my side during the writing of this book—even though he was asleep 90 percent of the time.

Contents

ACKNOWLEDGMENTS   vii
FOREWORD BY CURTIS M. RIMMERMAN,
   M.D., M.B.A, F.A.C.C.   xv
INTRODUCTION   xix

DAY 1

  Living: Pay Attention to the Red Flags   1
  Learning: Life Catches Up to You: Risk Factors   9

DAY 2

  Living: What Is Heart Disease?   24
  Learning: Heart Disease Is Not Limited to Coronary
    Artery Disease   36

DAY 3

  Living: Your Heart Is More Than a Pump   51
  Learning: Understanding the Circulatory System   60

DAY 4

  Living: Choosing a Cardiologist   65
  Learning: Getting a Second Opinion   76

DAY 5

  Living: How Do I Know I Have Heart Disease?   81
  Learning: How to Survive a Heart Attack   89

DAY 6

Living: Heart Attack Recovery   106
Learning: Recovery from Heart Bypass Surgery   119

DAY 7

Living: What to Expect Emotionally   128
Learning: The Family Impact   138

FIRST WEEK MILESTONES   147

WEEK 2

Living: Returning to Sex and Intimacy   149
Learning: ED Medications: Are They for You or Your Partner? 155

WEEK 3

Living: Women and Heart Disease   160
Learning: Pregnancy and Heart Disease   174

WEEK 4

Living: Congenital and Acquired Heart Disease   178
Learning: Gaining a Global Perspective   185

FIRST MONTH MILESTONES   193

MONTH 2

Living: Getting Control: Take Inventory   195
Learning: Getting Control: Making a Game Plan   203

MONTH 3

Living: Quitting Smoking   211
Learning: Lowering Your Cholesterol   223

MONTH 4

Living: Obesity   231
Learning: Losing Weight and Keeping It Off   238

MONTH 5

Living: Exercising the Right Way   255
Learning: Choosing the Right Equipment   262

MONTH 6

Living: Stressed Out!   268

Learning: Getting a Grip on Your Stress   273

SIX MONTH MILESTONES   279

MONTH 7

Living: Alternative Medicine   281

Learning: What Alternative Treatments Can Help—
or Hurt—My Heart?   290

MONTH 8

Living: Taking Your Heart Medication   296

Learning: Quick-Reference Medication Chart   303

MONTH 9

Living: Dining Out and Traveling   321

Learning: Living Alone   327

MONTH 10

Living: Keeping Your Costs in Check   333

Learning: Navigating the Health-Care System   337

MONTH 11

Living: Will I Need a Heart Transplant?   344

Learning: What's on the Horizon?   347

MONTH 12

Living: Healthy Cooking, Healthy Living   352

Learning: Organizations and Websites   362

GLOSSARY   367

BIBLIOGRAPHY   375

INDEX   381

Foreword

Heart disease is the number-one killer in the developed world. Despite this, the diagnosis of heart disease is not necessarily an imminent death sentence. In fact, it may be an opportunity to inventory your lifestyle and risk factors and to modify and eliminate detrimental health habits.

A diagnosis of heart disease can be a blessing in disguise. It can provide the impetus for a healthier you. Why is this so important? A sustained lifestyle-modification program has been proven to reduce the incidence of future heart attacks and heart attack death rates. Keep in mind that more people live with, than die from, heart disease.

As a "heart disease" patient, lifestyle changes include efforts to lower body mass index, blood pressure, cholesterol and triglyceride values, and blood sugar; engage in a regular exercise regimen; and stop smoking. These require an ongoing commitment to making healthier choices and developing good, sustainable health habits.

What is the role of medications in all this? Like lifestyle modifications, medications reduce heart attack and death rates. However, since drug therapy is only about 50 percent of the puzzle, relying solely on the benefits of medications can be a significant mistake. Instead, working closely with your physician to develop a joint program of lifestyle modifications and appropriate medication therapy is your path to success.

This book was written by someone who is successfully traveling such a path to good heart health. Larry Chilnick has written this book to inspire others to travel the same path. Not only does he interject his own true life experiences, which offers credence to the subject, but the information presented is based on carefully conducted research at leading medical centers around the world.

Larry Chilnick understands the experience of heart disease firsthand. I know Larry well, as I am his cardiologist. He has survived both a heart attack and subsequent coronary bypass surgery.

I first met Larry when he was overweight with sky-high blood sugar. His diet was a roulette wheel devoid of conscious planning. Exercise and Larry were like oil and water. He took his medications, but that was about it. He was clearly headed in the wrong direction, health-wise.

One day, Larry was in my office complaining of shortness of breath. His lungs sounded congested, and he had an early form of congestive heart failure. Congestive heart failure can be a dire development, especially in a patient who has already had a heart attack and bypass surgery, as Larry had. That was when Larry and I had one of several serious conversations as to what changes were absolutely necessary for him to make to lead a long, healthy life.

Larry eloquently describes his heart journey—both ups and downs—in this book. Even after he had surgery, his lifestyle efforts were a low priority. Finally, after deep introspection, he developed a renewed focus and will to live. In this book, Larry relates how he reprioritized his health and family. He now understands that without good health, a career is meaningless.

Larry's health transformation is truly remarkable. He has become a faithful exerciser. He now meticulously reads food labels and takes the time to research recipes. He allocates the time to cook healthy meals using fresh ingredients. Larry's weight has plummeted, as has his blood pressure. His diabetes is now well under control. Most important, he is happier and he has more energy and improved self-esteem. Larry exudes confidence and is tackling new projects left and right, on his terms and on his timeline.

Larry's story is a success. Yours can be, too. Read this book, follow Larry's journey, and learn from his mistakes and successes. Listen to and adopt Larry's recommendations. It's all about implementing a disciplined and sustainable heart-healthy game plan. You, too, can achieve this.

Curtis M. Rimmerman, M.D., M.B.A, F.A.C.C.
Gus P. Karos Chair in Clinical Cardiovascular Medicine
Medical Director, Cleveland Clinic Westlake,
Lakewood, and Avon Pointe
Cleveland Clinic,
Cleveland, OH

Introduction

○ More than 2,500 Americans die from heart disease each day.

○ More than 79,400,000 Americans have one or more forms of heart disease.

○ Every 20 seconds, a person in the U.S. has a heart attack.

○ Heart disease kills more women over age 25 than the next four diseases together.

○ More than 105 million adults in the U.S. have high, unsafe levels of cholesterol.

○ At least 250,000 people die of heart attacks each year *before* they reach a hospital.

○ Each year 152,000 heart attack victims are under age 65.

○ Six-and-a-half million Americans suffer from **angina** (severe cardiac pain).

○ There are 71,300,000 Americans with one or more forms of **coronary artery disease**.

Despite these grim statistics illustrating the threats to our health and economy from the spread of heart disease in baby boomers, younger adults, and the emergence of troubling high-risk symptoms among children and adolescents, heart disease is not the twenty-first century version of the plague. In fact, from 1994 to 2004, the death rate from coronary artery disease declined by 33 percent.

As a 60-year-old male with a family history of heart disease whose first heart attack occurred at age 48 and who had a quadruple bypass at age 54, I can assure you that heart disease *can* be overcome. In fact, in many cases like mine, you will lead a better, healthier life than ever before. This book will show you how you, too, can regain your optimum health, despite having heart disease.

The first step to recovering your health is to recognize that you need to develop both personal insight and medical knowledge. A vast majority of Americans suffer from what the former U.S. Surgeon General Richard H. Carmona, M.D. calls "health illiteracy." Overcoming health illiteracy and dispelling health myths that you have accepted over the years is the place to begin. In this book, you will learn everything you must know about heart disease to improve your life and the personal skills you must embrace to develop a positive "health-style."

Of course, this is not a simple task. It took me a decade of struggle just to recover my health and, as with virtually all chronic illness, there is no magic solution. It is easy to live badly with heart disease, but not easy to live well; yet you *can* regain your health over a period of time, and in this book, I will show you how. If one theme runs through this book, it is this:

You are not alone, and if you take charge, your recovery will be smoother and more successful. While this might be a cliché, it is true, and I am living proof of it.

When your cardiologist or surgeon puts you on a clearly planned path to health, you must stay on it. You have to *want* to stay on this road, a task that varies in difficulty for everyone. The challenges can be complex. For example, you may have had a **myocardial infarction (heart attack)** that damaged the heart muscle permanently. Or you may have **cardiovascular disease (CVD)** that puts you at risk for a stroke from a blood clot. Each day, you may be required to take multiple medications (I take ten) with **side effects** that range from **gastrointestinal distress (e.g., stomachache, diarrhea, constipation), erectile dysfunction (ED)**, or random headaches that can keep you in bed all day. You cannot get better unless you make some alterations in your lifestyle, such as losing weight and getting regular exercise. As you do this, you will develop personal insight into your health behavior that will not only help you, but will reduce health risks for your entire family.

Most cardiologists have multifaceted practices that include nutritional guidance, medication monitoring, and **cardio-rehab classes** led by specially trained nurses and other staff. As you gradually take advantage of these services, your cardiologist will become a big part of your life. However, cardiologists will tell you that a large percentage of their patients—especially middle-aged adults—are in denial. Other patients actually think that if they have survived an initial cardiac event, they are *more invulnerable* than ever. That was me, a cardio-idiot, and you do not want to be one.

How to Use This Book

This book does not have traditional chapters. Instead, your road to recovery is presented in days, then weeks, and months, with more information offered at each stage. This is a journey that you will find is best measured in time units. Anyone whose life has suddenly been transformed medically will be best served by absorbing information slowly. It begins symbolically, with the first day you are diagnosed and you are dealing with or recovering from heart disease. For example, in the **Day One** section, you can learn to assess your risk factors, understanding those you can, and those you cannot, control. You will also find a brief overview of various types of heart disease. Later, as you go deeper into the weeks and months, related information is presented in depth.

The days, weeks, and months also are organized into sections called "Living" and "Learning." For me, this is a logical way to understand what is going on in the journey to wellness. For example, in **Month Two**, you will find "Living" information discussing general steps to modify previous health behavior. The "Learning" section then provides concrete information about behavior modification, along with the specific resources you will need.

I like to think of the organization of this book as a good meal. The opening first days are the appetizers. The next four weeks are the soup and salad courses, while the rest of the months of the first year are a hearty meal. Dessert follows in the form of print and Internet resources, a bibliography, and a glossary.

The Benefits for You in This Book

○ Because no one can overcome heart disease alone, this book will help you build successful relationships with your family and your team of medical professionals. Just as management of diabetes relies on a team consisting of the physician, patient, nutritionist, and certified diabetes educator to maintain **glucose** balance, heart disease requires a team to treat and control it properly. Working with a cardiologist whom you trust and respect is vital. Key to a successful recovery is having supportive people at home who can adapt to the change in your diet or the effects of your medications.

○ It will help you recognize your current risk factors or those that got you into trouble in the first place. This book will help you to look at your past family history with eyes wide open.

○ As you go through the chapters, you will find the tools to rebuild your life to a healthy heart state. You will also find that learning to use these tools requires you to take ownership of the process. For example, you will need to know how to control your stress, maintain compliance with your medication schedule, and lose weight. You will also need to learn basic nutrition and to adapt your dietary patterns accordingly, possibly reducing salt and sugar intake. You might also want to learn how to cook, which usually results in a much healthier way of eating by helping you to control blood pressure and glucose levels and promote weight loss (**see Month Four**).

○ *The greatest benefit, however, will be the change in you!* You will learn how others have discovered that having heart disease does not mean life is over. It does not mean that you can't go back to work, play golf or tennis, have your favorite food again, enjoy an intimate relationship, or live out a normal life. In fact, regular or daily exercise is a key factor in recovery, so you can, as I have, be in better physical condition than you have been in many years.

Information You Can Use Every Day

How Your Heart Works

There are many other specific benefits in this book to help you during your first year of recovery. These include learning about the multiple causes and results of **coronary artery disease (CAD)**. Fully understanding the various disorders that frequently accompany heart disease, such as diabetes and hypertension, will also help you to balance your life to accommodate the multiple treatments you are undergoing. Of course, a wide variety of heart disorders, such as congestive heart failure, arrhythmias, and congenital defects, also are explained.

A lot of people know how to drive a car, but not that many know why the engine works to keep us going down the road. In general, we don't need that information. However, when it comes to heart disease, you must have a good basic understanding of how your heart works. There are many reasons, which are discussed fully in **Days Two and Three,** but one is obvious. Knowing how your heart works helps you pick up physical cues, like certain types of chest pain, that tell you when to seek medical help. In addition, your ability to communicate with your doctor will increase enormously. Physicians may unintentionally communicate with us using a great deal of medical jargon. They will show us an x-ray or a scan that we are somehow supposed to understand. Some physicians may only tell us what they think we need to know to be treated properly. You have to be on a level playing field with your doctor when it comes to communication.

Earlier, I referred to taking charge. This includes learning about the heart's anatomical structure and functions and how any damage to it affects your entire body. You have to know what degree of heart damage and level of risk you have in relation to how the heart actually works. By doing this—by becoming a better patient—you will have taken responsibility for your role in recovery.

Overcoming Bad Health Habits

Negative health behaviors developed over a lifetime can be overcome with the techniques and information in these pages. For example, do you snack in response to stress? Your health behaviors reflect on the health culture of your family. Learning how you can assess these behaviors and turn them around is another benefit found in these pages.

Do you smoke? It's the number-one negative health behavior responsible for those who develop heart problems: As difficult as it is to give up cigarettes, it can be done. In fact, if there is one negative health behavior you have to change, this is it.

Your Relationship with Your Partner

Heart disease can affect relationships in many ways. You are going to need your family to form a support group, but CAD can put unexpected strain on your personal relationships. Fear is a common emotion for both partners after an initial diagnosis or a heart attack. It takes time to adjust to a new lifestyle, but the healthy partner can overreact by watching every bite you take or by standing over you with a stopwatch to ensure that you are doing your exercises properly. You must remember that there are two sides to this story. You are adjusting to a life with heart disease and your partner is just beginning to learn how to manage life with your CAD. He or she also is terrified. This concern extends to sexuality, where function and libido may be affected psychologically and by your medication. Too often, couples don't recognize that when these sorts of interpersonal problems arise, seeking professional help is a must.

Women and Heart Disease

Heart disease among women is now so widespread that it is the leading cause of death in this population. Why has this happened? What can a woman do to mitigate her risk of further disease? What are unique symptoms for women, and which treatments are most effective? This and other CVD information relating to ethnic and racial populations is fully discussed in **Week Three** to provide a complete picture of CAD.

Alternative Medicine

Alternative medicine is widely talked and written about, but it's not easy to assess its value. Alternative treatments can range from simple vitamins and natural supplements to special diets, to yoga and tai chi, and to other approaches that advocates may claim are magic bullets. The reality is that there is a role for alternative medicine when it's combined with traditional medical treatment. This approach, advocated by such experts as Andrew Weil, M.D., is also referred to as **integrative medicine**. While there are many new treatments and medications introduced regularly, the magic bullet for heart disease is actually you and how you approach your first year and the rest of your life. (**See Month Seven.**)

Unique Challenges

There are some unique challenges you may have to face that this book will help you overcome. Living alone can make positive health behavior difficult. It doesn't have to be so, and some concrete ideas for a heart-healthy life in any environment are found in **Month Nine**. Anyone who has a disorder that requires a special diet or keeping track of medication can find this challenging if they live alone. Having lived alone for more than a decade, I know that you need practical ideas to combat heart disease in this situation.

Dining Out

What about eating out or traveling? It's fine to commit to a program created by your cardiologist and a nutritionist to help you maintain your health, but we live in the real world. It is not always easy to stick with a plan if you have to take clients out to lunch or you need to spend a few days on the road attending meetings where your meal choices are limited. Beyond sharing my personal experience and the solutions I've reached, you will learn how others have coped with this very difficult challenge.

The good news is that virtually everyone who has heart disease can find a path to better health. That is the goal of this book. Within its pages are the things you must know about heart disease in your first year, how to create a recovery plan, and how to stick with it. It has been said that anyone's life can turn on a dime. If you are reading this book, it is likely your life has recently turned 180 degrees, and you may be quite alarmed, if not terrified. Heart disease is not a pleasant diagnosis. But even though your life as you know it may have changed, it is not over, by any means.

living

Pay Attention to
the Red Flags

TWELVE YEARS ago, I was the poster boy for the sort of health behavior that results in everyone's worst nightmare: open heart surgery and the sort of close encounter with the grim reaper that you are better off without. Today, I hope I'm the poster boy for what the health-care community and you can do to turn your life around. However, you can only succeed if you are lucky enough to have the sort of medical and family support system that makes you understand why your life is worth struggling to preserve. I was, and still am, a lucky person. I had that support. Still, no matter how good the team is, if you aren't motivated, you need to be prepared to live out the rest of your days as a cardiac-cripple. It literally took me a decade to decide that I wanted to live again.

Many people with heart disease have stories similar to mine, and perhaps you do, too. If you do not, and perhaps you have just been diagnosed with heart disease, I hope you will recognize that you can avoid my real-life worst-case scenario.

Pay Attention to the Red Flags

Before you read further, keep this in mind: The main health behavior that probably saved my life is that I never smoked, or drank anything more than an occasional glass of wine or a beer. Largely this is because no one in my family smoked or drank. So if you smoke, you *must* stop now. Drinking, especially a glass of red wine, can be beneficial. Of course, check with your doctor. However, my family history was still a major factor in the events leading to my heart problems.

As a child, I grew up in a household where the concept of healthy living referred to playing pick-up sports. My parents were professionals who worked long hours, and dinner was almost always a carbohydrate-loaded meal, such as spaghetti and meatballs, frozen TV dinners, artery-clogging brisket, or matzo ball soup. We had so much junk food around the house that kids from the neighborhood would drop by to raid our cabinets. Still, as an active adolescent, through college, and into my 30s, I was very healthy. At age 45, I was 5'7" tall and weighed 140 pounds.

The first red flag that I missed, and that we all ignored, came in 1965 during my senior year in high school. My mother, at age 48, suddenly had a heart attack. While we were all shocked, she recovered and life went on. For the next 20 years, my family's health remained stable until my father developed kidney disease, which resulted in his death in 1983. The following year, my mother had a second heart event while visiting my sister in Los Angeles, resulting in a bypass operation. We learned then that she had been suffering from angina and other symptoms, but had ignored them because she was caring for my father during his lengthy illness: This was the second red flag that I missed.

Eight years later, in 1992, my mother (who now lived with us) had another event, and, after considerable debate, reluctantly agreed to a second bypass operation. The surgery had been accurately described as high risk, and it was. After the surgery, my mother spent six weeks in the intensive care unit. Then, six weeks after coming home, she had a massive stroke and died two days later. What is most remarkable to me now is that no physician mentioned the words "family history" and "high risk" to me until a year later. My mother had had heart disease for almost three decades, and neither my sister nor I was counseled or referred to a **cardiologist**: This was the third red flag.

Are you, or were you, in the same situation? Are you a proverbial cardiac time bomb, ignoring the red flags that tell you where the landmines are buried? You could be, since, according to **the American Heart Asso-**

ciation, 71,300,000 Americans have at least one form of cardiovascular disease (CVD) at any given time.

Fortunately, a year after my mother passed away, I was feeling lousy and went to see my family physician. I hadn't had a complete evaluation in years, and to my surprise, I had **high blood pressure** for the first time in my life. My **cholesterol** was practically orbiting Saturn at about 500 mg/dL, about 300 mg/dL above the high end of the acceptable level. "Get thee to a cardiologist" was the message.

This time, I saw the final red flag flying. It clearly indicated, "You are at high risk for a heart attack." This time it got my attention, 30 years after my mother had her first heart attack. From adolescence to middle age, I had done nothing to reduce my risk factors.

Was it lack of knowledge? Not really. The truth is more complicated, since I was a professional medical writer and publisher, and the creator of a 16 million–copy bestseller, *The Pill Book*. I had intellectual knowledge, but I had a much greater sense of denial and very little insight into myself. I never really connected what I read and wrote about to my own family history.

Where Was the Tough Love When I Needed It?

My newly acquired cardiologist welcomed me with what I now see was a much too gentle lecture and explanation of what I had to do. It was too simple: Change my diet, get nutritional counseling, which his practice provided, and stay active. He gave me a prescription for **nitroglycerin**, which I was to pop under my tongue if I felt angina pain (angina pectoris), and after talking to the nutritionist, I was on my way. "If you feel any severe chest pain, take one of these pills and get to a hospital," the doctor said.

Unfortunately, that was probably the worst thing I could have been told. The cardiologist didn't scare me, nor did he really emphasize the role my family history played in my level of risk. I simply vowed to stay out of his way. I was living under the deluded philosophy, "what you don't know can't kill you."

Studies indicate that stress has an effect on heart disease (see **Month Six**), and I am sure that what happened next pushed me over the edge. In the late spring of 1995, I had more than enough stressors in my life. My mother's drawn-out death and my draining divorce were the stressors you could see above the waterline. Work was a never-ending source of pressure. During this period, I was a publisher and vice president for new product development in a large, multinational professional book company. I was preparing a major presentation for the entire editorial board that would determine the next year's budget. The meeting had been cancelled several times, and my job was riding on this meeting.

The night before the meeting, as I rehearsed my talk, I began to experience the worst indigestion I'd ever had. Since I lived alone and didn't want to bother anyone else with it, I spent the night sucking on nitroglycerin, sleeping on and off. I knew it was not indigestion, but since I was conscious and breathing, I figured I was going to be OK.

This is also where I won first prize in the "What Were You Thinking?" contest; in fact, I made another of the worst mistakes of my life. The next morning, I got up and went to work. The moment I walked into the office, my assistant did a double take and said, "You have turned gray. Let's go to the hospital now!" Incredibly, I went to the meeting instead, managed to do my presentation, and *only then* went to the hospital.

It didn't take long for my cardiologist to confirm that I'd had a **myocardial infarction (MI)**, and he wanted to admit me to the hospital immediately. If the story is hard to believe thus far, it gets worse.

"I don't want to be hospitalized," I told him. "It's 24 hours from when I got sick, and I'm not dead. I'm out of here." After signing papers releasing the doctor and the hospital from liability, I left AMA (against medical advice), and went home. Unfortunately, no one picked up on one very salient point. *I was 48 years old—about the same age my mother was when she'd had her first heart attack.* That might have gotten my attention. Still, there was undeniable evidence that I was suffering from heart disease, even if I did not or could not understand just how serious my situation was. First, if I had gone to the hospital when I'd first felt ill, I would have been given an **intravenous clot buster** to mitigate any heart muscle damage. While the damage appeared to be minor, a complete diagnosis could have been made by a relatively simple procedure, **cardiac catheterization,** also known as an **angiogram.** Instead, later that week, I found another cardiologist who would, on the basis of lab tests, treat me medically (meaning lots of pills) and see me every three months.

Finally, Someone Gets My Attention

Ironically, it was not the heart disease that began to turn things around. It was my undiagnosed diabetes. Three years after my MI, I was experiencing shortness of breath. After a few simple tests, my internist walked into the exam room and delivered some unpleasant news. Not only was I now a **type 2 diabetic** (known then as **adult onset diabetes**), but the shortness of breath was really a symptom of angina. Rather than chest pain, diabetics may experience shortness of breath as a significant cardiac symptom. It was time for a complete cardiac assessment and time to pull my head out of the sand.

Unfortunately, my cardiologist had moved his practice to another state, and finding a new doctor whom I felt comfortable with was not easy. I tried four (see **Day Four**). My new doctor immediately informed me that he knew just how to take care of patients living in denial, and it was true. Eventually, he would become one of the key people who rescued me from the brink, but he could not easily change the effect of years of poor diet added to my family predisposition for heart disease.

After a number of tests, including a **nuclear stress test** and an **echocardiogram**, the results indicated I needed an angiogram, a diagnostic test that gives the physician a clear image of the heart's blood vessels. A dye is injected and a catheter is inserted in the femoral artery, which enables the radiologist to report blockages in the coronary **arteries**. The results were not unexpected and, again, an invasive procedure such as an angioplasty was recommended. However, since the past is the best predictor of the future, I bargained with the doctor. I bargained with my life; no angioplasty was performed.

For the next two years, I began to take medication to control my diabetes, as well as several new heart medications with unpleasant **side effects**. Despite warnings from my doctors, I did very little to alter my health behavior. My exercise was limited to playing softball occasionally in a company league. I took a new job with a lengthy commute that increased my stress even more, and my bachelor's diet makes me cringe when I look back on it.

In early February 2000, I went for a regular visit to my cardiologist. This time, he simply said, "You have no choice. The stress test says you've bought all the time you are going to have, and you are likely going to have another heart attack. You probably need open heart surgery, or at the very least, angioplasty."

I talked to three other cardiologists, and one nailed the case shut: "Look at it this way. You bought yourself five years. You should be in surgery today!"

I have asked myself frequently why I waited all those years. Why hadn't I gone to the hospital instead of going to work five years before? Why had I refused intervention before my health had deteriorated more? The answer is simple. I had to come to completely realistic terms with heart disease. I was unwilling to accept that I was sick and needed to make lifestyle changes. After my mother's experiences and subsequent battle with cardiovascular disease prior to her death, I was terrified. Despite cardiology's great strides in the 27 years between her first heart attack and her second bypass, she had died from a random postoperative complication that could have happened to anyone.

A few weeks after my cardiology appointment, I underwent a successful quadruple bypass, also known as a **coronary artery bypass graft (CABG)**, which I describe in greater detail in Day Six. To this day, I have virtually no memory of anything that occurred from the time I walked into the hospital until I awoke in the cardiac intensive care unit. Six days after the surgery, I was released and began the journey toward actually living well with cardiovascular disease.

There Is No Universal Prescription

I am a patient, not a doctor. Your cardiologist or primary care physician is the only one who can prescribe a heart-risk reduction, or heart disease prevention or recovery program for you. This book is designed to bring you the most important information you need to know about heart disease and the latest medical information. Heart disease is not a "one-size-fits-all" disease. In fact, as you will see in the following chapters, heart disease is really an umbrella term for at least a dozen specific diseases that can lead to another set of disorders. My experience as a patient is probably more extreme than many others'. My goal is not to prescribe a program for you, but to get your attention through facts and the stories of other patients and to give you tools for managing your heart disease.

While I will not prescribe in this book, I can help you identify the red flags that I missed in my own battle with heart disease. I also can tell you what has worked for me. Today, I have lost the weight my cardiologist recommended. My blood values—cholesterol, HDL, LDL—are all within normal range, something that hasn't happened in over a decade. My ejection fraction (the percentage of blood that the ventricle expels after a contraction) has risen by 10 percent, despite the minor muscle damage caused by my failure to get treatment quickly during my MI. Most important, *I feel good!*

As a medical writer and a patient, I have always felt that the best way to maintain good health is a combination of real-world experience that you can adapt to your own situation and the guidance of a medical specialist you trust. Helping you to fashion that winning approach is my promise to you, the reader.

My First Day

I consider the day I woke up in the coronary ICU after my quadruple bypass seven years ago and the several days I spent recovering in the hospital as the first day of the first year of my life with heart disease. I was lying in bed, hooked to the beeping, flashing machines, tethered to an oxygen tube helping me breathe, floating on a cocktail of pain medication, and trying to figure out if I was dead or alive. I vowed my life was never going to be the same.

A day later, I was transferred to the special coronary care unit, still hooked up to the oxygen line, a pulse-ox device on my index finger, and an intravenous line for meds and feeding. On my bed was a large, red heart-shaped pillow, a present from my surgeon. On it, he had drawn a diagram of my new heart with the bypassed arteries. Two other patients, also bound to machines or drips, greeted me with smiles and even a few jokes. They had heart pillows, too. It occurred to me that the cliché was true: I wasn't alone. That is when I began to become a patient, to listen to what I was told by my physicians, and to work with my "support family" of therapists, nutritionists, and my own actual family. This is the most important decision you must make on the first day of your diagnosis. The pillow sits on a chair next to me as I write these words, a daily reminder of my wasted years of potential good health and my wonderful new life.

IN A SENTENCE:

Everyone's path to heart disease may be different, but the sooner you recognize the red flags that indicate danger, the easier your road back to health will be.

Life Catches Up to You: Risk Factors

LATELY IT seems that heart disease is everywhere. We live in a society where it's reported that lifestyle, smoking, limited availability of health care, lack of nutritional knowledge, and obesity are just a few of the factors that have made heart disease, which includes several different cardiovascular problems, the number-one killer in the U.S. Among the statistics: One person dies of heart disease every 30 seconds. Men used to be viewed as the typical coronary patient, suddenly succumbing, seemingly without warning. Today, we know that women are part of that group. In fact, over the past three decades, more women than men have died from a variety of cardiovascular illnesses.

What does all this bad news mean for you, someone who has just heard the words: "You have heart disease"?

You Are More Than a Statistic

Stop for a moment and consider this question: Why do statistics tend to drive many of our actions, especially where health behavior is concerned? Each day's news offers a smörgåsbord of breakthrough studies, newly approved medications, sci-fi diagnostic technology, and dire statistic after statistic. Throughout this chapter, there are boxes with statistical data about heart disease. But these numbers are not the focus of this book. You and how you got into this situation are. In the case of heart disease, each individual's family history, concomitant disease, and personal circumstances differ so widely that you cannot see yourself as a statistic to which someone has assigned a predicted outcome.

This may not seem like a logical "First Day" message from someone who has lived the story I told in the introduction, but it is vital. For many years, I read the articles, watched the TV reports, and let them demoralize and depress me. There were times, I have to admit, that I wondered why I was going through it all. To be truthful, I asked myself: Are all these pills, side effects, and daily struggles worth it to gain a few more years, according to the latest scientific report?

Yes, because you are not a statistic!

Please, from this point on, spare yourself all the negative energy that I expended before I decided to get well. The sooner you begin on the positive path, the better you will feel and the more enjoyable life will be. If there is any reason at all to pay attention to today's data, it's to help you take control of your life and your own recovery. Learn to understand what a report means and whether it relates to you at all. Understanding the data may also help you make intelligent choices and enable you to talk to your cardiologist or other medical provider as a truly educated consumer.

Recognize the Risk Factors

OK, let's get started. You are probably asking yourself, "How has this happened and, more important, why has it happened to me?" Your head may be spinning with your recent diagnosis, and it's perfectly natural to be worried and quite scared. For some, discovering that you have cardiovascular problems can lead to guilt and anger. Most likely, your heart disease has its roots in risk factors that you were born with or that you may have developed over a number of years. Let's start with the concept of risk factors.

For heart patients, risk factors are disorders that influence your likelihood of developing a condition like cardiovascular disease. Now, it is not likely that you purposely took a chance at exposure to one of these risks. In reality, you collect cardiovascular risk factors and, with each one you add, your chances of getting sick are magnified. In general, most people with heart disease have some inherent predisposition to heart disease.

How do we know that this concept is accurate? According to the American Heart Association, "Major risk factors are those that research has shown significantly increase the risk of heart and blood vessel (cardiovascular) disease. Other factors are associated with increased risk of cardiovascular disease, but their significance and prevalence haven't yet been precisely determined. They're called contributing risk factors."

Major Risk Factors

There are three major risk factors that you cannot change. However, keep in mind that because you fit into one or all of the following categories, it doesn't mean you cannot overcome these risk factors or minimize their effects. One analogy would be athletic achievement. Some sports lend themselves to a certain body type. In professional basketball, for instance, the average height is 6'6". Sure, the taller the player is, the better he may be; however, there have been several extraordinary basketball players under six feet tall. For example, the NBA's Muggsy Bogues was a star at 5'3", and he was the shortest player to dunk a basketball.

The point is that when assessing your major risk factors, you have to play with the cards you've been dealt, but you can always improve your odds with hard work. Keep this in mind as we go through these major risk factors.

- ○ **Age** is the most significant major risk factor. Today, more than eight out of ten people who die from cardiovascular disease are over age 65.
- ○ **Gender** is the second major risk factor. Despite the increase in heart disease among women, men still are more likely to have heart attacks and to have them at a younger age. However, according to the American Heart Association, "At older ages, women who have heart attacks are more likely than are men to die from them within a few weeks." There are also indications that post-menopausal women are at greater risk, but not significantly so.
- ○ **Family history coupled with ethnic background** is the third major risk factor. If a member of your immediate family, especially

---

U.S. Surgeon General's Family History Initiative

In 2005, U.S. Surgeon General Richard Carmona, M.D., M.P.H., recognizing that "frequently, common disease can run in families," launched an online project to help track your health risk potential. Behind this effort was a survey that showed that 96 percent of Americans recognized the value of knowing their family health history, yet only one-third of us have ever actually tried to gather the information. "Family history is a powerful screening tool," says Dr. Carmona.

The surgeon general's office has created a computerized tool "to make it fun and easy for anyone to create a sophisticated portrait of their family's health." The site can be accessed at *http://www.familyhistory.hhs.gov/*.

---

your mother or father, had heart disease, you are at greater risk of heart disease. Your risk is also higher if you are African American, because this group has a greater incidence of high blood pressure, a risk for heart disease. Similarly, according to the American Heart Association, heart disease may appear in greater numbers in Native Americans, Native Hawaiians, some Asian Americans, and Mexican Americans "partly due to higher rates of obesity and diabetes."

Multiple combinations of contributing risk factors, the second category, are common among people with a history of heart disease. Confronting your contributing risk factors will be where you can give yourself a fighting chance to beat or, at the very least, keep ahead of the progression of your heart problems. In Month Two, we take an extensive look at how to reduce the effects of these risk factors, but, for the moment, consider where you stand with regard to the following contributing risk factors.

Contributing Risk Factors

The good news is that contributing risk factors are ones you can control. In some cases, the jury is still out on their significance. The bad news is that the more of these risk factors you have and the greater the level (e.g., high cholesterol, high blood pressure), the more the odds against you increase. If you have contributing risk factors, the dice are loaded against you, and every day that you delay confronting each risk, the closer to the abyss you get.

In the real world, we tend to have more than one risk factor. These are not listed in order of importance. They are cumulative, and the goal is to keep as many of them under control as you can.

1. Smoking

About 30 percent of the people who die from heart disease each year are smokers. Short of jumping off a ten-story building, smoking is about as suicidal as it gets, and it would be surprising to meet someone who doesn't know this. If you are a smoker who denies that you are at risk, you must get your head out of the sand now. Little that you can do to your body is more harmful. Smoking's damaging effects have been documented in literally thousands of medical studies.

Smoking has been definitively linked to atherosclerosis (narrowing of the arteries), lung cancer, blood clots, and harmful effects on cholesterol levels. Linked to atherosclerosis is **endothelial dysfunction.** The endothelial cells that line the inner sides of your blood vessels help control coagulation and a number of other vital functions. Studies have shown that smoking is one of a number of factors that compromise these cells and add to vascular disease risk.

It's not clear exactly whether tobacco is the direct cause of smoking's negative effects; however, cigarette smoke contains more than 4,000 different substances, and many are toxic. Nicotine, of course, is one of the most addictive drugs we've come up with yet. Simply put, it is hard to stop smoking, but you *can* do it (see **Month Three**).

Secondhand smoke has been recognized as a danger for many years, and now local businesses, restaurants, and even public parks have banned smoking. For a person with heart disease or risk factors for heart disease, secondhand smoke is even more dangerous. One myth is that pipe or cigar smoking is not as dangerous as cigarettes. Wrong. Pipes or cigars may be slightly less hazardous to your health than cigarettes, but that difference is not significant.

2. Obesity and Lack of Exercise

Obesity, in general, does not mean simply that you are fat or massively overweight. If you weigh only 20 to 30 percent more than the average weight someone your height and gender should be, you are obese. Not surprisingly, two controllable risk factors that go together are obesity and lack of exercise. There are differing opinions on what this means to each individual; however, there is virtually no disagreement as to how strong a risk these pose to your heart health. Twenty percent of the baby boomers who are obese also suffer from high blood pressure. Today, 61 percent of Americans are overweight. Worse, 15 percent of children between the ages of 6 and 19 are severely overweight or obese. The most accurate method of assessing your risk in relation to your height and weight is through the **Body Mass Index** (BMI), a universally accepted scale. If your BMI is between 18.5 and 24.9, you have a healthy/normal BMI. In the middle is a BMI of 25 to 29.9, which puts you in the "overweight" category. If you find yourself at 30 on the BMI scale, which is about 30 pounds past normal, you are classified as obese (see BMI Chart on 233).

This is where I found myself at one point before and then after my own myocardial infarction (heart attack) and coronary artery bypass graft. Perhaps learning that I fit into the "obese" category was one of the great shocks that motivated me to lose weight. I looked in the mirror and said to myself, "No way!"

Weight alone is not the only significant marker. "Love handles," ironically, are of great danger to your health. That's right, your waistline is a major indicator, along with BMI, of risk. Belly bulge is not simply a cosmetic problem; it signifies that you have too much visceral fat, which can be exceptionally harmful. Visceral fat is not that top layer of fat that you can pinch or hold onto (cutaneous fat); it's fat that accumulates in the stomach and in other vital organs near the abdomen, such as the liver. A 40-inch-plus waist for a man or a 35-inch-plus waist for a woman is considered a high-risk indicator. It's important to understand that even though we all know how hard it is to lose weight and keep weight off, an amount as small as 10 percent can make a difference in your heart disease risk.

As odd as this might sound, the hardest thing you may have to do during the first year of your life is simply to work some sort of aerobic exercise into your life. You may go to a gym or you may have a personal trainer. Depending on the exercise program and what your doctor has told you, now you have to make one fundamental change: *You must learn to lead an active lifestyle.*

Of all the changes you can make in your life to reduce the odds against you, this is perhaps the one that gets easier the more you integrate it into your life. Leading a healthy lifestyle is not about what exercise you do or which machines you use in the gym; it's about making a commitment to walk around the block a few times every day, to do more than watch TV when you can be working on a home-improvement project or playing a game in the backyard with your kids. As simple as this may sound, it works.

Your weight-loss goal doesn't have to be great. Losing 10 percent of your body weight or even ten pounds can make your life better and can help diminish your heart risk. The secret is to believe that you can do it, and then do it. In **Month Five**, there is a complete guide to heart-healthy exercise, preceded by suggestions for diet programs that have been successful for many patients (see **Month Four**). Yet it is going to be that simple change in your attitude or desire to turn your sedentary lifestyle 180 degrees that will help you reduce obesity as a significant risk factor.

> *One of my great physicians and friends, Ron Caldwell, M.D., of Asheville, NC, tells his patients, "Just do this 15 or 30 minutes a day—you will feel good!" He's right!*

3. *High Blood Pressure*

High blood pressure (HBP), also known as hypertension, is relatively common among patients with heart disease and the general population. According to the National Center for Health Statistics, "half of Americans aged 55 to 64 years old have high blood pressure." That's about 60 million people, which makes it the most common risk factor for heart disease. HBP develops when the heart is forced to work too hard. In untreated situations, the result can be heart muscle weakening, enlarging, and stiffening. Usually, the effects of hypertension lead back to a narrowing of the smaller blood vessels throughout the body, although a number of other diseases can be implicated.

High blood pressure is a particularly insidious condition because it is asymptomatic. You don't know you have it until you are tested for it, as it simply sneaks up on you, and the next thing you know, you've had a stroke, a heart attack, or your kidneys have been weakened. High blood pressure is not an equal-opportunity disease; it appears more frequently (not exclusively) in African Americans, Hispanics, smokers, and those with a diet high in sodium.

There are multiple estimates of how many people with hypertension are undiagnosed until something adverse occurs; however, the most important thing for you to remember is that HBP is damaging by itself, and that when added to risk factors you may already have, it can cause irreversible damage. Not knowing whether you have high blood pressure may shorten your life significantly, yet it is a risk factor that can be controlled.

Your blood pressure is measured in two ways, and is expressed in a numeric combination of millimeters of mercury, for example, "120 mm Hg over 70 mm Hg." Here's what this means. The first number, known as systolic blood pressure, refers to the heart when it contracts (see **Day Three**) and blood is surging through the aorta and pulmonary artery. The second number, known as diastolic blood pressure, refers to when the heart is at rest and the two lower chambers relax and fill with blood.

It's generally agreed that a blood pressure reading higher than 140/90 is a sign that you have hypertension and that you need some sort of treatment, whether through dietary adjustment or medication. A blood pressure reading of between 120/80 and 140/90 is a sign that you are at strong risk for developing HBP. This is known as pre-hypertension.

4. Diabetes

Type 2 Diabetes and Heart Disease.   Earlier in this book, I mentioned that if I hadn't been diagnosed with diabetes, I might never have known I was a cardiac time bomb. In my early 40s, I experienced breathlessness, and my doctor discovered that I had elevated blood pressure. When I showed up again a few months later complaining about my shortness of breath, my doctor checked my blood sugar and politely informed me that not only was I a type 2 diabetic, but the breathing problems were a sign of angina (i.e., transient chest discomfort).

Angina? How was that possible? I had no chest pain and I was basically an active and healthy person. Breathlessness among diabetics, my doctor said, usually masks the normal chest pain you would feel from angina. Luckily, I found a cardiologist and an endocrinologist to treat my diabetes.

You are not alone if you don't know about the link between diabetes and heart disease. The American Diabetes Association conducted a poll of 2,000 diabetics, and 68 percent had no idea that they were at increased risk of heart disease. Among ethnic populations who are at greater risk, up to 75 percent were unaware of their risk.

It's very important that you understand that type 2 diabetes and heart disease are linked in several ways, and that diabetes really is an important, if not a key, risk factor. According to the American Diabetes Association, two out of three diabetics die from heart disease and stroke.

As a diabetic, you have to be vigilant about your lifestyle. There are many excellent books about diabetes (including *The First Year: Type Two Diabetes,* by Gretchen Becker, in this series of books) that you should have in your library.

Traditionally, the most important aspect of self-monitoring for a diabetic has been the glucose intake level, but there now seem to be other important measures that can predict whether your diabetes has also increased your risk for heart disease.

Over the past few years, there has been confusion about the heart disease–diabetes link, perhaps because risk factors for both problems seem to dovetail. For example, certain fat-loaded foods can affect diabetes and increase coronary artery disease risk. The question that confuses patients and researchers is, in some ways, like the age-old chicken-or-the-egg quandary: Does type 2 diabetes lead to heart disease, or, if you have heart disease, are you more likely to get type 2 diabetes?

The short answer is this: If you have diabetes, you are putting yourself at greater risk for heart disease, but if you have heart disease, you are not necessarily at greater risk for diabetes. Ideally, you don't want both, but many people do have the combination. The reason for this is now pretty clear. Diabetes (more specifically, the high glucose levels that accompany it) causes the walls of your blood vessels to thicken and harden. This affects your blood flow and, in turn, can cut blood supply to your heart. This is why we categorize diabetes as a cardiovascular risk factor.

It is also not quite accurate to simply call diabetes a risk factor. If you have both diabetes and heart disease, you also have acquired a greater risk for high blood pressure and stroke and you are living with two complicated diseases that have to be monitored closely. With both diabetes and cardiovascular disease, the pressure on your arteries and buildup of plaque can lead to a clot breaking off and cutting off oxygenated blood to the heart or brain. To understand these connections, it's important that you understand the disease first.

What Is Diabetes? There are two types of diabetes: type 1, which was originally known as juvenile diabetes, and type 2, which, until recently, was known as adult onset diabetes. About 90 percent of diabetes cases are type 2 diabetes. The two types are significantly different diseases.

Type 1 diabetes is classified as an autoimmune disease. In general, type 1 diabetics have an insulin deficiency and must take insulin from the time of diagnosis. Type 1 diabetes occurs because the body's immune system attacks the pancreas, destroying the beta cells that make insulin, a hormone that regulates glucose. Without insulin, type 1 diabetics are at great risk, so they must inject synthetic insulin several times daily.

Type 2 diabetes, or diabetes mellitus, is the type that most people with heart disease have, so you should be familiar with it as you assess your heart risks. You can read more in-depth information about both forms of diabetes; however, understanding type 2 is most important for heart disease patients.

Until the past decade, type 2 diabetes was generally seen in people over the age of 65. Today, there is an epidemic of type 2 diabetes cases, and the age of the patient population is dropping. Shockingly, worldwide, 150 million people suffer from type 2 diabetes and 21 million of them—7 percent—are in the U.S. While 14.6 million Americans have been diagnosed with diabetes, another 6.2 million still may not have been diagnosed. Up to 176,000 people under the age of 21 have diabetes. It's estimated that one in every 400 to 600 children and adolescents has type 1 diabetes.

African Americans, Hispanic/Latino Americans, Native Americans, and some Asian and Pacific Island populations possess higher incidences of type 2 diabetes. There seems to be an increase in type 2 diabetes among children in these populations, too.

Diabetes also has genetic links. Studies of twins have suggested a high correlation between heredity and diabetes, and other studies have indicated familial predisposition. You may have heard that only overweight or obese people have diabetes. This is not necessarily true: Some data indicate that only 10 percent of obese people have type 2 diabetes. What they have, however, is a higher risk of developing diabetes, and weight loss reduces not only body mass, but also the amount of medication you may need. (In my case, a loss of 20 pounds enabled me to cut my insulin by two-thirds to only one injection per day.)

Type 2 diabetes develops when the body fails to efficiently convert glucose to energy to fuel bodily functions. When the body absorbs sugar properly, it does so through the action of the hormone insulin, which is created in the pancreas. Glucose transporters are sent out by the muscles to bring insulin to them.

In type 2 diabetes, insulin production is not the problem; the problem is that the peripheral tissues resist glucose uptake and use, so the glucose remains in the bloodstream. This is known as insulin resistance, and it is most closely associated with excessive body weight and visceral fat accumulation.

While diabetes is a significant risk factor, you can prevent or control it in several ways. Diet, weight loss, and medical intervention are the most common approaches. Diabetes, unfortunately, is one of the most serious risk factors for heart disease, and anyone with diabetes is probably twice as likely as someone without it to develop heart disease.

In general, most diabetics have been urged to closely monitor their "sugars," which actually refers to glucose levels in blood or urine. While monitoring glucose is still an absolute necessity, diabetics are also being urged to make sure their cholesterol levels are controlled and their blood pressure is normal.

The good news is that you can control your diabetes in much the same way that you can minimize the effects of your heart disease. This means monitoring glucose levels, following a rational and discretionary diet plan, and keeping your weight at a proper level. By doing this, your body can efficiently convert dietary sugar to glucose, which can be absorbed by your muscles and used for daily activity, instead of allowing it to build up and lead to blocked arteries.

Controlling the Diabetes–Heart Disease Link.   Beyond the normal treatments for your diabetes (i.e., insulin, medication, diet, and exercise), you can decrease your heart risk by controlling your lipids—that includes your cholesterol and the fats that are circulating within your system. This condition is referred to as diabetic dyslipidemia, and may be responsible for a stroke or heart attack.

What this means is that as a diabetic, you are more likely to have low HDL (good cholesterol) while your triglycerides are too high. Your LDL (bad cholesterol) manifests itself as particles that become plugs and clog your blood vessels.

The key to using this new information about diabetes to cut your heart risk is to have your doctor do a complete lipid panel, a simple blood test, to see where you fit into the new American Diabetes Association guidelines.

The American Diabetes Association recommends the following target levels:

Type of blood lipid	ADA target
LDL cholesterol	Below 100 mg/dL
HDL cholesterol	Above 40 mg/dL (men)
	Above 50 mg/dL (women)
Triglycerides	Below 150 mg/dL

Of course, your doctor or doctors will recommend the best combination of lifestyle and medication to meet these targets, and there are many good books on cooking and diabetic diets. The ADA publishes many of these books, and you can find them on their website, *www.diabetes.org*.

The *Be Smart About Your Heart: Control the ABCs of Diabetes* campaign of the National Diabetes Education Program (NDEP), in partnership with the American Diabetes Association, has been initiated to increase awareness among people with diabetes about the need to control blood glucose, blood pressure, and cholesterol levels to decrease their risk of cardiovascular disease. Visit NDEP's website at *http://ndep.nih.gov* or call 1-800-438-5383 to order printed materials.

The American Diabetes Association and the American College of Cardiology have started a national education program called *Make the Link!* to increase awareness among diabetics and care providers about the risk of heart disease in diabetics.

5. High Blood Cholesterol

If the American public is aware of any risk factor for heart disease, especially heart attack, it is the need to keep cholesterol levels in normal range. Whether through a media report of the latest scientific study or through a barrage of advertisements for breakthrough medications, we are reminded daily that the level of our "good" cholesterol (HDL, or high-density lipoproteins) or our "bad" cholesterol (LDL, or low-density lipoproteins) has to be carefully managed. This is especially true for LDL, which seems to have joined household germs and insects on the top-ten list of health-related bogeymen.

In addition, triglycerides (VLDL, or very low-density lipoproteins), which store fat that functions as an energy source for metabolic activity, also have to be carefully watched.

While media messages and commercial pitches may sometimes be over the top, the reality is that managing your cholesterol and other harmful substances you may have in your bloodstream is one of the most important ways you can control heart disease risk. Cholesterol and other lipids (or fats) bring our bodies the fats needed to create internal energy. They are essential building blocks of body tissues and organs, but they have to be carefully managed and monitored.

Staying on top of your cholesterol levels can also be a complicated process involving a combination of diet and multiple medications. An in-depth discussion on cholesterol and how to regulate it is found in **Month Three,** but here are basic issues related to your heart risk factors that you should understand as you assess your situation now.

"Unofficial" Risk Factors

In general, the medical community agrees that problems such as obesity, a sedentary lifestyle, family history, elevated cholesterol, and diabetes can increase your likelihood of suffering a heart attack or developing atherosclerosis and other heart disease.

However, I have learned in my journey with heart disease that there are some very logical and important things you must do to lower your risk that no one really discusses with you. I call these "unofficial" risk factors.

1. Not Taking Your Meds

Your doctor or, in many cases, multiple physicians may prescribe numerous medications for you. Truthfully, a lot of these medications have unpleasant side effects, and some physicians may dismiss these or diminish the importance of them. If you read the patient instructions that the pharmacist usually hands out, you may find a staggering list of side effects, cautions and warnings, **adverse effects**, and drug interactions that can certainly be daunting.

One thing to keep in mind: Most of these medications have similar side effects, including gastrointestinal effects like nausea, diarrhea, vomiting, or constipation. You may experience blurred vision, dizziness, and drowsiness. Some of the newer medications also have sexual side effects and may cause feelings of depression.

Over the years, you may find yourself taking more medications as new and more effective pharmaceuticals come on the market. Even if you do nothing else to reduce your risk factors, *you must take your medications as prescribed. Failure to do so will negate all the hard work you may have done in losing weight and changing your diet.* This is impossible to understate. Medications that increase HDL, lower LDL, and prevent increased heart disease risk may be promoted the way Big Macs and SUVs are, but they work.

You *must* work with your cardiologist when side effects appear. Don't hesitate to call and talk to him, rather than stop taking a med. Remember that problems like high cholesterol and hypertension do not have overt symptoms, and unless they are under control, you could have a sudden stroke or heart attack.

2. Not Learning About Your Condition

A great physician and friend in Boston, Harold Solomon, M.D., taught me this concept, and it has helped in my recovery as much as any treatment. Some people would refer to this as taking ownership of your disease. Simply put, this means learning all you can about heart disease. Read the newspapers, watch the wonderful documentaries on public television, read books, and surf the Internet. But that's only the start. It also means showing up for your appointments on time. Discuss this issue with your doctor.

The hardest thing for me to do has been to lose weight and change my diet. Taking pills on time has been easy. However, if you work at the hard parts of your recovery, you'll see results. Learn as much as you can, become the proverbial educated consumer, and you will recover much faster, feel better, and be the type of patient most doctors love to see walking through the door.

3. *Getting Stressed*

Another risk factor is the effect of stress. In **Month Six**, coping with stress is discussed completely. Some experts think stress can be significant; others see it in the same category as caffeine: The jury is still out. One reason for this disagreement is that stress affects people differently. Some people are stress junkies who thrive on it, drawing energy to meet deadlines and almost impossible goals. Others collapse under pressure.

Whether you are a hard driver or a nervous wreck from stress, if you have been diagnosed with heart disease, it is time to take a step back and learn to take time for yourself. You *must* find some way to change the lifestyle you've been leading. Don't bet that stress isn't a factor in the progression of your disease. Work on creating a less intense lifestyle.

IN A SENTENCE:

> *Although you may have inherent risks for heart disease, your contributing risk factors can be controlled and diminished if you take responsibility for this task.*

DAY 2

living

What Is Heart Disease?

AFTER READING the last section, you may feel that heart disease is best described in the words of the famous comic-strip possum, Pogo: *"We have met the enemy and he is us."* Truthfully, when you begin to learn about risk factors for heart disease, it does seem that predestination, inevitability, or even bad karma might also be accurate terms to describe the situation. This is partly true. Does it also seem that everyone is talking about heart disease or that you are more aware of it now that you've been told about your own condition? You notice newspaper articles filled with statistics or pay more attention when a new trend is revealed on the evening news. You may even pay more attention to the inevitable stories around the holiday dinner table about Uncle Jimmy's coronary, Aunt Edith's pacemaker, and the guy at the office who dropped dead in the gym. One thing you can count on is that your awareness level is way up there now.

Take your new awareness level and the knowledge that your lifestyle or DNA may be partly responsible for your heart condition and turn it into something positive. Realizing what can go wrong will also help you understand why what has happened to your heart is also affecting other parts of your body, like your legs and feet.

Here's another reason to learn more about heart disease: You may have one diagnosis, but you will want to know and understand how that might lead to further problems for you, and you'll want to minimize the risk of additional disease related to your primary diagnosis.

As you go through this book, don't overreact to what may seem like an overwhelming threat to your longevity and overall health. Learning is your best bet.

How widespread is heart disease? According to the American Heart Association

○ 72 million Americans have high blood pressure;
○ 7.9 million Americans will have a heart attack this year;
○ 8.9 million Americans will have angina attacks this year;
○ 5.7 million Americans will have strokes this year;
○ coronary artery disease causes 450,000 deaths annually and is the number-one killer among heart diseases;
○ about 325,000 Americans will have a heart attack and will die in the emergency room this year;
○ in 2004, coronary heart disease death rates (per 100,000) were 194.4 for Caucasian men and 222.2 for African American men; and
○ the death rates (per 100,000) was 115.4 for Caucasian women and 148.6 for African American women.

Throughout this chapter are statistics to give you some context to consider different disorders of the heart. Remember, however, that each statistic has different sources, some of which compete. As you continue learning about heart disease, keep in mind that your knowledge base and how you use it are the most important values of the stats. For example, The National Center on Health Statistics (a part of the National Heart, Lung and Blood Institute) and the American Heart Association report that "heart disease is the leading cause of death of American women and kills 32% of them." They also report that "267,000 women die from heart attacks each year, six times more than breast cancer."

What Can Go Wrong?

Calling "heart disease" an umbrella term for a number of different conditions that affect both the heart and the circulatory system is one way to look at the problem, but it's not quite accurate. "Heart disease" can

Symptoms of Heart Disease

- ○ angina (sharp chest pain)
- ○ shortness of breath
- ○ fatigue
- ○ edema (fluid retention)
- ○ loss of consciousness
- ○ light-headedness
- ○ palpitations

- ○ limb pain
- ○ abnormal skin color
- ○ ulceration
- ○ shock
- ○ vision problems
- ○ coordination problems
- ○ speech problems

mean heart muscle damage; arterial blockages; the heart's electrical system is on the fritz; the pericardial sac is inflamed; heart valves are inefficient, allowing blood to flow back into the heart chambers; or a major disaster, such as a myocardial infarction (a heart attack).

To some extent, heart disease is composed of many separate conditions that, as you will see, can also create other problems. If, for example, an artery is blocked, depriving the heart of oxygenated blood, the heart muscle will sustain potentially fatal damage. If the heart is damaged and can't push blood out, vital organs will fail, too.

Perhaps the nerves that control the heartbeat can become overstimulated or fail, causing an irregular heartbeat. This also can affect blood flow through the body, or a blood clot can block an artery in the brain, reducing blood supply to the brain cells, resulting in disability or death.

Heart disease can strike anyone at any age. One way to learn more about heart disease is to look at the overall picture before getting into the details. In the following pages, you will find an overview of the many different diseases of the heart and how they interconnect. In **Day Three**, you will find a complete discussion of these and other disorders (e.g., diabetes, high blood pressure) that often accompany heart disease.

Coronary Artery Disease

Of the scores of types of heart disease that can cause your circulatory system to fail, coronary artery disease (CAD) is by far the most common among adults. CAD is also referred to as coronary heart disease, and is a specific condition that occurs when the arteries supplying blood to the heart become narrowed. Arteries all through the circulatory system can become blocked in the same way, a condition called arteriosclerosis or hardening of the arteries. The eventual result is potentially catastrophic: severely reduced blood supply to the heart or to other vital parts of the body, causing wide-ranging damage, from stroke to heart attack. These conditions can occur in anyone, but are more likely to occur as you age.

How Do the Arteries Become Blocked?

Arteries are essentially tubes. The inside layer, the endothelium, is surrounded by a muscular layer, the tunica media, which is surrounded by the adventitia. The arteries are constructed so that as blood passes through, the walls expand with the pressure, keeping the blood moving.

If your bloodstream absorbs too much LDL cholesterol, plaque begins to stick to the inner coronary arterial wall. This eventually causes narrowing of the coronary (and other) arteries in a slow buildup, usually over many years. Plaque is composed of a number of substances, including cholesterol, fibrin, collagen, phospholipids, muscle tissue, blood cell components, and other debris wrapped in a calcium lump. Some plaque binds together and grows into lumps or small benign tumors called atheromas (see Figure 1, page 32).

For quite some time, it has been thought that narrowing of the arteries was the main reason for cardiac calamities. The analogy most people heard from their doctors was the "iron drainpipe that slowly accumulated rust as water and other debris floated through." Along with the rust deposits, your doctor may have said, the drainage system carried large objects, such as hair, soap, and an old toothbrush. All of this slowed the water flow, eventually allowing only a trickle through the pipeline. However, while this narrowing of the arteries does not necessarily cause a heart attack, it can create angina, or mild to severe chest-pain symptoms that may feel like a heart attack.

We now know that the simple accumulation of hardened plaque on the inner walls of the cardiovascular arteries is not the most dangerous development. It's widely believed (and proven) that softer plaque accumulating on the arterial walls is the culprit leading to heart attacks.

What happens is that the soft plaque that has grown into larger atheromas causes tears or ruptures in the inner lining of the arteries, which causes fissuring and bleeding. You may also hear this referred to as unstable or ruptured plaque.

The body immediately launches its automatic blood-clotting mechanism to close off the tear. This is done through fibrin (clotting fibers) that forms a patch, much like a tire patch. Ironically, the cure is what may cause greater damage. The new clot can begin to swell and, as it grows, it forms a blockage that shuts off arterial blood flow altogether, causing a heart attack or stroke.

How Is CAD Treated?

CAD is reasonably asymptomatic. You may begin to feel pain only when the disease has progressed. Activity can provoke arterial pain, yet some people feel pain when they are simply sitting and doing nothing. Today your cardiologist may suggest non-invasive or external studies, such as an electrocardiogram (ECG), a stress test, and nuclear scans.

Some of these tests may not be sensitive enough to detect small, developing blockages, so other invasive tests, such as coronary angiography, also known as arteriography or catheterization, are employed. These involve threading a very long, very thin, flexible hollow tube, called a catheter, into an artery in the arm or the groin. Once this is done, a radioactive dye is injected and x-ray images are taken to enable the radiologist or your cardiologist to determine how much narrowing is present.

Treatment changes for coronary artery disease are also developing rapidly. As a heart patient, it's important to keep in mind that your body is designed to fight off disease and to adapt to various conditions. One example is how the body protects itself, developing new arteries, called collaterals, that simply bypass your primary, clogged arteries.

Unfortunately, where CAD is concerned, it's likely that you will need treatments that range from dietary changes to a wide variety of medications, somewhat minor surgical procedures, or open heart surgery.

While most of us are at risk for CAD as we age, there are things that you can do to mitigate its development, *especially stopping smoking* and making lifestyle changes that are musts for anyone, with or without coronary heart disease.

Angina Pectoris

You may learn that you have heart disease when your physician tells you that the sharp, disabling discomfort in your chest is angina pectoris, a term that some say is derived from a combination of *ankhon* (Greek) and *pectus* (Latin) that translates to "strangling chest". Usually known as just angina, it normally presents itself as a sudden, sharp pain that spreads across your chest. Not everyone has pain. Some people experience pressure, squeezing, or discomfort in the chest. This is a red flag from your heart to send more oxygenated blood.

Angina is not a disease of the heart, but a constellation of symptoms. If your arteries have begun to shrink or clog and you experience the sensations associated with angina, you are fortunate. It is likely that it is not too late, but these warning signs are telling you: *Call your doctor immediately*!

Not everyone experiences the same symptoms, and many symptoms may not be angina, but may actually be something as simple as indigestion. A sharp chest pain that eases in a few seconds is usually not angina. However, *never* overlook a symptom that lasts longer than 10 to 15 minutes: You may be having a heart attack. If you have repeated bouts of angina within a short period of time, called crescendo angina attacks, and the pain seems to worsen each time, you may be experiencing a heart attack and you should call your doctor or go to the emergency room immediately.

Here are some of the symptoms you may experience:

○ a strong, painful pressure around your chest, neck, shoulders, jaw, or arm
○ a strong squeezing or burning sensation in the same areas
○ discomfort or a feeling of fullness in your chest that comes on suddenly
○ light-headedness, sweating, and shortness of breath
○ pain that spreads through the arm and neck and increases with exertion
○ nausea, gas, or feeling as if someone were sitting on your chest

A diagnosis of angina is not simply based on the signs or symptoms described above. For example, you may have angina, but the symptoms are being masked. Diabetics with CAD may experience shortness of breath, rather than chest pain. Your cardiologist may also perform an x-ray, an ECG, and a stress test to confirm the diagnosis. Your cardiologist will want to rule out problems that may mimic angina symptoms, such as stomach disorders or a pinched nerve.

What Brings on an Angina Attack?

Assuming that your circulatory system is compromised, angina can occur from both physical *and* mental stress and strain. The list of physical activities that may provoke angina includes an easy walk up a hill, climbing the stairs in your house, sweeping, lifting a box, sexual activity, and bike riding—anything that causes the heart to draw more oxygenated blood. Among the many people I've talked with about their heart disease, climbing stairs seem to be one of the most common activities that causes angina or breathlessness.

Your brain is a major consumer of rich, oxygenated blood. Not surprisingly, when you are stressed out, your brain sends a message to the heart for an increased order. If the heart becomes strained in the effort, it's likely that you'll actually experience angina. Obviously, if you are involved in an argument or love making that is causing an emotional spike, you may have angina symptoms. However, you may simply be sitting at your desk *thinking* about a problem at home, or your boss has suddenly dropped a new assignment on your desk and expects it to be done by the end of the day. You may not have moved an inch, but the next thing you know, you're sweating, breathing heavily, feeling pain across your chest, and debating which is more important, your life or your job?

From someone who has been in the same position and who made the wrong call, the correct answer is to contact your doctor or go to the ER.

How Is Angina Treated?

If you are diagnosed with angina, generally, your doctor will prescribe nitroglycerin, which, in the form of a tablet, is placed under your tongue. Usually, your pain will recede within a few minutes. Your doctor will immediately begin a comprehensive cardiac evaluation. Most patients (like me) always carry a small vial of "nitro," but if your angina or your nitroglycerin requirements intensify, contact your primary physician or your cardiologist at once.

Other medications used for treating angina include beta-blockers and calcium channel blockers. Beta-blockers are known primarily as high blood pressure medication. They reduce the pulse rate and the heart's demand for oxygen. Several calcium channel blockers have a similar effect on the heart. These and other lifestyle interventions are discussed fully in **Month Eight**.

Heart Attack

I've never met anyone who had a heart attack exactly like mine. As any 7.2 million people differ in many ways, the same goes for the 7.2 million acute heart attack victims each year. Heart attacks are now the number-one cause of death in men and women.

On certain levels, you may have many of the same general risk factors, such as family history, obesity, diabetes, high blood pressure, age, gender, ethnic background, stress level, and others discussed in **Day One**, yet no one has the same *combination* of risk factors.

Usually, a heart attack or myocardial infarction is not the dramatic event we see on TV or in the movies, where the victim is suddenly struck down, clutching his chest, gasping for breath, able to only utter a few last words. But it could be like that.

Very few heart attacks occur in the hospital. It is more likely that you will experience the symptoms of a heart attack at home or at work unexpectedly, and if you act quickly, you can mitigate the damage to your heart. On the other hand, you may actually have symptoms over several hours that slowly worsen, or even a feeling of doom that you can't shake. *If you know what to expect, then you can save your life.*

What Are Symptoms of a Heart Attack?

What does it feel like to have a heart attack? Despite the fact that there is no classic constellation of symptoms, there are several that most people experience:

○ Severe, intense chest pain in the center of your chest.

FIGURE 1

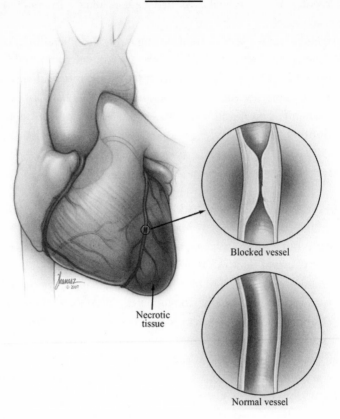

Blocked vessel

Necrotic
tissue

Normal vessel

○ A squeezing sensation, fullness, and pain. *When this lasts for more
than a few minutes—call 911!*

○ An uncomfortable feeling that makes you seem "full" (you'll know
when you have it).

○ Pain in your neck or jaw that spreads down your left arm, but can
include both arms.

○ Sweating; difficulty breathing; nausea; feeling disoriented, dizzy,
or faint.

○ Feeling of impending doom.

○ Women have similar symptoms; however, they may feel more pain
in the chest, upper body, arms, back, jaw, and stomach, along with
shortness of breath, sweating, and dizziness.

○ Others around you may tell you (as my assistant did before she
dragged me to the hospital) that you look pale or gray.

○ Periods of angina that occur in succession.

○ Pain or discomfort that lasts longer than 10 to 15 minutes.

○ Pain or discomfort that does not completely abate in response to nitroglycerin.

These symptoms are only the most common for a heart attack. I can't emphasize enough that even if you are doctor-phobic or don't think your symptoms are any big deal, *don't hesitate to get help. Don't take a chance with your life, as I did.* There are many of us who think we can pop a Tums, don't want to bother the doctor, don't want to believe this is really happening, or have cried "wolf" before.

In fact, you may have one or none of the symptoms listed and still have what's referred to as a "silent heart attack". A silent heart attack occurs far more frequently than you would think, and the nickname is a bit misleading. A study published in the *Journal of the American College of Cardiology* reported that 20 percent of men and women over age 65 actually have had a silent heart attack. What this means is that either they had no symptoms or the symptoms were not severe enough in the victims' minds to motivate them to contact a doctor. When they later had an identifiable heart attack, damage from the silent event was discovered. More important, if unrecognized, the damage goes untreated.

The elderly are not the only ones at risk. It's estimated that one in four of those who eventually suffer a full-blown heart attack have had silent heart attacks. If you are diabetic, if you've have had previous medical problems that have compromised your heart, if you are a member of a minority group, or if you have suffered a stroke, you're at increased risk for silent heart damage. Women are also at greater risk for fatal heart attacks because their symptoms may not be as easily identified, so they are not treated as quickly. This is why it is important that you do not ignore any symptoms that you may experience.

Cardiac arrest, complete stoppage of the heart's effective pumping capacity, is possible for someone at risk for a heart attack, and it usually strikes suddenly, without typical MI symptoms. However, the signs include

○ lack of response to touch or to attempts to rouse the victim

○ no sign of breathing within five seconds after the head has been tilted back to open the airway

*Acting quickly is the single most important thing to do when you sus-
pect you or someone else is having an MI.* It's estimated that 15 percent of
all heart attacks are fatal within the first hour, and most people wait two
hours before seeking help. To deal with this problem, the American
Heart Association and the National Heart, Lung, and Blood Institute
launched the Act in Time campaign to increase awareness of heart attack and stroke symptoms. Because minutes can make a difference, it's
vital to act at the first sign of symptoms.

When you think you or someone else is having a heart attack, you
should

○ Call 911. *Don't hesitate. Two-thirds of the people who die of a heart
  attack do so within the first hour after they began to feel ill. Tell the
  911 operator where you are.*
○ Wait for emergency medical services (EMS). EMS personnel are
  trained to begin treatment immediately, to call ahead to the hospital, and to transport the patient. (Patients who come to the
  emergency room are usually taken for treatment immediately.)
○ If you have no access to emergency medical services, have someone drive you to the hospital immediately.
○ Take a chewable aspirin.

What Causes a Heart Attack?

A heart attack happens when the supply of oxygenated blood to the
heart is blocked. This can occur when unstable plaque breaks off and
creates a clot that stops the blood altogether or allows only minimal
blood through to the heart. It can also happen when a coronary artery is
narrowed by coronary artery disease to the point that blood flow is reduced to a trickle.

When blood and other nutrients fail to reach the heart, the heart
muscle begins to pump erratically or irregularly (arrhythmia) and can
begin to die. This process (coronary occlusion) can begin within a few
minutes to three hours before the damage to your heart is permanent.
The heart muscle degrades and becomes scar tissue, and the pumping
ability of the heart will be reduced. (See Figure 1, page 32.)

> ### Symptoms of Heart Disease
>
> Not surprisingly, a heavy smoker, a recreational drug user—especially a user of cocaine—or someone who's been stranded in the frigid outdoors can suffer a heart attack even though he or she may not have coronary artery disease.

You may be told that your heart attack has been small or mild. This only means you have been lucky: The amount of heart muscle damage has been minimal. While the symptoms of small and more significant heart attacks can be similar, the potential for an uneventful recovery is greater in those with minimal muscle damage and a second heart attack is greater in those with severe muscle damage. Any muscle damage your heart may sustain can be the beginning of a downhill slide, and anyone who has had a first heart attack is at greater risk for a second heart attack.

If you have been diagnosed with coronary artery disease, if you have angina, and if you are still in denial over your life-threatening situation, then a heart attack is a wake-up call that should turn your life around. The risk factors outlined in **Day One** for coronary artery disease are the same ones that can lead to a heart attack. Primary among these are being male, age, family history of heart disease, prior heart attack, heart surgery, or angioplasty. Women often are at least ten years older than men when they have their first heart attack.

Simply stated, any heart-attack warning signs, especially those of an acute heart attack or myocardial infarction, should always be considered life-threatening. *Even if you are not sure about your situation, you should seek medical attention.*

IN A SENTENCE:

> *Heart disease can mean many things—for example, the heart muscle could be damaged by arterial blockages or the heart's electrical system could fail—and if heart disease is not recognized early and managed properly, disaster can strike at any time.*

Heart Disease Is Not Limited to Coronary Artery Disease

HEART DISEASE goes beyond coronary artery disease that evolves into angina, heart attack, or heart failure. There are a number of related disorders that may be congenital (those you are born with), viral, or structural, such as valvular problems. (Note: The following information is in alphabetical order.)

Arrhythmias

You may have experienced a type of cardiac arrhythmia (CA) that came and went quickly, also known as a palpitation, a brief, slightly scary feeling of throbbing in your chest, with a little anxiety thrown in for good measure. A palpitation, however, is not a true CA. When your heart muscles don't contract regularly—they contract faster or slower—you may be suffering from full-blown CA. *This can be a life-threatening condition.*

The far more serious arrhythmias occur when the sinus node in the heart muscle loses its ability to keep the heart beating at its regular 60 to 70 beats per minute. Once the heartbeat skyrockets over 100 beats per minute, you are technically in tachycardia. (If the rhythm is slower than 60 to 70 beats per minute, you are in brachycardia.)

The first thing you may feel is a slight series of palpitations; however, if that quickly develops into a strong, pounding feeling, possibly followed by dizziness and fainting, you are in trouble, but not necessarily near death. In fact, being too pumped up from exercise that has increased adrenalin in your body, or the caffeine from too many trips to Starbucks or a six-pack of Mountain Dew, can bring on a period of arrhythmia.

Another form of arrhythmia, fibrillation, can be quite serious, especially if your problem is the result of atrial or ventricular disruptions in your heart. In this case, the rhythms might either increase or decrease in frequency and strength. A rapid heartbeat, known as a supraventricular tachycardia, originates in the upper chambers of the heart. You might experience a fluttering sensation known as atrial fibrillation. In the lower chambers, the same sensation may occur as ventricular tachycardia.

The risk of experiencing tachycardia or brachycardia varies greatly, depending on the condition of your heart, any history of a prior heart attack, blood chemistry imbalances, or endocrine abnormalities. Your cardiologist may identify any of these conditions while listening to your chest with a stethoscope, or you may require more sophisticated testing such as an ECG, an echocardiogram, or other tests used to detect heart attacks and angina.

Because this is a life-threatening condition, you may need surgery to implant an artificial pacemaker or only medication may be required. As with any other cardiac-related condition or symptom, getting treatment rapidly is essential. *Don't hesitate. Call 911, call your doctor, or get to an emergency room.*

Bacterial Endocarditis

One significant but low-profile heart disorder is bacterial endocarditis (BE), which is relatively uncommon. However, it is just as dangerous and potentially fatal as many other diseases that can compromise your heart's function. Bacterial endocarditis is a serious infection that strikes both the heart lining (the endocardium) and the heart valves that are directly involved in blood flow.

Usually, BE is caused when bacteria in the blood flows through the heart and adheres to the valves and/or the heart lining, causing high fever and other typical symptoms of an infection. The infection may also be caused by bacteria within the mouth, intestines, or urinary tract. Most commonly, BE may result from a dental procedure, especially in someone who has pre-existing heart-valve abnormality, artificial valves, or prior bouts with BE. Dental procedures, even simple ones such as tooth cleaning, can release bacteria that can lead to BE in people with a structural heart defect. In most cases, BE will not develop unless the heart-wall lining has been damaged.

Treatment of BE usually requires high doses of antibiotics given intravenously over a period of two to six weeks. Antibiotics are given ahead of dental procedures to those at high rish of infection. This is called antibiotic prophylaxis, and its potential indications are important to discuss with your physician.

Cardiomyopathy

A very serious disease, cardiomyopathy, occurs when your heart muscle—the myocardium—becomes inflamed and fails to work effectively. If untreated, the heart can begin to fail, leading to arrhythmias and possible sudden cardiac death. In general, cardiomyopathy is diagnosed as one of three or four specific types.

Cardiomyopathy

Cardiomyopathy is not as common as other forms of heart disease, but it can become so severe that only a heart transplant will help you. Perhaps 50,000 people every year suffer from one form or another of cardiomyopathy.

The most common form, dilated (or congestive) cardiomyopathy, is often the result of another specific disease, such as high blood pressure, heart-valve problems, or a congenital heart defect. Because your heart wall is weakened, it stretches, and your heart fails to pump normally. From there, the problems cascade. You may develop arrhythmias and the normal electrical system that keeps your heart pumping blood through it can begin to fail.

FIGURE 2

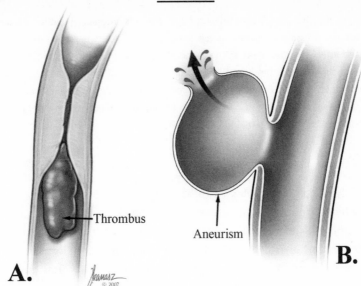

Because blood tends to coagulate when it slows down, this pumping failure can lead to a clot known as a thrombus (see Figure 2), which can break free and block a blood vessel. This is called an embolus (A). A number of things may then occur:

○ Mural thrombi can stick to the inner lining of the heart.
○ A pulmonary embolism can form when a clot breaks off from the right ventricle and travels into the lungs.
○ When a clot breaks off on the left side of the heart, it can flow into the circulatory system and form a cerebral embolism in the brain, or clots may occur in the kidney or even within the coronary arteries, abdominal organs, and legs.

Treatment is multifaceted, including blood thinners to stabilize clots, artificial pacemakers and defibrillators, and medications, including vasodilators, to lower blood pressure.

While hypertrophic cardiomyopathy appears in two forms, the basic problem is the same. The muscle that forms the left ventricle chamber in your heart enlarges, or hypertrophies. In one case, the wall that separates

One of the great dangers that can happen in the circulatory system is an aneurysm, which occurs in a single spot. Caused by a weakening or a diseased artery (or other vessel), the blood literally begins to form a bulge in the wall of the artery. If the blood bursts through the wall of the arteries, death from stroke or other complications can occur quickly. While usually occurring at the base of the brain, it can occur in the aorta. A variety of treatments including surgery and even stenting can help resolve this situation. (See page 39, Figure B.)

the left and right ventricles (the interventricular septum) expands, reducing blood flow from the left ventricle, known as asymmetrical septal hypertrophy. It's thought that more than 50 percent of these cases are hereditary, and also can cause leakage of the mitral valve. The other form, non-obstructive hypertrophic cardiomyopathy, is when the thickened septum does not prevent blood outflow.

If you have developed hypertrophic cardiomyopathy, you may experience breathlessness, fainting, or angina. General treatment of this problem is with medications such as beta-blockers or calcium channel blockers to permit the heart to more fully relax and fill with blood. Surgery is often indicated and performed to remove the thickened heart muscle, permitting unobstructed blood outflow.

It's unlikely that you will develop restrictive cardiomyopathy, since it is quite uncommon in the U.S. Restrictive cardiomyopathy occurs when the ventricles fail to fill with blood after each heartbeat because they have hardened. The heart demonstrates impaired relaxation. If you have swolen hands and feet or unusual exhaustion after physical activity, call your cardiologist. He or she may schedule an echocardiogram.

Another relatively uncommon version of cardiomyopathy is arrhythmogenic right ventricular dysplasia, which results in formation of fibrous scar tissue and is related to disturbances of the heart's electrical system.

Overall, it's important to remember that the health of your heart muscle is one of the most critical aspects of your ability to live a normal life. Damage that occurs to your heart muscle is not normally going to regenerate by itself. Its overall effect is to reduce your heart's ability to output blood adequately, robbing the rest of your body of the oxygen and nutrients you need to survive.

Congenital Heart Defects

According to the March of Dimes, the well-known institution whose focus is on reducing infant mortality, more than 32,000 infants (one in every 125 to 150) are born with heart defects each year in the U.S. The defect may be so slight that the baby appears healthy for many years after birth, or it may be so severe that the child's life is in immediate danger. (A complete discussion of children and heart disease can be found in **Week Four.**)

"Heart defects are among the most common birth defects, and are the leading cause of birth defect-related deaths. However, advances in diagnosis and surgical treatment over the past 40 years have led to dramatic increases in survival for children with serious heart defects. Between 1987 and 1997, the death rates from congenital heart defects dropped 23 percent," the March of Dimes reports.

Heart Failure

Heart failure, sometimes known as congestive heart failure (CHF), can quickly become one of the most serious, chronic, life-threatening cardiac conditions. When your heart fails to pump properly, especially as a result of other cardiac conditions that rob it of oxygenated blood (e.g., coronary artery disease), it can cause congestion in the lungs and other organ sites. It is different from cessation of the heartbeat (asystole) or a heart attack (which can also precipitate CHF), as the heart does not stop working; rather, it has to work harder to pump blood efficiently. Eventually, the heart weakens, the chambers (especially the left ventricle) enlarge, and the result is a failing heart.

CHF is also a complex disease, and many sources break it down into a variety of classifications, such as right or left heart failure, or by measuring the level of symptoms that you may experience. Tests such as an echocardiogram, heart catheterization, a chest x-ray, an MRI, a nuclear stress test, and an ECG are common diagnostic tools.

The most common symptoms of CHF (see below) may be similar to symptoms of other cardiac diseases, such as heart attack, arrhythmias, valve disorders, and cardiomyopathy. CHF is a life-threatening problem, and because it may have subtle symptoms or symptoms that mirror other conditions, don't hesitate to get help if you experience some or all of these symptoms, especially if you have family history of CHF or heart disease:

O shortness of breath when walking or lying down
O sudden breathing disturbances at night
O quickly becoming exhausted
O increased heart rate
O disorientation, dizziness, or memory loss
O swollen hands or feet
O a constant, hacking cough or coughing up bloody mucus
O weight gain
O nausea and vomiting
O loss of appetite
O irregular or rapid pulse
O frequent nocturnal urination or reduced urine (which, in men, also could suggest prostate disease)

Prolonged periods of CHF can cause physiological changes, including the following:

O Remodeling: The enlargement and thinning of the left ventricle, which, in turn, leads to increased oxygen demand, mitral-valve regurgitation or leakage, and decreased ejection fraction. This process will eventually set off a complicated series of actions, such as inflammation of the heart, damage to the cells, and further damage to the ventricle or to the entire heart.
O Tachycardia: The heart, already strained as it tries to keep up with the demand for more blood, begins to beat more rapidly than normal.
O Hypertrophy: The heart walls may thicken in an attempt to maintain the increased force of blood flow.
O Due to the reduced amount of blood reaching organs throughout the body, severe effects can follow. For example, kidney failure often coexists with CHF.

Treatment of heart failure is usually a two-pronged approach, a combination of medication and lifestyle and dietary modifications. Cardiac surgery in the form of valve repair or replacement may be reduced or prevented by examining the cause or reducing lifestyle causes. It is critical that you follow your doctor's instructions, monitor yourself, and report back to your physician.

In general, ameliorating medications include ACE inhibitors that expand the blood vessels to reduce the stress on the heart, multiple diuretics that help relieve the congestive (excessive blood or tissue fluid) aspect of CHF, beta-blockers used judiciously in specific types of CHF, and drugs to control heart rhythms, such as digoxin and vasodilators. In some cases, balloon angioplasty, along with stenting, surgery, pacemakers, and heart-transplant surgery may be necessary.

Pericarditis

Pericarditis is a very specific heart disorder that occurs when the pericardium becomes inflamed. The pericardium is the thin, membrane-like sac that contains the heart and protects the blood vessels that extend from the heart. The pericardium is composed of two thin layers with a tiny amount of fluid between them that keeps the layers fluid and flexible. Inflammation, or pericarditis, causes increased fluid, which, in turn, constricts the heart, minimizing its effectiveness.

Pericarditis can either be acute or chronic; however, in many cases, the cause is unknown. A viral or fungal infection, heart attacks, spreading cancer, radiation treatment, an injury, or complications from surgery can result in pericarditis. Pericarditis is often seen with inflammatory arthritis, such as rheumatoid arthritis and some forms of lupus.

Pericarditis may take several forms:

O Constrictive pericarditis, which occurs when the pericardium becomes so hardened that it begins to squeeze the heart until it loses its elasticity and can no longer receive and pump blood effectively. It can be fatal.

O Viral pericarditis, the initial symptoms of which are similar to those of a chest cold or upper respiratory ailment. It's possible that you may contract mumps, chicken pox, flu, mononucleosis, or another virus that will lead to this type of pericarditis.

○ Bacterial pericarditis, a rare form of pericarditis that stems from a bacterial infection. The use of antibiotics has reduced the incidence of this potentially dangerous condition. Bacterial or suppurative pericarditis often appears as a complication of another disease, and recovery is likely when the underlying problem has been treated.

○ Fungal pericarditis is usually found in people with various chronic illnesses, such as cancer, or complications from surgery.

○ Uremic pericarditis, an offshoot of kidney failure, which can be treated with dialysis.

Your doctor may treat pericarditis with anti-inflammatory drugs, analgesics, or antibiotics, depending on the cause of the inflammation. In rare cases, fluid can be reduced through a minor surgical procedure, and bouts with pericarditis are usually cleared up in one to four weeks.

Hole in the Heart

Patent foramen ovale (PFO) is a hole in the heart, and is actually more common than you might think. About 10 percent of the population has an undiagnosed PFO that usually isn't evident until another problem, such a stroke or a TIA (mini-stroke), develops. A PFO can increase your likelihood of a stroke.

The foramen ovale is a small, flaplike opening in your heart that forms between the left and right atria (the upper chambers of the heart) while you are in the womb. Most people may have PFOs at birth; however, they close after birth. The foramen ovale permits oxygenated blood to flow within the heart, as the fetal lungs are not mature. If the foramen ovale is not fully closed (i.e., patent), infrequently a clot may form when blood leaks through the hole. Rarely, the clot may break off and travel to the brain, causing a stroke.

Often, PFO is seen during a confirmatory echocardiogram. In general, no treatment is begun and closure is rarely necessary unless some other problem appears, such as a clot that puts you at risk for a stroke. Most infants are not affected by PFO, and research is continuing in this area to see whether PFO is linked to migraine headaches or other conditions, such as certain valve disorders.

Rheumatic Heart Disease

Rheumatic heart disease (RHD) begins with, and is a complication of, rheumatic fever. Rheumatic fever most often is a result of an acute fever caused by the streptococcal virus, more commonly known as strep throat. In the early part of the twentieth century, rheumatic fever was one of the leading killers of young children and adolescents. Today, it has virtually disappeared in the U.S. as a result of better diagnosis and the availability of antibiotics, but it still exists throughout the world. Estimates run from 5 to 30 million cases among children, leading to 90,000 deaths each year.

Once inflammation from the strep infection spreads, the joints, heart, brain, and skin can become involved. The most serious effect of rheumatic fever is potential damage to the heart valves, which may not be identified immediately. In this case, the valve's ability to open or close may be impaired. This condition, which can remain with you for life, may progress to valve deterioration and congestive heart failure.

Preventive measures for both RHD and RF are simple. When a serious sore throat or strep infection occurs, make sure that a throat culture is obtained. If it's positive, ensure that it is treated immediately with penicillin or some other antibiotic. *One of the key risks of RF and RHD is previous episodes of the disease, so it is vital to get immediate treatment. The more often it occurs, the more likely it is your health may be compromised.*

Silent Ischemia

Silent ischemia is sometimes called a silent heart attack, but this is not accurate, even though the condition may actually lead to an MI. Ischemia is a general term that describes what happens when oxygenated blood fails to reach a part of the body because blood flow is restricted by a narrowed artery. Silent cardiac ischemia is when the blood supply to the heart is temporarily cut off and, despite some potential angina, there is little pain. Although you may experience irregular heart rhythms, you usually do not recognize any problem—thus, silent ischemia is the result.

SCD in Athletes

Sudden cardiac death rarely makes the front pages unless the victim is a celebrity or, in many cases, a young athlete. In some cases, it may be both, as in the case of "Pistol Pete" Maravich. Maravich had a long, successful career in the NBA. Averaging 44 points per game in college, he seemed to be indestructible until an injury forced him to retire in 1980. In January 1988, while playing a pick-up basketball game, Maravich suddenly collapsed and died within minutes. He was 40 years old.

Maravich did not die from a heart attack, but from a rare congenital condition that, under the right conditions, shut down blood flow to his heart, killing the muscle almost immediately. Basically, Maravich was born with only a single vessel feeding his heart enriched blood. Eventually, his heart tissue decomposed and could not carry on. It was not a condition that could have been identified during a routine physical.

Pistol Pete was not alone. Each year, perhaps 1 in 10,000 runners and fewer than a dozen young athletes, mostly football players, die suddenly. Other reports claim that between 1 in 100,000 to 1 in 300,000 such deaths occur.

Some deaths are not SCD, such as the heart attack suffered by running guru Jim Fixx. In Fixx's case, he had a long family history of heart disease, and his death from an MI at age 52 came ten years later than his father had lived.

SCD in athletes almost always occurs like Maravich's did, the result of a congenital defect. It may, however, be brought on by the high level of exercise that causes electrolytes and endorphins to be released, affecting heartbeat and undetected blockages.

Sadly, few athletes who suffer SCD are revived; however, use of CPR and portable defibrillators give the victim a chance.

According to the American Heart Association, 3 to 4 million Americans may have episodes of silent ischemia every year, and it is possible that silent ischemia may cause a sudden heart attack. If you have had a heart attack, coronary artery disease, or diabetes, or if you are obese, you may be at greater risk for silent ischemia. If you are a smoker, if you have high blood pressure, or if you overuse alcohol, you may also increase your chances of an episode. For this reason, your cardiologist may order an exercise or stress test.

Treatment for silent ischemia is essentially the same as for any other condition requiring improved blood flow to the heart.

Sudden Cardiac Death

Sudden cardiac death (SCD) is a frightening concept. The heart simply stops without any warning. You may not necessarily have a heart attack or know that you have cardiovascular disease. What happens is that the cardiovascular system shuts down so quickly that the brain is denied oxygen, the victim collapses, and the heart stops. Within a few moments, brain function begins to deteriorate, followed by death.

SCD is not isolated. According to the American Heart Association, about half of all deaths from coronary heart disease—930 Americans per day—are the result of a sudden coronary event. In more than 90 percent of those who die of SCD, two or more major coronary arteries are occluded or narrowed and the condition is undiagnosed. Drug use—both illegal and prescription—also is found in multiple cases.

Other potential causes of SCD include interruption of the electrical system of the heart, rapidly spreading infection, sudden loss of oxygen (strangling), sudden embolism in the lungs, and accidents such as electrocution or drowning. Often, SCD is mislabeled as a massive heart attack, which is a misnomer because the cause of a heart attack is death of the heart muscle, which is not usually the case in sudden cardiac death.

Can you survive SCD? While surviving SCD is a contradiction in terms, it is possible to come back if you are fortunate enough to be with someone who knows cardiopulmonary resuscitation (CPR) or has access to a defibrillator. If the victim is revived within a few minutes, brain damage could be minimized. In most cases, the person may survive if the underlying causes are corrected. It's generally accepted that beyond ten minutes, resuscitation may not be possible.

Valvular Disease

Valvular disease or cardiac valvular disorders are relatively common, especially among those who have had heart attacks. Some estimates indicate that between 3 and 4 million Americans have some sort of heart-valve abnormality. Other sources believe the number is closer to 8 million people. About 95,000 valve surgeries are performed every year, and approximately 42,500 deaths occur from valve disorders each year.

There is some evidence, according to the American Heart Association, of a genetic pattern within families with heart-valve disease. These studies "suggest that unknown genetic factors contribute to death due to mitral valve disease and death due to non-rheumatic aortic valve disease." The researchers emphasized that these are preliminary and that more research, especially among ethnic groups, is required.

The heart's basic structure consists of four chambers: the upper left and right atria and the lower left and right ventricles. The atria and ventricles are connected by unique valves that allow blood to flow out and that close after each heartbeat to prevent backflow. The valves are not exactly valves, but are more like flaps, and each valve flap is called a "leaflet" or "cusp."

Heart valves can be damaged by an infection or a disorder such as rheumatic fever. Damage to the valves keeps them from opening fully to allow blood to pass or causes incomplete closure so blood returns to the chamber it just came from (regurgitation). Heart-valve damage frequently is the result of a congenital defect that can be treated with medication or surgery.

You may hear the term mitral valve prolapse (MVP), which is the most common valvular disorder of the left side of the atrial-ventricular structure. In this case, when the left ventricle contracts (or is in systole) the blood is supposed to flow out through the aortic valve into the aorta to refresh the oxygenated blood in the body. In MVP, the flaps do not fit exactly right. They may be too large, and what is described as a ballooning-out effect occurs, allowing some oxygenated blood to flow back into the left atrium. Your cardiologist or physician may hear a clicking or murmur when you are examined with a stethoscope. In general, MVP may cause symptoms such as chest pain, palpitations, and fatigue. Treatment may include medications and, in extreme circumstances, surgery, but *it's very important that you inform your doctor or a dentist that you have a valve problem prior to any procedures*. Dental work can cause risk of infection, as can surgery, and your doctor may decide to give you antibiotics to prevent any valve infections that harm your heart. This warning also extends to pregnant women whose doctor may administer a preventive course of antibiotics during delivery.

On the right side of the heart, the tricuspid valve can be affected in a similar manner. Usually, the problems of the tricuspid valve are less serious than are those of the mitral valve (see Figure 3).

FIGURE 3

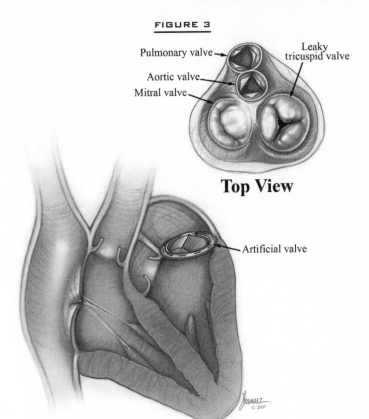

Pulmonary valve
Aortic valve
Mitral valve
Leaky tricuspid valve

Top View

Artificial valve

The pulmonary valve, which enables blood to flow from the right side of the heart into the lungs, also can develop abnormally or can possess the same sort of regurgitation flow problems as other defective valves.

The aortic valve may also have a similar defect, which prevents blood from completely flowing out into the aorta from the left ventricle. The same sort of regurgitation can occur because the aortic valve has developed with only two leaflets instead of three, a condition called a bicuspid valve. In addition, if the valve is harmed or becomes stenotic (the blood passage becomes severely narrowed), the heart itself can be injured from "pressure overload."

Treatment in this case can include use of a special balloon catheter to open the valve; however, valve repair or replacement for MVP and other valve anomalies also are used. Fortunately, this has been a successful method of treatment.

Artificial tissue valves (see Figure 3) are made from tissue taken from the pericardium of either cows or pigs. These have been in use for some time. In some cases, human valves from cadavers are used. There are also several types of mechanical or artificial valves that your doctor will discuss with you if you are faced with a valve replacement. He or she will explain the pros and cons of each valve type. There are many variables, such as your age and the amount of damage to your heart from the compromised valve. You may have to take blood-thinning medications, but depending on other conditions, such as your overall health, associated heart conditions, kidney problems, and a multitude of other factors, the decision is usually individualized.

Each year, new guidelines are released to improve the treatment of valve disease and to seek methods of early detection and prevention, among them increased monitoring of heart diseases such as endocarditis and coronary artery disease.

Vascular disease, which includes stroke, atherosclerosis, aneurysms, varicose veins, and other disorders, along with diabetes and hypertension, may be part of your overall diagnosis.

IN A SENTENCE:

> *Cardiovascular disease is a constellation of disorders that either are a result of a diseased heart or, conversely, lead to a damaged heart, resulting in multiple systemic failures.*

living

Your Heart Is More Than a Pump

WHAT DO you need to know about your heart? After all, it seems to have failed you. Do you need to know as much as a cardiologist? Will a general understanding of the physiology of the cardiovascular system suffice?

The answer is simple and definitive: The more you know about the anatomy of this extraordinary organ and the amazing system in your body that it supports, the better your life as a heart patient will be. As you take the initial steps to recover your health, it's a very good idea to understand, in some depth, how the heart and your circulatory system function as a team to keep you up and running.

Anyone who has a damaged heart knows that when the heart cannot perform its basic functions, the rest of your body is impaired and virtually every other organ is compromised. Over the years, I've consulted many reference books about heart disease, finding that you either need several years of medical school to understand them or they are too simple. In this section you will learn important details about the structure and function of your heart that will help you better understand your condition.

How the Heart Works

Your heart, a muscle with nodes, chambers, and valves, is the central engine in a 70,000-plus-mile system of veins, arteries, **capillaries**, and blood that services 300 trillion tissue cells in your body. When all is well, the heart is an extraordinary organ that pulses blood through your body in a carefully regulated cycle. This is what is commonly called **the cardiovascular system,** and it is energized by naturally occurring electrical impulses and chemicals in the heart.

There are many analogies that have been used for the heart's role in the body. The common one is to liken it to a pump—taking in low-oxygen blood and pumping out high-oxygen blood. But that is too simple—especially if you have heart disease and know better. A mechanical pump is easy to fix; a heart is much more complicated. Your physician or surgeon needs more than a few tools to take care of your heart and to restore it to its highest functional level.

My experience in learning about heart disease has led me to visualize my heart as a sophisticated, complex machine. In the best of all worlds, an effective and healthy heart should maintain what is called homeostasis within the body. When this effectiveness is impaired, it can cause the machine's operation to become threatened and, in turn, can reduce its ability to bring the nutrients in your blood to their proper destinations in the cellular system. Therefore, although one of the heart's most important functions is to pump blood through it, when we are looking at it from the point of view of someone who has *heart disease,* the analogy is too simple.

A Perfect Machine

Take your hands, close them together into a single fist and hold them up. This is essentially the size and shape of your heart. Generally, the heart weighs between 7 and 12 ounces, depending on the sex and size of its owner. It rests in the middle of your chest, slightly off center, tilted toward your left hip. The rib cage in front and the spine in the back provide important protection from injury. Despite its size, your heart is a tough little machine, vital and powerful.

As organs go, the heart's construction is relatively simple, but amazingly well designed to do its main job: circulation of life-sustaining, energized blood that keeps your body running at the level you need. The heart is supported by a surrounding sac called the pericardium. Beneath that are three layers that form the heart wall.

The outermost layer of the heart, and the inner layer of the pericardium sac, is the **epicardium**, a thin connective tissue that protects the heart.

The middle layer, the myocardium, is often referred to as the heart muscle, although it actually is the wall of the heart and it contains the heart muscle. It plays the most important role in transporting deoxygenated (low oxygen) blood into the heart's chambers and sending oxygenated blood out into the body. It is made of muscular fibers, or myocytes, that contract in unison to energize the heart so it can alternately compress to pump blood and relax to allow more blood to flow in from the circulatory system. The myocytes are critical because they control the relaxation and contraction function of the heart muscle.

Each myocyte cell is stimulated by electrical jolts from cells produced by the heart's sinus or sinoatrial node (also called SAN cells) and the atrioventricular node. These bundles of fibers within the muscle generate electrical impulses that initially power your heart to contract and relax (beat), allowing blood to flow through the chambers. Each impulse begins in the sinus node in the right atrium, is transmitted through the myocyte cells, and then is passed on to the ventricles through the atrioventricular node. The power surge continues through the His-Purkinje system, which is bundles of fibers spread throughout the heart muscle. This all occurs in one one-hundredth of a second!

Bundles of Kent

The heart has many bundle-like structures that come into play when needed. One is the Bundle of Kent, which acts as a bridge between the atrium and the ventricle in response to a specific rhythmic problem, Woff-Parkinson-White syndrome, a disorder of the conduction system.

In effect, we have an invisible wiring system attached to a sort of natural pacemaker that creates electrical stimulation throughout the heart tissue. We refer to this as our conduction system. The heartbeat actually consists of a momentary contraction, then relaxation that takes about one second. If you listen to your heart through a stethoscope, you'll hear the famous "lub-dub" sound. Next time you see your cardiologist, ask to hear your own heart. It is (usually) quite reassuring.

While this system is usually steady and regular, it is designed to increase with stress or other emotional stimuli. However, when we create a situation in which inadequate oxygenated blood flows to the heart because of arterial blockages, for example, the heart muscle begins to function less efficiently.

Finally, the inner surface of the heart is called the endocardium and, like a fitted sheet on your bed, it comes in smooth contact with all the surfaces within the heart. The endocardial tissue is similar to the elastic endothelium tissue that lines the blood vessels. One of its functions is to act as a barrier between the blood contained within the heart chambers and the myocardium. This ensures that the myocyte cells are not flooded or destroyed.

Inside Your Heart

The vital blood-pumping work of the heart—driving the circulatory system (see Figure 4)—takes place within the multi-layered structure described above. However, you will see that the real genius of the heart is in how all the various structures manage to work in perfect synchronicity to achieve blood cleansing and recirculation throughout the body. Normally, it's a well-adjusted machine unless something goes wrong. A breakdown can be a slow, unnoticed process unless you are aware of signs that all is not well.

To understand the basis of the circulatory system, think of a washing machine where you throw in your dirty clothes, then transfer them to the dryer. Your clean, fresh clothes are ready to use again. Or think of your car that you hop into and fill with gasoline, which is essentially like the nutrients you consume in your diet. We turn it on, and the gas-fed ignition system sparks to life, sending power to the engine that propels you to your destination.

FIGURE 4

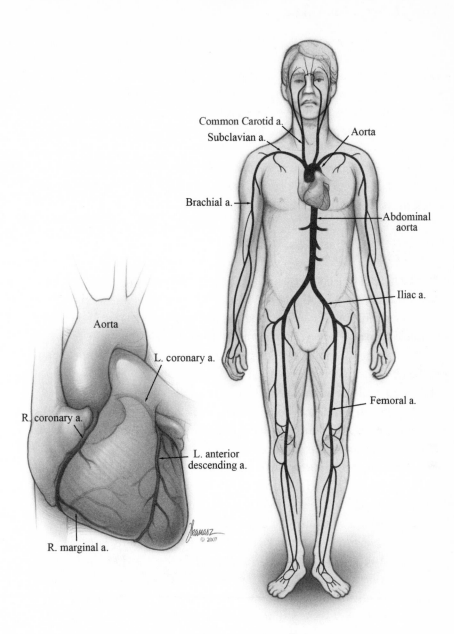

The Heart Chambers

Within the heart wall are four chambers that serve two separate purposes. On top are the right atrium and the left atrium. Below are the right ventricle and the left ventricle (see Figure 5A).

Essentially, the job of the left atrium is to gather the oxygenated blood as it flows in from the lungs and then pass it to the left ventricle, which expels the newly oxygenated blood back into the bloodstream, through the aorta.

The right atrium receives oxygen- and nutrient-depleted blood from the bloodstream, which is then passed to the right ventricle and released back to the lungs for re-oxygenation.

The Heart Valves

The heart is designed to avoid flooding the vessels with blood. The heart has two different sets of flap-like valves that open and close so that blood will flow in only one direction. One set of valves connect the atria and the ventricles and are known as atrioventricular valves (see Figure 5B). A second set of valves between the ventricles and their arterial or venous connections to the circulatory system prevents blood from backflowing as it is pumped off toward its destination. These are known as the semilunar valves.

Oxygenated blood that comes into the left atrium passes through the mitral valve into the left ventricle and is pumped out through the aortic valve into the aorta. The aorta is your body's largest artery, and is the premier conduit for your refreshed blood as it is carried throughout your body. The wall of the left ventricle is the strongest part of the heart muscle, and the pressure is so strong that if it were pointed out of your body, the blood would spurt as high as six feet.

Blood that flows into the right atrium from the veins is oxygen-depleted as it returns from its trip through the body. It is then pushed into the right ventricle through the tricuspid valve. Blood in the right ventricle is pumped through the pulmonary valve into the pulmonary trunk and the pulmonary system (lungs) to pick up oxygen.

It's important to remember that the heart, as described above, is only a part of the cardiovascular system that has you on this journey of renewal. Let's take a look at the rest of the nuts-and-bolts side of the heart picture.

FIGURE 5

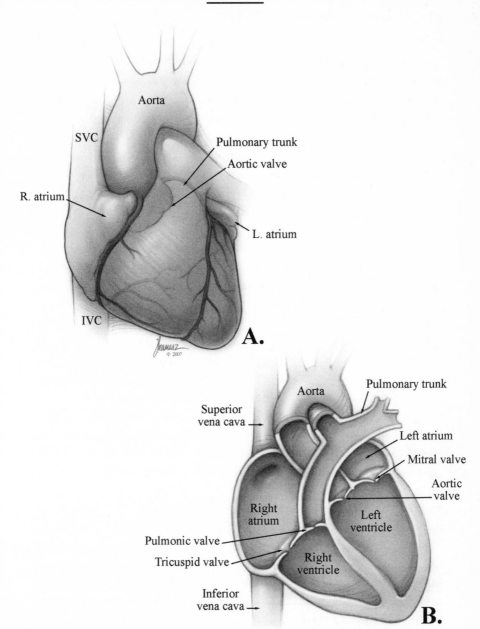

A.

B.

What Makes the Heart Beat?

Every good machine needs a power source to spark it to life and an internal system to get it up and running smoothly. The heart is no different. As I mentioned, the heart has an electrical conduction system that provokes the opening and closing of the valves to and from the atria chambers, forcing blood through the ventricles and into the bloodstream.

For the heart to function efficiently, we need a regular heartbeat. Technically, the heartbeat is produced by the contraction and expansion of the heart in a regular rhythm. The heartbeat is what is actually measured when someone takes your pulse, which is why the heartbeat is also one of the few parts of the cardiovascular system that we actually feel. This may be another reason why the heartbeat is used in language as a tangible expression of strong emotion. Two obvious examples: "You are so beautiful you make my heart beat faster" or "I was so scared I could hear my heart beating."

Is this true? Can you actually hear your heart beat at the sight of someone you love? Actually, it's possible. Our normal resting heartbeat is about 60 to 80 beats per minute, but can easily jump to 100 beats per minute and provoke palpitations, shortness of breath, sweating, weakness, dizziness, fainting, and chest pain. Common events, such as exercise, anxiety, stress, medication, dehydration, fever, excessive caffeine, nicotine, recreational drugs, and a number of medical conditions, also can provoke rapid heartbeat.

The heartbeat is actually the effect of the blood flowing through the heart chambers in a synchronized manner. When the heart beats, we feel the heart muscle contract and force out the blood that has entered the heart through the two chambers. This is called systole. When it relaxes, this is called diastole. These are the two terms we use to describe blood pressure: a combination of the pressure exerted by the blood flowing out of the heart and any resistance it meets because the arteries may be blocked or narrowed. It's generally agreed that a blood-pressure reading higher than 140/90 is a sign that you have hypertension and that you need some sort of treatment, whether through dietary adjustment or medication. A blood-pressure reading of between 120/80 and 140/90 is a sign that you are at strong risk for developing high blood pressure.

When your blood pressure is abnormal, that is a clear red flag for your cardiologist.

Another important sign of heart-muscle difficulties related to the heart chambers is the ejection fraction. This is a measure of the percentage of blood pumped out of both ventricles during the contraction or pulsing phase when they are at full capacity. Understanding this is very important because your cardiologist will mention it as a good or bad sign (this is another example of how knowing the jargon can help you in your own treatment). If your ejection fraction is about 55 to 60 percent, then your heart is functioning normally. It can even rise as you work out, but if your heart is damaged in any way, it could be substantially lower.

A recent report from my cardiologist stated that my ejection fraction had gone up significantly. Not only was I happy because of the positive health implication, but I knew that this was a result of my daily exercise regimen. While the workouts (in my case, 30 minutes a day on the treadmill) may be a pain, this news is the best positive reinforcement you can get!

IN A SENTENCE:

> *The heart is a sophisticated organ that functions like a finely tuned engine and that has to be maintained properly for the greatest benefit to your body.*

Understanding the Circulatory System

UNDERSTANDING THE basic anatomic structure of the heart is only part of what you should know about your cardiovascular system. As miraculous as the heart structure may be, its role as the engine driving the entire **circulatory system** is just as remarkable and critical to your heart health. In fact, when the circulatory system develops problems, the effect on your heart can be instantly devastating, and you may have had no warning. Even more amazing, your body's constantly circulating blood runs through about 75,000 miles of blood vessels!

Unlike the heart, there are no odes or poetic tributes to the circulatory system. Its main task, carrying blood throughout the body, doesn't seem too spectacular. In fact, you'll find common analogies that are fairly obvious. One compares the veins and arteries to a superhighway; another compares your blood cells to little UPS packages being transported through the streets that branch off a superhighway. Another sees the entire system as a figure eight, with your heart at its central crossover.

As far as the circulatory system is concerned, you don't need a visual image or a clever analogy to help you understand what it is and how well it works. We can, however, pick up from our comparison of your heart to an engine that enables your body to receive the vital nutrients it needs to sustain your daily activities.

Blood Cells

Our blood cells are often overlooked in the various descriptions of the heart, heart disease, and the blood's superhighway system, but, despite their size, they have the responsibility for performing a wide variety of essential tasks. Your own growth and health depend on the health of your cellular system. All tissues in our bodies are composed of cells, and virtually all our body's functions are carried out by cells. There are a wide variety of cells, depending on their duties in the body, and they are reproduced in only one way: cell division. That means that if we lose certain cells, we are vulnerable to disease and we don't function at our maximum capacity.

Your body has about 5 million red blood cells that carry oxygen from the lungs through the body, depositing it in other cells that need replenishment. At the same time, they pick up the waste products, such as carbon dioxide, from those cells. The red blood cells return the carbon dioxide to the lungs, where it is exhaled.

Our white blood cells (leukocytes) are critical in the battle against germs or infection. They are the first line of defense against infection. White blood cells have a short life span, from days to weeks, and their numbers increase if you develop an infection. In fact, if you develop a very high white-blood-cell count, it can be a symptom of something significantly amiss, such as leukemia or another form of cancer. There are also different types of white blood cells that may join together to fight disease, including B-cells, helper-T cells, plasma cells, and several others that play multiple roles.

More About Your Blood

Did you ever wonder why you stop bleeding when you cut yourself? Within your blood vessels are a third type of blood cells, called platelets, that help blood coagulate to seal damaged blood vessels. At the first sign of a cut, the platelets link to each other at the edges of the cut to form a blood clot. Unlike a clot within a blood vessel that can lead to a heart attack or stroke, this is more like a blood plug.

These cells are also only one part of your blood. About half of your blood is composed of a liquid called plasma, which is generated in the liver and carries the blood cells and other blood components through the body.

The last component of the blood-cell system is bone marrow, which is a soft, naturally occurring material found in the interior of the bones. Red blood cells are produced in the bone marrow and the spleen.

Circulation: A Two-Way System

So far, we've talked about how the heart is built, how it works as a sophisticated machine to send blood through your body, and the millions of cells that come together to form blood. As you will see, the circulatory system is another remarkable aspect of your cardiovascular system.

> Essentially, the circulatory system is composed of three major parts: arteries, capillaries, and veins that carry blood away from and back to the heart. Without this system, our cells cannot gather nutrients, water, and oxygen and remove wastes such as carbon dioxide.

Arteries

The largest artery in your body is the aorta, which rises directly from the left ventricle in the heart. Oxygen-filled blood from the left ventricle flows into the aorta, which branches off to give enriched blood first to the brain, then to the arms, chest, and abdomen. At this point, when the descending aorta reaches the level of your navel, it divides and branches into two iliac arteries that continue carrying blood to your pelvis, legs, and feet.

As the arteries get farther and farther away from your heart, they also become smaller and ultimately convert to arterioles that can reach virtually anywhere in the body. The arterioles are a key part of the system that regulates the flow of the blood, keeping about 10 percent of our total blood volume circulating in the arteries at any time.

The main arteries and veins are elastic and are composed of layers of tissue, including a layer of smooth muscle that absorbs the pressure from the pulsing blood. This smooth muscle structure maintains blood flow at

---

The Pulmonary Artery

Because the heart has to have the strength to send blood throughout the body, it also has to send fresh blood to itself. It does this through a part of the circulatory system called the **pulmonary arteries,** which are the route your blood uses to go from the heart to the lungs for refreshment. Originating at the base of the right ventricle, the pulmonary artery splits into two separate vessels leading to each lung. Once oxygenated, the blood leaves the lungs, returning to the heart. The two pulmonary veins feed blood into the left atrium, on through the left ventricle, and out the aorta. The **coronary arteries** branch off from the aortic arch, and, in turn, feed blood into a web of capillaries that deliver it directly to the heart muscle.

---

constant pressure, even as the arteries shrink in size. If all is well, the blood simply flows through the arteries and doesn't leak out of the vessels.

Ultimately, the arterioles connect to the tiny capillaries, which is the means by which the blood is distributed into the cells. In fact, the capillaries become so narrow that the cells literally have to flow through them in single file! Even more amazing, it's estimated that your body may have 300 trillion cells and, since your blood has to come in contact with all of them to keep them alive, capillaries make up most of the body's blood vessels.

Structured as a sort of web, the capillaries' role differs in various parts of the body, depending on the metabolic activity of the tissues they reach. When your blood flows into the capillaries, it may release oxygen, pick up carbon dioxide, and allow an exchange of gases, nutrients, and other waste products. In some cases, such as in the **connective tissues** in the muscles, large amounts of oxygen are required to function, so capillaries are spread throughout them.

Veins

The venous system is the remarkable path that your blood takes on its way back to the heart. Veins are spread throughout the body, just as the arteries are. At the end of each vein is a tiny venule that connects to the capillaries carrying wastes and deoxygenated blood from the arteries.

Like a network of widening roads heading for Main Street (in this case, the heart), the venules join together to form a network of increasingly larger veins.

Two major veins receive blood from the body and connect directly to the heart: the **superior vena cava,** which returns blood from the head, chest, and upper extremities, and the **inferior vena cava**, which returns blood from veins below the waist. The veins are constructed somewhat the same as the arteries are, but are less elastic and thinner. Once the blood is in the superior and inferior venae cavae, it flows back to the heart and then through the right atrium, into the right ventricle, and to the lung. Once cleansed and reoxygenated, it flows into the left side of the heart and the blood's journey begins again.

Veins are where blood is drawn from when you need blood tests for diagnostic purposes, since they do not pulse, as your arteries do.

IN A SENTENCE:

The circulatory system is a clever complex of tiny vessels carrying precious red and white blood cells from the heart throughout the body, where they perform their functions and return in an endless loop.

DAY 4

living

Choosing a Cardiologist

UNLESS YOU'RE in the emergency room after a sudden heart attack, any treatment for heart disease, even recovery from scheduled heart surgery, actually begins *before* you undergo medical procedures. Sounds contradictory, but it's not. If your primary care physician or another doctor has told you that you should be in the care of a heart specialist, you first need to choose the right cardiologist *for you*. Once a diagnosis is made, you have several other choices to make. If surgery or another procedure, such as an angiogram, is indicated you also have to decide who, what, where, when, and how, and you must make an informed choice that leaves you comfortable and secure. It's often said that the most important purchase people make is their home or car, but in reality, making a decision about who will help you with your health care is an even more vital purchase.

Your options for selecting a cardiologist before a crisis and after you find yourself in the emergency room after a sudden heart attack or in your doctor's office complaining of chest or neck pain are vastly different. *These last two situations are ones that you categorically want to avoid.* The information below, like most of this book, is dedicated to ensuring that you do not end up in a crisis. In **Day Five,** you will find emergency

---

What Is Cardiology?

Cardiology is a subspecialty of internal medicine, and requires special training and certification. In general, cardiologists deal with diseases of the circulatory system and the heart, but some only treat children with congenital heart problems or the elderly. Interventional cardiologists specialize in treating patients with non-surgical methods, such as angioplasty and stenting. Many cardiologists are involved in research and many also perform electrophysiology procedures, such as inserting pacemakers and other rhythm-control devices.

---

response details; however, in this chapter, we'll assume that you have examined your risk factors or you have been referred to a cardiovascular specialist *before* you are in a crisis.

Although I'm sure your primary care doctor has explained to you why you are being referred to a heart specialist, you've probably had some tests that suggested to him or her that this is the proper course. You may not realize that when you go for a physical or you meet with a doctor, he or she is assessing specific indicators, such as blood tests that come back with elevated cholesterol or other blood values that indicate potential arterial blockages. Vital signs, such as blood pressure, pulse, breathing, temperature, and basic reflexes are part of this exam. Along with this, a urine test may show elevated glucose levels and a potential for diabetes.

Your doctor will palpate, or press down, on various places on your abdomen to determine whether or not you have swelling, tenderness, or any other abnormalities. While this may seem unnecessary to you, an internist or family physician adds information gained from this to the other information picked up during the exam, such as your general overall health, weight, skin condition, and even your real age compared to the age you may look. When your doctor listens to your chest, his goal is to hear any abnormal heartbeat, make sure your lungs are clear, and check your abdomen to see whether your bowel sounds are normal. A complete physical will include many other tests for vision, spinal, and hearing problems.

In my case, my family physician, who had seen me for many years, decided that my high glucose levels, elevated cholesterol, and high blood pressure indicated that I should see a cardiologist. In retrospect, she was smart: She also diagnosed my denial and lack of motivation to change my health behavior. By sending me to a specialist, she recognized that, in the hands of someone who dealt with patients like me daily, there was a chance for me. She was right, and she likely saved my life.

Finding a Cardiovascular Specialist

When you first discover you may have some sort of cardiac problem, the importance of finding the right doctor is probably not going to be the first thing that pops into your mind. That's understandable, but it should move up the list quickly. If you do have some sort of problem, the right cardiologist is going to become your new best friend. Whether you spend a lot of time together, you and your cardiologist will have to interact, respect each other, and partner. Ultimately, you will have to put your complete faith and your life, in some cases, in his or her hands.

It's likely that you ended up in your first (or present) cardiologist's office when someone else, most likely your primary physician, gave you a name. Is this the right way to go about choosing a cardiologist or any other specialist for a major health issue? Today, several factors can affect your choice of a specialist. The primary one may be that your insurance company only allows treatment by certain doctors within its network without additional charge. More doctors are accepting virtually all insurance plans, so you may find the doctor you are seeking is within your plan. The same goes for HMOs, managed care programs, Medicare, Medicaid, or workers' compensation, where certain physicians are recommended or second opinions are required.

There are many specialists in practice today, so you should have plenty of choices. However, with out-of-network doctors, you will likely have to pay some fee (often up front). This is not simply about the doctor wanting to make more money, but because they cannot legally accept your insurance if they are not in your network. If they did it for you, they would have to do that for every patient.

There may be another limitation on your choice of a cardiologist. The doctor you want may not be taking new patients at the time, or the wait for an appointment may be too long. In that case, there may be other

What Does "Board Certification" Mean?

One way to evaluate your choice of a cardiologist is to review his or her train-ing and determine whether the doctor has gone beyond the basic training that all doctors go through on the road through medical school, internship, and res-idency. Many doctors who decide to specialize in related areas enhance their skills by seeking board certification. Twenty-four specializations related to dif-ferent aspects of medicine are part of the American Board of Medical Spe-cialties (AMBS), which was founded in 1933 "to create uniformity in physican certification and to increase public awareness of the value of specialty certifi-cation. ABMS advocates for safe, quality healthcare through its efforts to es-tablish and maintain high standards for professional physician certification."

In order to become board-certified, most physicians spend a year or more in specialized training, which is sometimes called a fellowship, after which they must undergo strenuous written and oral tests administered by a board of physician examiners in the chosen specialty. Each medical specialty has its own requirements, and some may demand greater training than others, due to the nature of the specialty (e.g., certain areas of surgery).

Almost all cardiologists are board-certified in internal medicine. If they have the initials F.A.C.C. after their names, this means they have become fellows of the American Academy of Cardiology, and with three more years of training, they may then "sit" for board certification in cardiology. Recertification is re-quired, generally every ten years. This exam is administered by the American Board of Internal Medicine (215-446-3500, 800-441-2246, or www.abim.org). For more information on board certification of surgeons, contact the American Board of Surgery (215-568-4000 or www.absurgery.com).

cardiologists in the same practice who can treat you. This happened to me, and it turned out that the younger doctor had more time for me. We formed a bond that was a key aspect of my recovery. Another upside of this situation is that doctors within a practice usually do consult with each other about cases that may not be straightforward. If no immediate appointments are available with your cardiologist of choice, you certainly can ask them for a referral to someone outside of the practice.

Word of mouth is a common way that people find a doctor, and it is not necessarily a bad reason to see someone *if the person who is recom-mending the doctor has had actual contact with them*. Although you have to remember that there are many other factors to consider in these cases, such as the doctor's practice focus and experience, many specialists get a large percentage of patients from word-of-mouth recommendations.

Another way to get valid referrals is through the local or state medical society, which can provide a list of local cardiologists and answer background questions you may have. Lists of specialists are available from **The American Board of Medical Specialists** (1-800-776-2378) and other organizations, such as the **American Heart Association** (www.americanheart.org). A local hospital also can give you names of staff cardiologists and tell you how to contact people in its cardiovascular program.

Ancillary health-care professionals also can be a good source of referrals. Many cardiac patients spend considerable time with physical therapists, nutritionists, and other members of cardio-rehab programs. They can be wonderful sources of information and suggestions, although sometimes their recommendations can be biased. Today, many medical practices and virtually every hospital or clinic has a website. Spend some time online (see **Month Twelve**) looking at both the doctor's credentials and information about the facility.

Making the Choice

What is the bottom line once you have a few doctors' names to consider?

Consider, above all, the doctor's training and experience. You may think that a young doctor might be a better choice because he or she is closer to the cutting edge of technology and research breakthroughs, but this is not necessarily the case. You'll want any doctor you see to be board-certified (see Box "What Does 'Board Certification' Mean?") in his or her specialty. In addition, almost all physicians participate in CME (continuing medical education) courses each year and have to accumulate a certain number of credits each year to remain licensed.

Medical education should only be one part of your search criteria. You want to find a doctor who also has as much hands-on experience as possible. If this person is a surgeon and you are having open heart surgery, you will want to know how many procedures the surgeon has done.

If the answer is 200, fine, but if the answer is 2,000, your choice is obvious. In medicine, *always* go with experience.

Another thing to consider is that many treatment methods today are fairly standard from facility to facility and from doctor to doctor. One reason you can expect this is a legal-medical principle called standard of care. The standard of care refers to the type and level of care health-care consumers should expect to receive. Many malpractice suits are based on whether the standard-of-care criteria have been met. In your case, this principle really means that the doctor you are looking for can and should be giving you the best possible care using the most commonly accepted treatment protocols. Thus, the treatment offered will not vary all that much from doctor to doctor, so your choice is often based on personal feelings.

Beyond training, what should you consider?

Some intangibles count more than others, and it's likely that you may base your decision on one of them. Remember that when you become a patient of a cardiology practice, you are being taken care of by a team. Make sure you know what other resources are available through this practice. If your cholesterol levels are out of whack, does the practice have a lipid clinic to give you advice and monitor you? Is there an on-site cardio-exercise or rehab facility? If at all possible where cardiovascular treatment is concerned, you'll want to be in a practice where a team is assembled, rather than only the cardiologist you chose.

Some other questions to keep in mind are:

Your Relationship with the Doctor

- ○ Do you like the doctor? If you don't, your motivation to comply with a treatment plan may be undone. There is no reason that you cannot change doctors. After all, your health is at stake.
- ○ Does this doctor inspire you to regain your health?
- ○ Do you feel comfortable going to the doctor's office? Does his or her style fit your personality?
- ○ Does the doctor listen to you? Don't hesitate to let a doctor know when you don't understand something.
- ○ Does the doctor respond to your questions, even if they come from the Internet or from a family member?

The Office

○ Do you have to spend hours waiting in the office on a regular basis? This could indicate that the doctor is overbooked or the staff is not responding to you. However, the practice of medicine today is filled with paperwork and forms that can stretch a staff's capabilities.

○ Can you reach the doctor or the on-call doctor in off hours?

○ Can you get to the office easily for regular visits?

○ Is the practice affiliated with a hospital you'd want to go to if necessary?

○ Does the staff help you willingly and correctly with the paperwork?

Treatment Plan

○ Is the doctor conservative or aggressive in his approach? Does the doctor suggest that the first thing you do is surgery when you want to try something else?

○ What about alternative therapies? What's the doctor's attitude compared to yours? (See Month Seven.)

○ Is the doctor involved in any way with a pharmaceutical company that could create a conflict in treatment? Some doctors have recommended procedures in which they have a financial stake without disclosing this fact.

○ Can the doctor get you into a research drug trial program if that can help?

○ Does the doctor have a wide circle of relationships with others who can help you if a certain procedure is required?

The First Visit

Once you have an appointment with a cardiologist, here are a few things to bring to your first visit:

○ a written narrative of why you are visiting the doctor (a few paragraphs will do)

○ a written narrative detailing specific signs and symptoms (use one or two words for each)

> ## Lesson Learned
>
> One lesson I've learned since I became a heart patient is that sometimes bigger is better when it comes to your cardiology choice. For several years before moving to Cleveland, I was treated at a large cardiology center in Asheville, North Carolina. It was a group practice with at least two dozen cardiologists, many ancillary therapists, a full-fledged lipid clinic for nutritional counseling and regular blood testing, and facilities for most typical non-invasive tests. It was well run, efficient, and if you had a 1 p.m. appointment, you were usually taken at that time. That experience was key to getting me back on the track to recovery, which then became a full-scale journey at Cleveland Clinic's Heart Center through Dr. Rimmerman.
>
> Not everyone can be fortunate enough to live near such a practice or world-famous care center, but if you have a choice, a larger practice has, in my experience, been the way to go.

○ a detailed list of both past medical history (e.g., hypertension, diabetes) and past surgeries, including dates, locations, and findings. It's best to have the surgical reports from your past doctors.

○ copies of major test reports, such as past heart catheterizations; these should be organized chronologically; if available, CD-ROMs and hard copies of x-rays in addition to copies of the radiologist's reports are quite helpful

○ a list of current medications, including dosages and frequency

○ a list of medication allergies and side effects

○ a list of social issues: tobacco, alcohol, illegal substances, marital status, children (with ages), exercise regime, educational level, occupation

○ family medical and surgical histories (first-degree relatives: parents, siblings)

When you go to see a new doctor, your share of the responsibility for your health care does not disappear. You have to be willing to meet the doctor halfway, not simply sit and expect a genie to pop into the exam room with all the answers. If anything, your responsibility will increase, and you must become more proactive in your own care.

Over the years, I've learned that there are some tangible things you must do to maintain a successful relationship with a doctor. At many practices, a physician assistant (PA) or a nurse practitioner will probably meet with you first. After your blood pressure and weight are taken, you'll likely be asked some questions about medication and your health history. You may also have an electrocardiogram (ECG). This helps your new cardiologist establish some baseline indicators. Most practices have adopted (or will soon) an electronic medical records (EMR) system in addition to the traditional paper chart, which will be updated at every visit. If you are able to give the PA or nurse complete information, it will help the cardiologist to ask more informed questions, leaving more time during your visit for you to discuss what's being recommended.

Be Prepared

While your primary care physician may say he or she will send your medical records to the specialist, make sure they have been sent before you go for your visit. Have a list of medications (or bring the bottles) that you are taking. Other *musts* for the first exam or consultation include the following:

○ Jot down some notes on your past health problems or related information. What sort of symptoms have you had? Have you been sick or hospitalized?

○ Do you exercise regularly?

○ What sort of tests have you had recently, such as an ECG or x-rays? These may seem obvious, but once you are in the exam room, half dressed, and probably stressed, nervous, or anxious, you want to be able to give your doctor all the information needed for an accurate diagnosis.

○ A doctor once told me, quite correctly, that the past is the best predictor of the future where health is concerned. Take a few minutes to jot down a few notes about your family's health history, going back at least two generations. This will help your doctor immensely.

○ I've found the easiest way to recall family health events is to make up a short time line. Indicate whether your parents, grandparents, or siblings suffered from heart disease (heart attacks), high blood pressure, diabetes, obesity, or other risk factors discussed in **Day One.**

You can count on two things happening during your first visit to a cardiologist: You will be very nervous and you may not understand some of the things your doctor says. Neither you nor your doctor is at fault. The truth is that if you are not nervous, you are in denial, and if you think you understand the doctor, you probably aren't listening to it all. Having visited cardiologists for more than a decade as a patient and as a journalist, I always learn something new and add to my knowledge and behavior-modification information bank.

This possible disconnect from what you are told and what you hear and absorb is why you are urged to bring the information listed previously with you. Another reason is that before you even get out of the waiting room, you'll be handed a clipboard with several forms to fill out. These are even more ubiquitous today because most physicians' offices use the electronic medical records systems along with paper charts. This is where the written lists mentioned come in handy. Not only will you save time trying to fill in all those questions on a confusing form, but it will make it easier for your doctor to get a better picture of your medical profile.

Call ahead and ask for the office to mail, fax, or e-mail the forms to you so you can fill them out and bring them with you to save time. Have your insurance information and contact information for your referring doctor with you. Consider bringing someone with you (not a child) to help you remember what will be said to you after your exam and to take notes. Your doctor may not want that person in the exam room; however, it is entirely proper to have someone with you in the office when you find out the doctor's initial diagnosis.

When the nurse or physician's assistant takes your vital signs and goes over your history, this is an ideal time to ask questions. If the nurse can't answer them, ask her to tell them to the doctor. Your cardiologist will try to put you at ease with a few quick questions that you think you've already answered! Your doctor's goal is to assess a number of factors to make a diagnosis. Most doctors use a process called a differential diagnosis, which is a systematic method of reaching a conclusion. Patients often assume doctors have some sort of checklist, but what they really do through the questions they ask you is eliminate possibilities until they have narrowed their diagnosis to the most likely cause. Let's jump forward for the moment and assume that your cardiologist has given you a diagnosis and that you have to make a decision about the recommended treatment. You have always heard that a second opinion is a must. Is this true? We'll look at this next.

IN A SENTENCE:

> *Connecting with the right cardiologist is vital to your long-term health, so make sure that you are comfortable with both your doctor and how the practice is run.*

Getting a
Second Opinion

MY QUADRUPLE bypass was performed at Morristown
Memorial Hospital, a suburban medical center in central
New Jersey, about 20 minutes from my home. I made that
choice for two reasons. First, my cardiologist was affiliated
with the hospital. Second, cardiovascular surgeons there had
performed more than 1,600 coronary bypasses that year,
more than the Mayo Clinic. When I finally pulled my head
out of denial and accepted my doctor's diagnosis, I had several options for surgery. I lived 45 minutes from Manhattan,
where there were several top medical centers, or I could go
to Boston, where I had multiple professional and personal
friends who practiced at the numerous hospitals affiliated
with the Harvard Medical School. As it turned out, the doctors who ran the cardiovascular program at Morristown had
trained together at Johns Hopkins Hospital, one of the top
three heart centers in the country.

When it came down to a decision, I chose Morristown
and a great surgeon, John M. Brown III, M.D., who, as I
learned from my research, had (and still has) the lowest rate
of mortality in cardiac bypass procedures in New Jersey. This
was a lucky choice because the Morristown Memorial heart-
care recovery program is designed to begin *before* you have

any procedures. As much as anything, this helped get me to actually cross the hospital's threshold on the day of my surgery.

Before I was admitted, I met with a social services worker (which is standard) to go over the technical and medical things I needed to know about my pre- and post-operative period, such as insurance coverage, medications, and other practical information to smooth my stay at the hospital.

She also offered a videotape that went through the details of the surgery with a great demo of the operation.

Along with about ten other people who were about to undergo various heart surgeries, I attended a sort of "pre-op" mini-support group, where the leader talked and answered questions that turned out to be very accurate. He also did a good job of reducing the considerable fear levels in the group, at least on the surface. The group consisted of non-emergency patients who were anxious to know what we really faced. We practiced exercises for post-operative recovery, such as learning how to blow into a contraption called an incentive spirometer that measures and helps increase lung power. We were given reams of resources to contact if we needed them, and this, too, proved to be helpful later. I had a lengthy pre-surgery meeting with Dr. Brown. Your surgeon may have a very different style from your doctor or cardiologist. When I met with my surgeon for the first time, he was thorough, showing me the images of my blocked arteries and fully explaining what he was going to do. However, as we left, there was an exchange that made me laugh and feel totally confident, or at least more at ease.

Me (at the end of the meeting): "Well, I feel confident; I've been told by everyone that you are one of the best around."

Dr. Brown (straight-faced): "I *am* the best."

Instead of being taken aback, I thought to myself, "That is what I really wanted to hear." I firmly believe that the more confident you are of your surgeon's ability, the more likely the outcome will be positive. You need a surgeon who listens to you and who has a great track record.

Among the many myths that surround medical care is that you have to go to a great teaching hospital or a major academic medical center for proper care, especially for something like heart disease. For many diseases that require special care, most large, local facilities will have similar success rates. One reason is that many of the physicians, nurses, therapists, and other staff have trained in these major centers, and the other is that the surgical procedures are, in most cases, consistent from case to case.

Should You Get a Second Opinion?

Should you simply agree with what your surgeon or new cardiologist recommends, as I did? Heart disease is life threatening, and it's your life. Part of building confidence in the doctors who will care for you will come from a second opinion that, most often, confirms the initial diagnosis. Unless you are in the emergency room and your angiogram or other indicators show that you are in a critical situation, you *should* consider seeking a second opinion. In some cases, your insurance may require it, especially workplace-oriented programs such as workers' compensation (see **Month Ten**). Your own doctor also may want to have another doctor consult if he or she feels that some other health problem (e.g., diabetes) may affect your ability to undergo surgery.

You may feel awkward about getting a second opinion; after all, you may have feelings of loyalty to your cardiologist and you may assume that any surgeon he recommends is the best possible choice for you. Getting a second opinion will not and should not offend your doctor. It's not the same as shopping for a better deal on a car. Doctors are professionals, and this occurs all the time. In fact, if your doctor resists, that is a red flag. The best way to approach this process is to ask your primary physician or the internist who referred you to your cardiologist for another referral.

Other important points when you go for a second opinion are:

○ Let the new physician's office know that this is a visit for a second opinion. The office will tell you ahead of time what you need to bring with you, such as x-rays and a medical history.
○ Bring a series of questions with you that you want answered.
○ Recognize that while you may like the second doctor better than the first, if the opinions are the same, it is unlikely that he or she will take your case.
○ You should not be disappointed if the new doctor does not tell you what you want to hear. There is a point of diminishing returns and the objective is *not* to find someone who will tell you what you want to hear.

With today's technology and the wide exchange of data and outcome information among different medical specialties, many doctors approach diagnosis and treatment similarly. Sometimes you will find physicians and surgeons who prefer to try a conservative or non-invasive approach, such as using an injection in an orthopedic case or prescribing a combination of medications for heart disease.

What happens when your doctor's diagnosis and the second opinion differ? In most cases, the physician giving a second opinion will explain why he or she has a different opinion. It is unlikely that he or she will call or write your primary physician and express reservations. That, too, is considered unethical. This is where you have to step up, take responsibility, and become a patient. That requires the following:

○ Discuss the situation with the primary care doctor or internist who first identified your problem. He or she should be able to give you an objective view and allay your fears.

○ Do the research. In recent years, information on the Internet has become more dependable and far more ubiquitous. With new search engines (see **Month Twelve**), there are multiple websites that can answer questions or give you leads.

○ Talking with family members is something you will be doing anyway; however, do not get caught up in the Uncle-Joe's-second-cousin's-gardener-had-a-similar-thing-four-years-ago-in-Czechoslovakia syndrome. Your family and relatives may mean well, and you may even have a close relative in the medical field, but no one knows your entire medical history, your test results, prior medical treatment, and other factors that have led to your diagnosis. Appreciate their care and comfort, but take only advice that you're convinced is from a reliable source who knows your case.

Finding Out More Online About a Physician

Numerous websites offer information on the background of particular physicians. Beware of these. Many are simply advertising sites that often provide little free information, but tantalize you with half-facts and make you pay for inaccurate information. In some cases, these sites contain information that's been placed there by physicians or medical

---

Questions to Bring to a Second Opinion

When you go for a second opinion, you should bring a list of questions. Some of these are pretty straightforward, and you should not be afraid to ask them. For example, ask about the physician's training, his medical education, where he or she did residency, and board certification. What kind of additional training did he or she do that can help indicate whether he or she is up to date? Perhaps the doctor has won awards that he or she will be more than happy to tell you about.

Bring with you all your family and medical history information, including your medication list, and also, if you feel the need, have a friend or relative come with you to help you take in everything that's said. Because this is a second opinion, you may want to compare what both doctors have told you, and it is easy to become confused. Take notes and don't be afraid to ask questions. Two of the most common feelings people carry into the doctor's office are embarrassment and a sense of intimidation. You need not feel this way. Virtually all physicians are asked to consult or give another opinion, and they want you to feel comfortable.

We live in an age where doctors are very careful to make sure their patients understand everything, but they cannot do that if you don't ask them to show you your x-ray and explain it, or answer your question about a medicine's side effects. Ask the doctor to write things down and to give you a copy of the letter that is sent to your own physician with his or her conclusions.

---

groups and may not be accurate or up-to-date. The best way to get accurate information about any physician is to contact your local and state medical societies or the American Board of Internal Medicine (www.abim.org).

IN A SENTENCE:

> *Getting a second opinion is your right and a proper option, but in the end, it is your comfort and trust in your choice of cardiologist that really counts, so don't let yourself be pressured into a decision that does not feel right.*

How Do I Know I Have Heart Disease?

GENERALLY, MOST cardiologists let you know in their office that you have heart disease. Unfortunately, some people are diagnosed in an emergency room or in the intensive care unit. In the best of all possible worlds, your heart problems will be diagnosed before any part of your cardiovascular system is seriously compromised, but some of us (such as I) tend to lean toward denial. On one level, you know something is wrong but don't want to know what it is; on the other hand, you know what is wrong, but you don't want to deal with it.

While a definitive diagnosis of heart disease can only be made by your physician through a number of steps (discussed below), you have a primary responsibility in this process that can't be emphasized enough. As you know, your constellation of risk factors, especially family history, described in **Day One**, is the first sign that heart disease may be in your future. In effect, you know that you may develop heart disease at some point in your life, and waiting for a random visit to your doctor to find it, or stalling until a significant symptom, such as breathlessness or chest pain, appears is not just practicing denial, it's Russian roulette. When a doctor finally does link the symptoms to CAD, you could become sicker sooner. Diagnosis really begins with you. The question you should ask if you suspect that anything is wrong or if you have significant risk factors is, *How do I know I have heart disease before it's too late to reverse it, or to stop the damage now?*

Diagnosis—Level One

It's unlikely that the cardiologist or any physician will simply accept your diagnosis of a heart problem or even the suspected diagnosis from your primary doctor. It is possible that your symptoms may be so severe that you will be sent directly to the hospital; however, let's assume that this is not the case, and that you are on what you might call diagnostic level one, which includes the physical exam and risk assessment.

Anyone who has ever visited a new doctor knows he or she will be asked to answer a number of personal and family history questions, sometimes several times. Some doctors will send you forms to complete before you come in. In addition to insurance data, you will be asked for in-depth health, social, and personal information that will include background on family members, your work, significant complaints, other medical problems, medications you are taking, previous illness, and a range of other questions. It is likely that this process will be repeated by a specially trained physician assistant/nurse who will enter it into electronic medical records (EMR). Then the cardiologist will go over the information with you, but a bit more informally.

Following the history, you will also be given a complete physical examination that will include certain non-invasive tests. The physical includes common procedures, such as temperature, weight, height, pulse, listening to your chest and lungs for proper rhythms, blood pressure, electrocardiogram, chest x-ray, and possibly some blood tests, but those may be done under fasting conditions (i.e., when you have had no food for 12 hours).

If, after your initial exam, you have symptoms that are common to heart disease, you might think your doctor would tell you that it's heart disease of some sort. This is not how the determination is made. The process is actually the opposite. Your doctor will use a systematic approach known as the differential diagnosis, although the result may be the same: to discover why you have these symptoms and whether they indicate that you have heart disease.

The questions that your doctor asks and the diagnostic tests described here are designed to rule out different diseases as the list is narrowed. Sev-

Blood Tests

Routine blood testing is usually done by your personal physician, and can often be a tip-off to potential heart disease. A phlebotomist at the doctor's office or a blood lab will draw several test tubes of blood that will be assessed for key markers. Your cardiologist wants to know what your lipids are: HDL, LDL, triglycerides, total cholesterol.

If a heart attack is suspected, then your cardiac enzymes, which are proteins found in your heart that seep into the bloodstream after a heart attack, also will be addressed. They are usually a sure sign that you have some sort of cardiac damage. Your blood may also be tested for oxygen levels and clotting ability.

Beyond cardiac-specific tests, your doctor may order glucose testing to determine your risk for diabetes, electrolytes such as potassium and sodium, carbon dioxide levels that measure kidney and adrenal functions, and the acidity level that may also indicate diabetes.

Infections may be suggested in a complete blood count (CBC) test that examines white blood cell count, hemoglobin, iron, and platelet count.

eral diseases may have similar or the same symptoms, so your doctor will move on to the second track of diagnosis and testing, despite the fact that the physician has a pretty good idea of what is wrong. Your doctor's goal is to paint a picture of your cardiac system, illustrating clearly where you may have blocked arteries, weakened heart muscle, or a compromised electrical system to keep you pumping along. Usually, several tests are done in a first group and then, based on the results, more may be ordered.

The American Heart Association offers an exceptionally important suggestion when it comes to this initial examination: "Be honest, and don't be afraid to look bad. For instance, if you or family members smoke, eat a lot of high-fat food, or don't exercise, tell the doctor. Your doctor can't make an accurate diagnosis without full input from you. Think of the doctor as your healthcare partner. You have to work together to be successful."

Diagnosis—Level Two

I have had virtually every test discussed in this section. In fact, over the years, I've had each of them several times, and I still have some on a regular basis. The first few times I had some of them, I was hardly a happy camper for several reasons, the most important being that I knew the results were not going to be encouraging. As the poster boy for cardiovascular disease denial, the tests represented facing reality. Having survived and having been fortunate to recover, I now see the regular check-up tests differently. Today, the tests have become an opportunity to see how well I'm doing and a challenge to leave with a simple "Come back in six months" from my doctor.

Chest X-ray

Usually done in the doctor's office, it's a garden-variety x-ray by an x-ray technician. Your doctor will look for signs of an enlarged heart caused by fluid or congestion that could indicate pneumonia or evidence of congestive heart failure. Usually, the cardiologist interprets the x-ray, but in consultation with radiologists.

Electrocardiogram

Known as an **ECG**, this is usually done in the office by a nurse or physician assistant before you actually see the doctor. You will be asked to lie on your back and allow several electrodes wired to the device to be attached to your chest, arms, and legs. The ECG quickly prints out a strip of paper that shows (through tracing) how well your heart may be beating in terms of rhythm and electrical conduction. The results are an important indication of what may be causing your symptoms. For example, it can show that you've had a heart attack, thickening of the heart wall or ventricles, and rhythmic disturbances. The ECG reading can indicate to the doctor whether you need more tests or what treatment might be appropriate immediately.

Holter Monitor

This portable ECG continuously records your heart rhythms over a 24-hour period. A small monitor is hooked to several wires that are attached to your chest. You can put the Holter in a pocket or in a special pouch, and as you go through the day, you keep track of your activities in a small written diary. When you give the Holter back the next day, your doctor matches the recording with the activities. In general, your doctor will want you monitored this way if you've had a heart attack, have heart rhythm problems, or experience other unexplained chest feelings, such as palpitations or feeling faint.

Echocardiogram

Sometimes called an **echo**, this test is common. If your doctor orders it, do not become alarmed. The echo is an ultrasound test similar to those administered during pregnancy. It shows abnormality in the heart structure, determines how well it's pumping, and measures the heart muscle mass by sending out sound waves that reflect off the heart through a device held to your chest. The result is a complete picture of your heart function. The echocardiogram also measures the ejection fraction of your heart. This vital information (see **Day Four**) shows whether the proper amount of blood is being pumped into and out of the heart.

Stress Tests

These tests determine how your heart reacts to physical activity as you walk on a treadmill. In some cases, you may be asked to ride a stationary bike. There are actually two types of stress tests: the exercise stress test and the thallium stress test. The goal of both tests is to determine how much blood is pumping in your coronary arteries as they try to feed the heart during the stress of exercise. The difference between the tests is how much information each provides and how they are done. A stress echocardiogram also may be recommended.

The exercise stress test is relatively simple. You are hooked up to an ECG machine. Your doctor takes your blood pressure as you begin to walk and during the test. As the machine goes faster, the floor plate tilts upward gradually, like walking up an increasingly steep hill, and the speed increases to raise the stress on your heart. The doctor will tell you when to stop, or you can stop when you feel that you can't go any further or faster. This stress test will help in diagnosing suspected coronary artery disease and how much exercise you can safely do. It can also assess your future heart attack risk. This test usually lasts 10 to 15 minutes, and you will be given specific instructions beforehand, including what you should eat or drink and what to wear. Make sure you have those instructions and that you understand them. During and after the test, your doctor will be able to identify the source of pain in your chest and will note how well your heart's rhythms are performing, your suspected extent of coronary artery disease, and your overall cardio fitness.

After this set of tests is completed, your doctor may decide that your risk for a heart attack or heart failure is high, and that some more intense tests are necessary to begin developing a treatment plan as soon as possible. Some of the tests discussed here are the same or similar to those you will have for a suspected heart attack in an emergency situation. Another form of stress testing is the thallium stress test, sometimes called a nuclear stress test or a myocardial perfusion imaging test. This test enables your doctor to have more definitive information regarding the amount of blockage in your coronary arteries, the extent of damage to your heart muscle, how well your blood is flowing through your arteries after certain heart procedures, such as a bypass, and how much exercise your heart can safely bear. Thallium, a low-dose, safe radioactive element, is injected in your bloodstream during the test at the point when your doctor determines you are at your maximum exercise tolerance. After you come off the machine, you are taken into another room, where you lie flat and as still as possible and a gamma camera takes an external picture of your heart arteries as your blood mixes with the thallium. The camera captures how much blood is reaching the various parts of the heart when it is under stress from the exercise by the amount of thallium seen. If no thallium is seen, it's likely there is absent blood flow, equating with heart damage.

After resting for another two to three hours, a second set of gamma camera pictures is taken that shows the amount of blood circulating when your heart is resting. By comparing the exercise and resting thallium test, the result delivers a definitive picture of your heart and cardiac arterial health. Your doctor can determine how blood is flowing through the arteries and whether your heart is getting enough blood. Of course, seeing how well your heart performs when you walk on the treadmill will help your doctor decide how serious your heart disease has become and whether an invasive procedure is required. It's possible that you may not be able to exercise on a treadmill or bike. In that case, a substance called dipyridamole or adenosine is injected into a vein and a gamma camera is used to produce a picture of the blood flow through the coronary system. These medications simulate exercise and represent an excellent alternative.

Cardiac Catheterization

Cardiac Catheterization (also known as **angiography**) is both a diagnostic test and part of a treatment that is usually done on an outpatient basis in a cath laboratory at a hospital or a heart treatment center. This procedure is also used in treating a heart attack, and its use in that case is more fully described in Day Five. This test is done by your cardiologist and provides definitive information he or she will need to make a definitive diagnosis. The actual procedure takes approximately 20 minutes once initiated and you will, again, be unable to have food or fluids before the test. Make sure you totally understand what you have to do before the test begins. Prior to the test, you will be given some relaxing medications, but you will not be asleep during the procedure. It is important that your doctor be able to communicate with you as the test is being carried out. Once you're in the cath lab, you will lie on a table with an x-ray machine above you. You will be hooked up to an ECG and other machines that keep track of vital signs such as pulse and blood pressure. Fluids will be gently administered through an IV.

The catheter is a thin plastic tube that is inserted into an artery in the groin; however, it's possible that the brachial artery in your elbow or your radial artery in the wrist may be used. The tube is threaded over a guide wire that is removed when the catheter is in the artery. As your physician monitors the path of the catheter through your arteries, using an x-ray, he or she advances the catheter up into your coronary arteries, then into the heart chambers, giving the cardiologist a clear picture of the pressures within the heart, perhaps taking a blood sample. The doctor then moves the catheter into the region of the cardiac arteries. At this point, a small amount of dye to provide contrast in the x-ray is injected, and images of the inside of your arteries are studied. You don't feel this because your blood vessels don't have nerve endings.

Your angiogram (the complete picture of your cardiovascular system) will show your doctor where you have blockages and how serious they may be. Blood pressure, flow rate, heart muscle damage, and other data will confirm the type and level of intervention you will need. After this test, you'll be taken back to a room, where you will rest for several hours, allowing time for your small incision to seal and for you to recover. Specific instructions, including your activity level, will be provided before you leave.

The cardiac catheterization procedure is also used in the treatment of clogged arteries by balloon angiography and implanting arterial stents, which is discussed in Day Five.

A number of other tests are used in the diagnosis of heart disease, but those described above are the ones your doctor will turn to first. In some instances, a computed tomography (CT or CAT) scan and a **magnetic resonance imaging** (MRI) are used to get a different look at the heart. In general, CT and MRI are used when an x-ray does not provide enough information. These tests also are non-invasive, so they provide a greater safety level for certain patients.

IN A SENTENCE:

> *Today cardiologists make accurate diagnoses of heart disease on the basis of experience coupled with rapidly evolving technology, helping them rectify problems before serious damage can occur.*

How to Survive a Heart Attack

WHAT IF you have a heart attack while at work, while driving a car, or while mowing the lawn?

As a person with heart disease, you must understand what's involved in emergency care and treatment of a chronic cardiac condition. Basic cardiopulmonary resuscitation (CPR) and other first aid skills are taught virtually everywhere. Everyone should be able to perform CPR. If you or someone whom you are caring for is having a heart attack and CPR is called for, it is the first line of treatment.

How Do You Know You Are Having a Heart Attack?

From one point of view, this is an easy question because there are a series of well-known symptoms, but men and women can have different symptoms and, in some cases, only a few symptoms or none at all. It is not unusual for diabetics to have silent infarcts (heart attacks) that can occur without any pain and that can produce significant heart-muscle damage.

While some specific symptoms indicate that you may be having a heart attack, the definitive diagnosis can only be made by a doctor, so you *must* be seen by a physician. In some situations, common heart attack symptoms might only last a few moments, only to return again in a short while.

Here is the general list of symptoms that the American Heart Association recognizes as warning signals of a heart attack:

- ○ Pain across the chest
- ○ Uncomfortable pressure or a feeling of fullness in the center of the chest that lasts more than a few minutes
- ○ Feeling of impending doom
- ○ Mild or intense pain or a burning feeling spreading to the shoulders, neck, or arms
- ○ The proverbial elephant's foot on your chest
- ○ Pain in the upper abdomen, neck, jaw, or inside the arms or shoulders
- ○ Lightheadedness, fainting, sweating, nausea, or shortness of breath
- ○ Anxiety, nervousness, and/or cold, sweaty skin
- ○ Paleness
- ○ Increased or irregular heart rate

In general, women have symptoms similar to those of men, and women (see **Week Three**) may be more likely than men to experience nausea or vomiting, back and jaw pain, and shortness of breath.

Here is a message that comes from someone who could have gotten help quickly, but for all the wrong reasons did not. If only having one or two of these symptoms won't overcome your reluctance to move quickly, think of it in this context: If I am feeling these symptoms *and* I have a family history; I smoke; I am overweight, obese, sedentary, and diabetic; *and* I have had a stressful day, then perhaps something is wrong and I should call 911! It's not only the symptoms that should spur you to action, but your total health picture.

Getting to an emergency facility as rapidly as possible and receiving the correct treatment is the goal for anyone showing signs of a heart attack. Improving this process has been the focus of an effort to increase public awareness. In 2006, the American Heart Association; the National Heart, Lung, and Blood Institute; and other groups joined together

What to Do in an Emergency

○ Dial 911 or your local emergency medical assistance number. The paramedics know what they are doing and their job is to get help to you quickly. Don't tough out the symptoms of a heart attack. Do not try to drive yourself. If you don't have access to emergency medical services, have a neighbor or a friend drive you to the nearest hospital. Police or fire rescue units may also be a source of transportation. Try to have someone wait with you until the ambulance arrives. Get help ASAP! Minutes matter!

○ Besides the psychological reason for having someone with you, there are the obvious practical ones, such as contacting relatives, helping with paperwork, and answering questions. For example, it's vital that someone know your allergies. Some people are not only allergic to medications, but they also may be allergic to the dye used in a clot-clearing catheterization procedure. Consider wearing a Medic Alert bracelet or keeping a list of allergies in your wallet.

○ If your doctor has previously specifically recommended that you take an aspirin if you think you're having a heart attack, do so. Seek emergency help first by calling 911. Take the aspirin as your doctor has advised. If you haven't talked to your doctor about taking aspirin when you're having a heart attack, don't take the aspirin.

○ Take nitroglycerin, if prescribed. If you think you're having a heart attack and your doctor has previously prescribed nitroglycerin, take it as directed. Do not take anyone else's nitroglycerin, as that could put you in more danger.

○ Begin CPR. If you are with a person who might be having a heart attack, and he or she is unconscious, tell the 911 dispatcher or another emergency medical specialist. You may be advised to begin cardiopulmonary resuscitation. Even if you are not trained, a dispatcher can guide you until help arrives.

to launch a new program called **"Act in Time"** to "increase people's awareness of heart attack and in the importance of calling 911 or for other help immediately." They issued a new set of guidelines for faster response to those having a severe heart attack or who have heavily blocked arteries that are keeping oxygen from the heart.

The main goal of this initiative is to get patients into a catheter lab for **angioplasty** within 90 minutes after they arrive in the emergency room.

The *New York Times* reported (Nov. 13, 2006) that a delay of even another 30 minutes raises the victim's risk of death by 42 percent. While
90 minutes may seem like a long time span to get someone whom doctors suspect has had a heart attack ready for an angioplasty, the procedure requires both preparation and teamwork at the hospital. Under
these recommendations, the ER team would preemptively alert the cath
lab to a potential procedure, rather than wait for a cardiologist to come
in for a consult or give the written orders.

The issue of speed in initiating treatment cannot be overemphasized.
The moment the oxygenated blood flowing to your heart is reduced significantly or is cut off, your heart muscle begins to deteriorate and, eventually,
to die. The more muscle is damaged, the less chance you have to survive
and recover. Heart muscle does not regenerate. You as a patient may be
able to recover somewhat, but the best care for your heart is to prevent
damage. In the case of a complete, sudden cutoff of blood to the heart
caused by a total blockage, you may die, and it can happen within minutes.

> Forty percent of people who have a heart attack die before they get to the hospital.

Like an operating room, the cath lab is staffed by an experienced
team of physicians, nurses, and technicians. The new guidelines would
set up a system to activate that team quickly and would require a cardiologist on site at all times. There is no reason why you can't talk to your
doctor about the issue of speed so that in an emergency, you know
where he would prefer for you to go if you are not in deep distress. Otherwise, that decision will be made by the paramedics who are called to
save you. The sooner you do seek help, whether or not you think you are
"really" having a heart attack, the better off you will be.

Acute Response

Once you have reached the ER, or when you have gone from the doctor's office to the hospital, the first step will be to ensure that you are
stabilized, which includes administering oxygen and assessing your
blood pressure and heart rhythm. A laboratory analysis is performed
immediately, as is an electrocardiogram. Medications may be given to

you to enhance your blood-thinning ability, which is another compelling reason to get to the hospital quickly. The doctors treating you will be concentrating on maintaining blood flow to the heart and minimizing the amount of muscle damage.

Although you may be fearful, because you will have been given strong pain medication, you may, instead, experience a sense of dissociation or a surreal feeling. On the other hand, your pain may have subsided and you won't feel as bad as you did prior to coming to the hospital. You may want to leave to get back to the important things you had planned for that day. The second reality is that you have no idea how serious your situation may be. To make decisions, your doctors will need blood tests, ECGs, and other tests. If at all possible, have a family member present who is aware of your condition and who can help you make decisions that require consent for surgery or other procedures.

One thing is absolute: The ER is not like it's shown on television, with general chaos everywhere, patients flying in and out, doctors jumping from one room to another, saving gunshot-wound victims while conducting clandestine trysts in the supply closet. The ER system today is based on a concept called triage, which is the process of sorting victims, as of a battle or disaster, to determine medical priority in order to increase the number of survivors.

The modern ER is attuned to patients who come in with chest pains. Rochelle Rosen, M.D., who practices emergency medicine in Pittsburgh, told me, "We are very aware that speed is primary, and there are multiple nurses to cover each patient. Some ERs actually have a separate reception area for patients with chest pains; however, in most cases, the triage nurse will get any patient with chest pains back into the ER very quickly, hook them up to an ECG and a heart monitor, and administer oxygen and possibly an aspirin or nitroglycerin, depending on what you've already taken."

If you are being brought to the hospital in an ambulance, the paramedics will already have you hooked up to an ECG.

Medications

If one of several drugs called a thrombolytic (i.e., TPA) or clot buster is administered, it will in most instances dissolve the blood clot threatening your heart. Although there is some controversy over their use, clot busters work well in about 75 percent of cases. There are also varying protocols, as different thrombolytics work in different ways, such as time of action and condition of the patient.

Three other medications fall under the clot-busting category: clopidogrel (Plavix), heparin (a widely used blood thinner), and tirofiban (Aggrastat). Tirofiban is one of a category of medications, called glycoprotein IIb/IIIa inhibitors, often used as part of an angioplasty procedure, usually with aspirin and heparin for further anticoagulant effect.

Beyond medications to reduce or break up **plaque**, several other drugs may be given as a first line of treatment. Often, these are indicated because you have a concomitant condition, such as high blood pressure (see **Month Eight**).

The class of drugs referred to as beta-blockers includes such well-known medications as atenolol (Tenormin), propranolol (Inderal), and metoprolol (Lopressor). High blood pressure can be identified in many heart patients; however, a heart attack can increase previously normal blood pressure and a beta-blocker can help control an increase in blood pressure.

Calcium channel blockers, also known as channel blockers or calcium antagonists, are used to reduce angina, high blood pressure, **cardiac arrhythmias**, and chest pain. Among the most common are verapamil (Calan, Isoptin), diltiazem (Cardizem), amlodipine (Norvasc), and nifedipine (Procardia). Nifedipine has been the subject of some concern by the AHA and the National Heart, Lung, and Blood Institute, which "recommends to doctors that short-acting nifedipine should be used with great caution, if at all, especially at higher doses in the treatment of high blood pressure, angina, and myocardial infarction."

Angiotensin-converting enzyme (ACE) inhibitors are usually given on the day of the heart attack. These vasodilators enlarge or expand the arteries and lower blood pressure, effectively reducing the workload imposed on the heart muscle.

Other drugs sometimes are administered in the event of a heart attack. For example, cholesterol-reducing agents known as statins, which include Lipitor, Zocor, Mevacor, Crestor, Lescol, and Pravachol, are widely used in patients whose lipids are elevated, but there is evidence that they are protective for high-risk patients to prevent a heart attack or to control further buildup of plaque.

Clearing a Passage to the Heart: Balloons and Stents

In virtually all cases of heart attack—some reports indicate 90 percent—angioplasty or percutaneous coronary intervention (PCI)) is considered in the first hours after a heart attack is diagnosed. In general, PCI is the first line of treatment for heart attack victims.

The goal of PCI in heart attack treatment is to break up clots, clear the blocked artery, save the heart muscle, and get the heart pumping more effectively.

Drug-eluting stents (see Figure 6) are approved by the FDA, giving doctors a new tool for preventing restenosis or re-closure of the arteries. Often, this closure is caused by scar tissue that formed within the arteries after a PCI. Stents are controversial, and you should discuss them with your doctor; however, in an emergency situation, the most important priority is to keep or restore blood flowing to the heart.

Once your arteries are open, blood flows through them and damage to your heart is minimized. Your heart can be saved and your recovery will be greater. This is something that I did not fully understand when I had my first heart attack. This lack of knowledge, combined with my own reluctance to admit that something bad was happening, likely has changed the course of my life. Had I gone to the hospital when I first sensed something was wrong, I would not have gone through much of what I have had to endure.

Barring the need for heart surgery, the first procedure recommended in the ER will be a balloon angioplasty that will widen the blocked artery. Your doctor can follow the progress of the catheter because a contrast material is injected that shows up on an x-ray that your doctor uses as the catheter is advanced through your arteries.

This procedure is frequently performed in patients who have had heart attacks, either immediately or later, when arterial blockages may have increased. A very small balloon is compressed and wrapped around the tip of the tiny catheter, which is inserted into the clogged area of your artery through the plaque. Once in place, the balloon is inflated to press the plaque against the wall of the artery. While this may provide immediate relief to the heart attack patient and save your life, in most cases, balloon angioplasty and insertion of a stent are done at the same time, reducing the rate of restenosis.

FIGURE 6

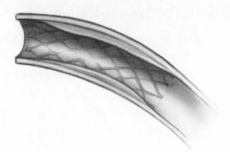

Stenting at the time of the balloon procedure has become common because a number of patients' opened arteries re-closed, sometimes as soon as the patients were moved to the recovery room. In some cases, the only treatment was a bypass, which, in an emergency, is not ideal. The stenting procedure is preferred as first-line treatment. While the rate of immediate restenosis after balloon angioplasty has varied, some estimates range from 10 to 50 percent over several months. Once simultaneous stenting with angioplasty became common, the rate dropped to about 10–15 percent.

The stent is a small wire mesh tube mounted on the balloon and inserted into the clogged artery to support the damaged, traumatized arterial wall. Stents are designed to be implanted permanently, and it's not uncommon to have several inserted in different locations.

Your cardiologist or another doctor who is doing the angioplasty and stenting will begin by making an extremely small incision in the femoral artery in your groin (or the radial artery in your arm) and threading the catheter into the blocked artery (see Figure 7). Once the combined catheter and stent are properly set, the stent is opened by inflating the balloon, which is then deflated and withdrawn. The artery accepts the stent and, after a few weeks, the stent becomes part of the artery.

Beyond stents for the coronary artery, stenting is used in other parts of the body to treat atherosclerosis. For example, carotid artery stenting is a widely used but relatively new procedure that clears blockages in the carotid artery that feeds blood to the brain. If these remain blocked, they can cause a permanent stroke or mini-strokes called transient ischemic attack (TIAs) that can last for several hours but that do not necessarily cause permanent brain damage.

FIGURE 7

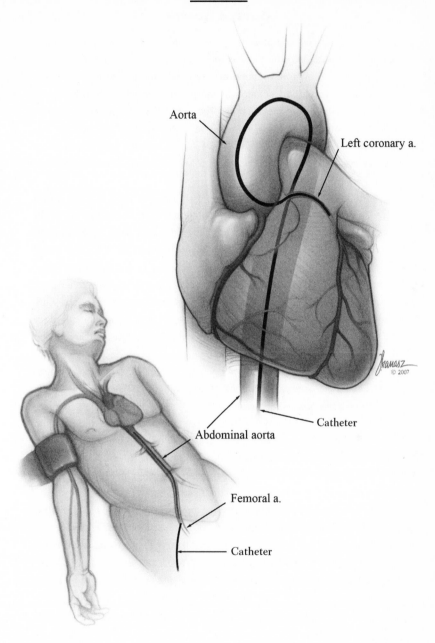

Aorta

Left coronary a.

Catheter

Abdominal aorta

Femoral a.

Catheter

Coated Stents

In the late 1990s, several pharmaceutical companies began looking at the idea of actually coating the stent with a blood-thinning medicine, Plavix, a process that is known as creating **drug-eluting stents (DES)**. Initially, this seemed like a very good solution to the problem for patients, who could avoid surgery by stent implantation. The first DES procedures began in 2002, and within four years, approximately 6,000,000 procedures had been done. In 2003, over 625,000 stent implants (twice as many as coronary bypass operations) were done, largely as a result of the introduction of the DES that year.

Unfortunately, a trend began showing up in the next two years that linked the DES in a small number of cases to creation of blood clots, termed "stent thrombosis," which could be fatal. This has launched a major controversy in the cardiovascular world, referred to in one publication as "the stent wars." One side argued that the DES had been approved on the basis of studies that were "too small, too short, and in low-risk patients." On the other side, proponents suggested that the cases that produced negative reactions were in high-risk patients who were never the prime, low-risk patient indicated for the DES. It was estimated that "60% of the patients who get them in practice are sicker with more complex blockages."

The controversy has gone back and forth and remains, at this time, controversial. During the writing of this book, I spoke with more than 25 different clinicians who used drug-eluting stents and bare metal stenting. Many of them were ambivalent about using the DES because the patient needed to be on Plavix for at least a year, if not longer. Clinicians pointed out to me that the cost of the drug—$4 per day—could lead to noncompliance. Another negative is that if emergency surgery was needed by a patient on Plavix, the blood-thinning effect would make surgery more risky.

One report published in the *Journal of the American Medical Association* by a leading Cleveland Clinic cardiologist, Deepak Bhatt, M.D., "found that coated stents had five times the risk of clots than the plain metal ones." However, this was not a direct study but an analysis of pooled results of 14 randomized studies. Other medical experts see stents as a risk-to-benefit issue. Elizabeth Nadel, M.D., director of the National Heart, Lung, and Blood Institute, told the Associated Press in 2006, "the benefit of having a drug-eluting stent is tremendous."

The issue of drug-eluting stents will probably not be settled immediately, since there does seem to be great benefit in many cases. What is more likely is that the product will evolve. New stents already are scheduled to reach the market in 2008.

What should you believe about drug safety? Serious or fatal reaction to a medicine may occur in persons who have an existing medical condition that was not detected before the clinical trial began. No two patients are alike, and absolute safety is never guaranteed anywhere in life. Even some brands of peanut butter were recently recalled. How many PB&J sandwiches have you had with no bad effect (perhaps too many calories!)? The point, in the case of drug-eluting stents, is that you should never agree to any procedure without fully discussing it with your doctor, although in the case of an emergency, this may not be possible, so if you are at risk you should do your homework.

Prior to September 2004, the basic treatment for blockages in the carotid arteries was an endarterectomy, which involved opening the artery in the neck and clearing out the plaque. The danger during this operation is the possibility of stroke, which is lessened through stenting. When the FDA approved the device, however, the regulations limited it to patients who have had strokes or TIAs and significantly blocked carotid arteries (50 percent or more), those with blockage of 80 percent or more with or without a history of TIA or stroke, and those whose medical condition makes endarterectomy risky. Like any coronary artery stenting, carotid stenting is not indicated in patients who take blood thinners, who have a history of bleeding, who are allergic to the stent's metal (nickel-titanium alloy), or who have some other problem that prevents the catheter from reaching the carotid artery.

Another area where the stenting procedure may be used is to repair a thoracic aortic aneurysm that occurs when there is a weakness in the aortic wall. If the aorta is compromised by expansion, it can break through the inner lining. The general treatment for this condition has been an open chest repair surgery; however, some patients can now be treated by the use of stents. In these cases, the catheter is used to guide one or more stents to the site of the aneurysm, where it is inflated to support the arterial wall. This procedure is limited to certain patients, depending upon aneurysm site and location.

While coronary artery stenting is effective as an emergency procedure, it is also used for patients whose arteries may have restenosed and

FIGURE 8

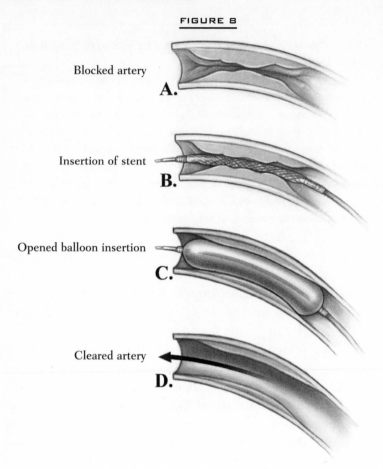

Blocked artery

A.

Insertion of stent

B.

Opened balloon insertion

C.

Cleared artery

D.

in stable patients with angina. Some studies indicate that stenting is not effective in patients who are stable three days after a heart attack. One physician familiar with this says, "A recent study in *Journal of the American College of Cardiology* showed the benefit of stents for not only the infarct-related artery, but also for lesions at a distance. This means again that the individual situation is what has to be considered in every case."

Coronary Artery Bypass

If stenting is not possible, you may be taken to the operating room for an emergency coronary bypass operation, which is sometimes called a

CABG ("cabbage"). It is essentially the same procedure that you would have as an elective or non-emergency treatment for coronary artery disease. Bypass surgery is one of the most successful advances in modern medicine, transforming survival rates for patients like you and me. It's widely recognized that we in the U.S. have a high death rate from CAD; however, we rank below more than a dozen countries, including much of Eastern Europe and Scandinavian countries such as Finland. One reason that we are doing a slightly better job than other countries is our increasing awareness of risk factors such as smoking and diet. This growing population requiring bypass surgery, along with the safety of the procedure, has driven the expanded use of this technique as an emergency option and as elective surgery.

Calling coronary bypass surgery elective does not mean it's in the same category as a facelift or fixing a nagging carpal tunnel problem at your convenience. I had my quadruple bypass about five years after my heart attack. I chose to avoid surgery as long as I could because it had not been successful for my mother, who died six weeks after her second bypass. When all my treatment options, such as medication or stress reduction, failed to stabilize my heart condition, a stress test confirmed what my cardiologist had made clear: The bypass was my only way to avoid a potentially catastrophic heart attack. (Did I mention that I still got four "second opinions"?) The only thing elective about the surgery was when the surgeon could schedule it. The bottom line is that coronary bypass surgery or angioplasty may not be the first-choice treatment, but when one of them is recommended and your doctor explains clearly why, don't put it off, as I did.

The procedure usually takes between three to five hours; however, you will have few memories of it. Once you are given a sedative and prepped for surgery, much of your anxiety will fade.

If the diseased arteries that feed blood to your heart cannot be opened by angioplasty, the CABG operation enables you to have new connections around the blocked blood vessels. These new routes are created by harvesting the saphenous vein from your leg or the internal mammary artery (inside your chest wall). This is possible because your legs have multiple veins that can be used if more than one graft is needed (see Figure 9). A new connection is created when pieces of those veins and arteries are spliced to re-route sections of your coronary artery after the blocked

FIGURE 9

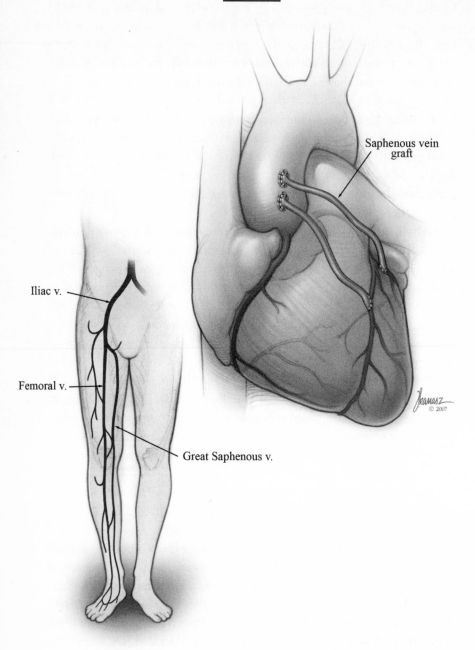

Saphenous vein graft

Iliac v.

Femoral v.

Great Saphenous v.

FIGURE 10

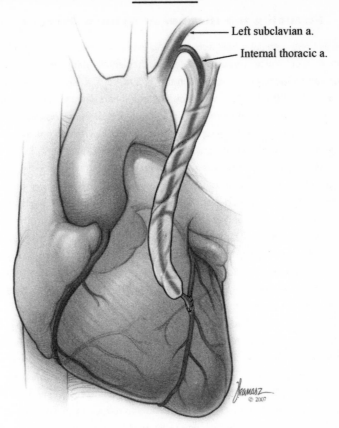

Left subclavian a.

Internal thoracic a.

sections are removed. This creates detours or grafts. This procedure can be repeated several times, creating new pathways from the aorta feeding the heart. The number of bypasses performed is usually determined by the number of clogged arteries.

Before the bypass procedure, you will be given anesthesia. A breathing tube is inserted after you are asleep and before the operation commences to help keep your lungs clear. Medications are circulated in the bloodstream to cool the body. After you are unconscious, the surgeon opens your chest along the breastbone with an incision called a sternotomy. Depending on the circumstances and the surgeon, your heart can be stopped and you will be hooked to a heart-lung machine that assumes the role of your heart and lungs to keep you alive during the surgery. Your heart stops beating for the duration of the bypass. It's also possible to keep the patient's heart

Reducing the Number of Bypass Surgeries

Like all great medical breakthroughs, CABG took years of research, including both accidental discoveries and determined scientific study before it became a safe and widespread procedure in the 1970s.

Given the 900,000 to 1 million deaths from heart disease each year in the U.S., clearly we have far more to do in the area of prevention. As any nutritionist will tell you, we are learning more each day that certain things in our diet really do make a difference between life and early death. Not only have major cities like Manhattan and Cleveland banned trans fats (saturated oils used in frying that contribute significantly to clogged arteries) in restaurants, but many companies have followed suit. For example, Kraft foods actually removed trans fat from Oreos™ and reduced or eliminated it in about 650 other products, after being sued by a group, www.bantransfats.com. This group also sued McDonald's, alleging that McDonald's had misled its customers by stating that it had switched to non–trans fat cooking oil when it had not. The suit was settled when Mickey D's made a $7 million donation to the American Heart Association for a trans-fat education program.

The Oreo™ lawsuit had a huge domino effect, the group reported. The publicity that the lawsuit received created public awareness about the trans-fat issue and triggered an avalanche of events, including an FDA labeling rule that went into effect in 2006, requiring all nutritional labels to carry trans-fat amounts.

How does all this relate to cardiac bypass? The answer is simple, and it is an important social issue. Had you been able to reduce major risk factors, especially smoking and poor diet, you likely would not find yourself in an emergency room with a heart attack so serious that it requires open heart surgery. The good news, however, is that people are no longer depending on the government to take action. Reducing health risks has become a grass-roots movement that has shown great signs of progress in just a few years.

beating and off the pump. You will be given blood-thinning agents to keep your blood from clotting. Your doctor identifies which coronary arteries are blocked (see Figure 10), takes the newly harvested vessels, discards the blocked sections, and creates a new connection at each end. CABG is the most common surgical heart procedure: 365,000 were performed in the U.S. alone in 2007, according to a *New York Times* report. This is a drop of one-third in the past decade, largely due to the increase of stent procedures to about 1 million in 2006.

When the surgery is complete, the blood is allowed to recirculate, and you are taken off the heart-lung machine. The action of blood-thinning heparin is reversed by another drug, protamine. Once the heart is functioning on its own, you'll be sent on to the cardiac intensive care unit or the intensive care unit, depending on how your hospital is configured.

The final word on emergency treatment for a heart attack is that speed is of the utmost importance. Recognize and learn the signs of heart attack, make sure that your family and members of your support group also know them, and think about what you will do if you think you are having a heart attack. Nothing could be more important.

IN A SENTENCE:

> *Surviving a heart attack is a combination of speedy emergency treatment followed by the correct procedure, such as a bypass or angioplasty, depending on the level of damage.*

living

Heart Attack Recovery

FOR ME, one of the most surprising things about having a heart attack has been how many other people I've met who have shared my experience. While I was recovering, it seemed to me that everywhere I went I met another baby boomer who had had a heart attack of some kind. I'd meet guys on the train platform waiting to catch the 7:15 into Manhattan, or I'd run into a parent at the soccer field whom I hadn't seen in a while, and would learn that they had just gotten out of the heart unit at the local hospital. I even met several people on the golf course who became part of regular rotating "cardio-foursomes." In retrospect, this was also the first awareness I had of the health-care crisis that is facing us globally.

What did not surprise me about the people I met was that no one had actually had a "simple heart attack," if there is such a thing. Rather, their MI was part of a constellation of problems that included many disorders mentioned frequently in this book, such as obesity, high blood pressure, and diabetes. We all shared at least one other important thing: We were trying to follow a cardio-rehab program, some with, and some without, success. The key to these programs and why we varied was our ability to learn behavior modification. The common reality for the majority of those of us who have had heart attacks has been different negative health behaviors.

In **Day Seven,** there is information about what you and your family may face emotionally when you are recovering from heart disease or surgery. In order to really change your health behavior, there are also practical changes that you have to consider and implement that are just as critical. *You can do it—I have.* You do not want to have another heart attack, and after the first one, you are at greater risk for a second. In most cases, you can undo or at least mitigate the damage you have done to yourself. Finally, when you do truly make giant steps toward recovery—changing your diet, getting regular exercise, reversing your stress, and meeting other challenges—you will feel a lot better than you ever have felt! This is no small accomplishment.

What Will You Be Able to Do After Your Heart Attack?

Some label recovery as "return to normal activities." This is too simple. Curtis Rimmerman, M.D., my own cardiologist, sees the process this way: "Obviously, it must be individualized. I often equate heart surgery to a speed bump to the rest of your life. Life is a marathon, not a sprint. The heart and body must recover, and why not re-engage in a step-wise manner? It makes the most sense and does not equate with illness severity or permanent disability."

Recovering from a heart attack or cardiac surgery is a life-long activity for you now. You will do a few things in the hospital to prepare, but recovery really begins when you are given the green light to leave the hospital, which, in most cases, is five to six days after your MI.

Before you leave, your doctor will tell you what you should be doing, especially in the context of how serious and/or debilitating your heart attack might have been. Among the new friends I met, all of us had different programs with different goals. But I found that we also had different attitudes, and no matter what your rehab program may be, your overall attitude will make a vast difference between success and another emergency visit to the hospital. It's easy to read this statement as preachy, but please don't take it this way. The emotional after shock of a heart attack can be so strong that you simply may not feel like doing anything remotely related to exercise. After more than a decade of living with heart disease, two heart attacks before I was 50, and a quadruple

---

Will I Ever Lead a Normal Life Again?

No matter what your doctor tells you, this question may be on your mind. Despite my denial, it was always lurking there, and even today, feeling the best I've ever felt, I still think about it. The medical aspect of this question is more easily answered; after all, most people survive their *first* heart attack.

The big question is how many lifestyle changes you are willing to make. Only you can answer this question. You may have to redefine "normal." After all, your version of "normal" may have contributed to your heart attack. The good news is that whatever improvement you make—and you can—your new normal will be better. It has been for me, and it can be for you.

---

bypass, my recovery now is truly driven by a change in my attitude and desire to survive.

How Will You Feel?

After your heart attack, you will likely feel that your entire body has had a stunning blow, as if you'd been hit by a car or wounded in some way. Whether you had an unexpected heart attack or knew you were at risk, you are now among the newly diagnosed. You have to cope with your situation and draw on a great deal of strength and motivation you may not know you have. As corny as this may sound, it is true. Right now, you have a damaged organ that, like any part of your body, will take time to heal. The heart eventually forms scar tissue—over perhaps the next few months—and gradually your activities will be increased and resumed.

Coming Home from the Hospital

The most common feeling you will have when you are in the hospital and when you are discharged is exhaustion. You will also be given a great deal of medical and physical therapy advice during the initial weeks after you are discharged from the hospital. You will be set up in some sort of cardio-rehab program (described below). You can do what I did, which was to ignore most of it and make your long-term path more difficult. In my case, I was still in denial, I didn't feel that sick, and I made the mistake of going back to work quickly—within a few days. Do not even think about doing that. Listen to your doctor. Do what you are told to do.

Your First Days at Home

It's time to get that R&R. Your first goal should be to rest so that your other activities during the day do not make you too tired. Bedtime is the place to start. *Getting a good night's sleep is critical to most heart patients.* Sleeping well gives your body a chance to regroup, reenergize, and reinvigorate your muscles for exercise or small tasks you are going to do tomorrow. That goes for naps, too. No one expects you to be as spry as you were. You will probably feel exhausted, much weaker than you were, and not able to do much for yourself.

Congratulations—this is probably the first time in your life when your doctor will tell you to lie around and relax! Your body is weakened further because you've been in a hospital bed for a week or so. Sleeping in a hospital for any undisturbed period of time is difficult at best and usually impossible. You have to eat when you are told to eat. You probably have lost a substantial amount of your muscle strength, and this is where you will begin to regroup when you get home.

> Many books refer to recovery and cardio rehabilitation in "stages" or "steps." While you may be able to do more as time passes, there are no predetermined periods. Your body and your motivation will determine how quickly you recover.

Your rest and relaxation program should be discussed with your doctor so you know what to expect. If you can't sleep, you have cause for concern. Notify the doctor. If you find that you *are* sleeping at night, but not getting out of bed until noon, or you're taking several naps during the day, it can be a sign of another problem, such as:

○ a physiologic disorder such as anemia,
○ your medication may need adjustment,

○ a drug interaction, or

○ an emotional reaction, such as depression (see **Day Six**).

In any case, call your doctor if your sleeping patterns change. You are not getting the benefit of this critical rest and recovery period after your heart attack.

Establish a Schedule

Resting, however, does not mean you aren't going to get up and move about. Because recovery is as much psychological as physical in this early stage, one of your first steps should be to establish some sort of daily schedule that includes being up and dressed by a certain time. Sometimes just being able to dress yourself and make breakfast is a great boost when, just a few weeks before, you were in a cardiac intensive care unit. Sometimes recovery is about how far you've come when you look back.

Besides getting yourself moving in the morning, creating an initial routine that gets you moving about is critical. Taking a walk every day is one of the best things you can do for yourself. Start slowly. Pick a goal, maybe to the mailbox and back for two weeks. Then go farther, to the end of the block and back. Join the mall walkers. I cannot emphasize how much walking did for me both physically and emotionally. It gives you a goal and a mark to measure your progress.

Make sure that your doctor or a physical therapist works out a schedule with you that covers your walks and household tasks. These might include simple, mundane things such as doing your laundry, sweeping the floor, or making the bed. Yet, you can unknowingly add strain to your heart as it repairs itself, and so home activities should increase incrementally. More activities, like driving, yard work, and shopping will follow in a few weeks as your doctor allows. *It is impossible to overemphasize how important this first part of your recovery is. You must not only take care of yourself, but draw on inner strength to rebuild.*

If you can, this is an especially good time to enlist a family member or a friend to join you in your walks to help you avoid the inevitable feelings of "I'll do it tomorrow" that might be floating around, especially if you are experiencing some depression, which often occurs during recovery.

Cardio-Rehab

Even as you begin the first days of recovery at home, you should begin to make what probably are the hardest changes. This will get you to your second goal: getting back to work or to a life that is close to what it was before. Your hope should be a *new life, not just a better life,* and this can be accomplished through a full cardiac rehabilitation program, which will lead to a new lifestyle. Your revitalization through a combination of exercise and a proper diet will help make you a believer, as I am now.

In general, most people with heart disease can benefit from basic cardiovascular rehabilitation programs. Among those are people who have (or who have had)

○ angina pectoris,
○ cardiomyopathy,
○ chronic heart failure,
○ congestive heart failure,
○ coronary artery bypass graft surgery,
○ congenital cardiovascular disease,
○ peripheral arterial disease,
○ PCI (balloon angioplasty),
○ pacemaker implant,
○ heart transplant,
○ recent heart attack, or
○ valve replacements.

Your doctor will decide whether or not you qualify for a rehab program. There are no specific age or gender parameters, as you can see from my own story below; however, you can be assured that good cardio-rehab programs are safe and beneficial.

In most cases, your cardio-rehab program will be designed specifically for you by your doctor, a social worker, physical/occupational therapists, nutritionists, and medical specialists who will deal with other related problems, such as diabetes. You may meet with them individually or in a small group; however, their goal for you is simple: to ensure that your heart disease improves and that your overall cardiovascular functions are enhanced.

How much of yourself you put into your rehab program will define your success. The American Heart Association guidelines for a cardio-rehab program recommend the following:

○ Counseling to help the patient understand and manage the disease process
○ An exercise program
○ Nutrition counseling
○ Helping the patient modify risk factors, such as high blood pressure, smoking, high blood cholesterol, physical inactivity, obesity, and diabetes
○ Providing vocational guidance to enable the patient to return to work
○ Supplying information on physical limitations
○ Lending emotional support
○ Counseling on appropriate use of prescribed medications

As important as starting a rehab program is how you deal with other problems that have added to your risk profile. The number-one change *must be to stop smoking.* All data about smoking shows two things: Continuing will contribute to your death, and stopping can reverse or minimize the damage you have done to your lungs.

Cardio-rehab goes beyond exercise. You learn about your heart condition and what you can expect to be able to do and not do physically, and you learn about nutrition, how to eat well, as well as other skills you should adopt for life. These aspects of cardio-rehab that take place early in your recovery will serve as a launch pad for the next phase of your recovery.

There are several other things that you have to ask your doctor about when you begin rehab.

○ Find out about the cost and how much your insurance will pay.
○ Learn who is involved and what each team member does.
○ Investigate ways that you can get specialized services, such as a psychological counselor, a smoking cessation program, or spiritual counseling.

The rehab class launched me and helped me build motivational tools to help me come back for more. The moral of this story is not that recov-

My Story: Rehab Reality

I have been through cardio-rehab programs twice. To be honest, the first several days of both were not fun. The first time, my motivation was not great, but the second time was a different story because my goal included recovering enough to get on a plane and fly to Mississippi for an important professional obligation. While my clients had no problem in rescheduling the meeting, I had learned from my first rehab, and my attitude had changed.

My cardio-rehab classes were held in a wing of my cardiologist's office, a relatively common setup. If you are given the choice of where to have your rehab, don't worry if it is not near to your cardiologist's office. Make it convenient for you because convenience is important to help ensure your participation.

My first day of rehab was a shock. I had assumed it was just going to be show up, walk on a treadmill, and be done. Not quite. It looked like a normal aerobic workout room: treadmills, stationary bikes, and the like. But the staff of nurses and therapists was a tough group. There was no TV to watch, and from the moment I walked in, every step I took was monitored with blood pressure and ECG equipment. Having never really exercised in any sort of program, and not being in shape, I found it was a challenge.

The key to a cardio-exercise program is to increase your heart's capacity to handle stress. In this program, the staff made sure that that happened. Once I was on the treadmill or the bike, I maintained the pace they felt was safe, even though I might have thought it was too hard. Every 15 minutes, my blood pressure was recorded and pulse checked. I finished with stretches and a cooling-off period. Fortunately, I returned each week and eventually realized that, doing this along with limited exercising at home, I did feel better.

Yet my physical recovery was not the greatest benefit from the rehab class. Unlike people I met on the train platform who had had heart attacks, everyone in the rehab clinic was in the same boat. No matter how young or old, they had joined a new club. At that club I met people like my new buddy Marvin, ten years older than me and a heart and cancer survivor who was indestructible. We met while walking on adjacent treadmills. Over the weeks, Marvin inspired me (actually, embarrassed me) to keep up with him. We exchanged family stories, along with other helpful information. Within a few more weeks, we were on the golf course.

More than anything, the group setting for the physical aspects of cardio-rehab helped me in my recovery. I learned how to exercise safely and properly, along with how to measure my progress. As someone who strongly preferred sports or activities to exercise, I was actually motivated to get a membership at the YMCA and to use it for at least another six months after my rehab class ended.

ery is simply following a program; it is that recovery is what you make of it. It's the things you put into your program—smoking cessation, weight loss, compliance with your medications—that will make it successful.

Going Back to Work

Work after a heart attack is not as simple a subject as you might think. While the decision is clearly one to be made with your doctor, there are some important issues to consider. Workplace stress has been definitively identified as a risk factor in the development of heart disease. One study of British civil servants found that workplace stress more than doubled the risk for heart attack and other cardiovascular complications.

Other studies have looked at the effect of "justice" or "fair treatment" by superiors. Those who felt they were treated well at work appeared to be at lower risk for heart disease. Some studies are limited and anecdotal; however, a large study of British workers disclosed that workers who "perceived a higher sense of justice were at 30 percent lower risk for cardiovascular incidents."

Scientists have cited the lack of data matching the relationship of stress at work to heart disease. In particular, data are scarce in women and in countries where work hours and conditions differ from those in the United States and the United Kingdom.

Another question to ask yourself about work is this: Did work make you sick? According to the National Institute for Occupational Health and Safety (NIOSH), part of the Centers for Disease Control and Prevention, little is known about occupational risks for coronary heart disease; however, specific toxins are known to affect the heart most prominently, including carbon disulfide, nitroglycerin, and carbon monoxide. You may encounter carbon monoxide in the workplace from vehicle exhausts, which can be very toxic.

NIOSH also lists exposure to heat and cold, along with occupational noise and stress that can affect blood pressure, as hazardous to your health. Even shift work, which can upset natural circadian rhythms, has been implicated, along with a high level of physical activity.

No matter what your occupation, this information raises important issues that should go into your conversation with your doctor. Many

My Story: Making Changes

Making the decision to return to work is an opportunity to consider what you do and who you are professionally. What has your career done to you? I was both a stress junkie and a workaholic, and I went back to work too soon after my initial heart attacks in my late 40s. I had a home office, and I always had a briefcase full of work with me. I spent time in the evenings with my family, but once things quieted down, I was on the couch with the TV on, reviewing a lap full of papers. I felt I had to do this. It was behavior I had learned from my parents, and I was probably hard-wired.

Five years later, after quadruple bypass surgery, I saw the world differently. The idea of *living* had attracted my attention.

I made a fundamental decision that the executive life was no longer for me, and I reinvented myself. I turned to the things that I enjoyed, including teaching and consulting, and I began to turn my health around. Not everyone is in a position to do this, or so you might think.

Where work and heart attack is concerned, if you cannot categorically state that your job did not contribute to your heart attack, then you have to consider alternative work. It is a matter of life and death.

There may be occupational counselors connected to your cardio rehab program or vocational counseling may be available. My new professional life, work that employs skills that I used in a former workplace, has made me healthier and happier. A friend once told me that "the best jobs are the ones you make," and you can adopt this philosophy and shape a new, saner, post-heart-attack work life.

guidelines are offered about returning to work, but, like all other aspects of heart attack recovery, they are suggestions at best. From a medical point of view, the amount of damage to your heart muscle may make the decision for you. The results of your cardio rehab program also can be a factor. In some cases, going back to your old job may be something you don't want to do. Ask yourself whether it is safe to go back and whether you would place others at risk, should something happen on the job.

One of the first things you may want to discuss with your doctor is the actual benefit of going back to work. Many people who have heart attacks thrive on work and are, as I was, stress junkies. If you feel your occupation has contributed to your heart attack, but you still love what you do, you may want to work with a counselor to learn how to control the stress or make it work for you. Your doctor, however, has to know the details of your job.

Ensuring That You Have a Job

Statistically speaking, eight in ten people under the age of 65 do go back to work, so it's likely that you will be back to work within a reasonable period of time. There is no average, but you can be back anywhere from a few weeks to a few months after your heart attack. Before you go back to work, contact your employer to let them know your condition. Keep them apprised of your recovery and when, realistically, you may return. Consider setting up a schedule that involves a gradual return to work. There is no reason not to make an arrangement to go into work for a few hours every day.

On the positive side, your job can become a place that also helps in your rehab simply because you are back with people you know. Human contact, after weeks recovering alone, can be stimulating and can help you deal with any mood swings that occur.

Keep this in mind also: Do you need to pass a physical for the job or do you need a certificate from a doctor? Make sure all necessary paperwork is done before you return to work. We live in an age of corporate self-preservation, and if you've never been on medical leave or in a situation that might affect your insurance coverage, talk to the human resources department. You may be unhappily surprised at the releases or waivers of responsibility you might be asked to review.

Most employers cannot simply fire you for having a heart attack; however, depending on the employer and the state in which you live, your employer may have some discretion on whether or not you return to work at all. Today, many employees are simply work-for-hires, even if you get benefits. One attorney discussing this subject told me, "Today, an employer can fire you for any reason, even if someone says something about you that is totally false." *Do your homework.*

Getting Better on the Job

Changing your diet will be a major aspect of your new post-MI life. If you are going back to work after a heart attack, you can't go back to eating poorly, if that has been one of your problems. This is where behavior change has to be made, and a time when you must get professional assistance. Work with a nutritionist and ask to have a program tailored for you that fits with your job circumstances and other responsibilities. In **Month Four,** you'll find a complete approach to post–heart disease diet, but this is another area that you can change—if you really want to change.

Your new heart-healthy diet should be adopted and followed as much as possible at work. If you are able to bring your lunch, you have more control over your choices. Today, companies have recognized that overweight and sick employees lead to an unhealthy bottom line. If your company is one of these, the cafeteria will usually have a salad bar and other options, such as fat-free dressings, low-fat yogurt, and other dairy products, cereals, and vegetables. If your company doesn't have this sort of program, explore starting one. You have to be your own advocate.

While lunch and breakfast are easy to manage, what about those mid-morning, mid-afternoon "walls" when you used to reach for a candy bar for a shot of sugar? The hottest things on the market are "100-calorie snack packs" that are essentially packages of your favorite treats shrunken into a lower-calorie version. Of course, fruit or vegetable sticks are always a good idea.

The biggest problem most of us have at work is the sedentary nature of our jobs. Start by finding a way to get in 15 to 20 minutes of walking (which I supplement with regular exercise at home). Every time you take a walk at lunchtime or as an afternoon break, your heart gets a dose of oxygen-rich blood, your blood pressure lowers, and you relieve stress. Try the stairs instead of the elevator and take advantage of any at-work programs, like Weight Watchers or exercise workshops. If you link what you can do at work to developing a healthy lifestyle that carries over to home, you can be more motivated overall. Where the workplace is concerned, you can be a leader and you can convince others to join you in regular activities.

Getting Back in the Office Pool

As you go back to work, you may find that your friends, like your family, treat you as if you are about to break. My experience has led me to be as up-front as possible. People are naturally curious, and many of your colleagues who are the same age may be thinking that you seemed to be in better shape than they are, and that this could happen to them.

Worry about yourself: That is the most important part of going back to work. Remember Dr. Rimmerman's advice: "I often equate heart surgery to a speed bump to the rest of your life. Life is a marathon, not a sprint. The heart and body must recover and why not re-engage in a step-wise manner? It makes the most sense, and does not equate with illness severity or permanent disability."

Recovery from a heart attack and heart surgery, as you'll see in the next section, is one of the most challenging life events you can imagine. You will go through a wide range of emotions, daily and even hourly. You may possibly have physical symptoms or random pains that will make you wonder if you are having another heart attack. It may take time for you to get back on a normal schedule. You may need medication to help you sleep or relax.

There is no "normal" in heart attack or surgery recovery. You may feel guilt for scaring and upsetting your family and children, or you can be angry at yourself for putting yourself at risk.

One thing we all share is fear. No matter how tough you think you are, how immune to harm, or how thoroughly you are in denial, you will have some level of anxiety or discomfort when you begin your recovery.

Your recovery journey is an opportunity, over time, to erase those feelings. Your doctor may lecture you, the rehab staff will push you, and all sorts of resources will be offered to you, but you have to bring the most important tool for fixing yourself. You have to find motivation somewhere to change many behaviors that have put you in cardio-rehab. You are likely part of a generation that is entering a high-risk period for pretty much everything. However, you are lucky because you are reaching this age despite your damaged heart, at a time when technology and cardiac medications can increase your likelihood of survival. You are, in an odd way, very lucky. Luck presents opportunity. Take advantage of it.

IN A SENTENCE:

> *Recovery from a heart attack requires a mixture of physical and emotional rehabilitation; however, more than anything, it requires motivation and willingness to modify your negative health behaviors.*

Recovery from Heart Bypass Surgery

THEY CALL it a "cabbage," which sounds just like the vegetable, but it's actually CABG—medical jargon for a coronary artery bypass graft, the most commonly performed heart surgery. Sometimes called the gold standard of coronary operations, CABG is performed each year on more than 350,000 patients in the U.S.

Early in the first year after your diagnosis, your doctor could decide that angioplasty, medication, diet, or exercise may not be enough to prevent another heart attack or further progression of your heart disease. This scary conversation also could take place a few years after your heart attack, as mine did. Either way, your cardiologist has determined that your coronary arteries now are too blocked to do anything else; bypass surgery will keep your heart receiving good, oxygenated blood.

Your doctor may show you your catheterization film. If not, ask to see it. Discuss it fully with your doctor until you understand what the images on the film mean.

Earlier, we talked about getting second opinions. Unless you are in the emergency room and the surgery is needed immediately, you should understand completely what this procedure is about and what to expect afterwards. (I got four second opinions, and each doctor agreed with my cardiologist.) Make sure that you get other opinions and that you feel comfortable with them.

Your Heart Is Linked to Your Head

You should go into surgery with a positive feeling. In retrospect, I wish I knew that how I felt *before* surgery would affect my recovery *after* surgery. As unlikely as this may sound, how you feel and your knowledge of bypass surgery are crucial. This is especially true at this time, when your head is spinning with emotions beyond those provoked by the level of your heart disease or a heart attack. Physicians, psychologists, and, especially nurses who care for surgical patients have long recognized that preoperative stress and denial can affect recovery. It's all about your attitude!

It's expected that you will have an emotional reaction to the news that you need a CABG or other major surgery. One study examined the feelings of a group of preoperative men that revealed strong feelings of apprehension, including fear, worry, anxiety, and suspicion, along with positive and hopeful feelings that increased as the surgery drew closer. Fear was linked to both the reason for surgery and what might happen during surgery, such as anesthetic complications, physical disfigurement, and death. Also not surprising (it happened to me), when anxiety levels are high, patients can demonstrate apathy. In general, most people do become positive as the surgery looms, primarily because they have hope of a cure and rehabilitation from their disease.

You may also find yourself under a great deal of stress when this news is dropped on you, even if you expected it. Multiple studies have shown that stress can affect your immune system. When you have surgery, especially open heart surgery, you are at risk for pneumonia or infection, and your immune system has to work well. Studies show that senior citizens who are under stress, perhaps as a caregiver to a spouse, should *not* receive flu and pneumonia vaccinations until they are less stressed.

Having the Surgery

Because your CABG may be needed soon after your diagnosis, you will be relieved to know that this procedure has a high success rate. Full

Why Do They Call It a CABG?

All industries have their own jargon; however, we tend to hear more *doctor-speak* because we see doctors in person frequently and we seem to have a fascination with medical settings for our prime time and afternoon soap operas. Shows like *ER* and *House* are essentially the same story over and over, and the dialog is pretty much the same: lots of shouting medical-sounding orders with *stat* (immediately) at the end of every sentence. You really have no idea what they are saying, and you may wonder why they talk this way.

Doctors have to memorize an enormous amount of complicated information. Many use **mnemonics**, which is a system of memorization that works several ways. Coronary artery bypass graft is a prime example. The initials CABG, when spoken together, sound like "cabbage." Doctors in training also learn many, many phrases and short rhymes that help them memorize diseases for recall and diagnosis.

Another reason for use of jargon is that it's simply faster. Doctors have to do reams of post-procedure reports. In the past they were written, but today they are dictated and transcribed for electronic medical records.

Surveys show that poor communication between doctors and patients has had a negative effect. Doctors are being urged to limit *doctorspeak*. In defense, many patients have taken it upon themselves to learn the lingo. There are numerous websites, such as www.aspexdesign.co.uk/jargonm.htmv, that have become encyclopedias of medical jargon. Today, thanks to the Internet, you can learn the M.D. lingo and even trip up your own doc on occasion.

recovery from CABG, while different from that after a heart attack, can be achieved through the same determination and motivation when coming back from an MI.

Prior to the day of surgery, you will have a number of tests, including a chest x-ray, an electrocardiogram, blood tests, urine tests, and, perhaps, a chat with a social worker or the hospital chaplain, if you wish.

In most non-emergency cases, you are admitted to the hospital on the morning of surgery, prepped, and given a sedative to help you to relax. After that, you are not going to remember very much about the surgery. Honestly, this is a good thing because no matter how much reassurance you have been given, you are going to be nervous. One thing I found very helpful was to keep in mind that my surgeon was very experienced.

Cardiovascular surgeons who perform bypass operations tend to do many of them each year. In my case, the surgical team at Morristown Memorial Hospital, a mid-size facility in central New Jersey, did over 1,200 bypass surgeries per year, which was more than any other hospital in New Jersey.

The next thing you are likely to remember is awakening in the cardiac intensive care unit (also called the CCU) or a similar unit. In my case, the first thing I saw was a nurse sitting at the end of my bed welcoming me back to consciousness.

You may not be all that aware of what's going on—you will still be sedated—but you will be surrounded by IVs dispensing medications that help keep your blood from clotting and reduce pain. Multiple monitors that check your blood pressure and heart rate will be hooked up through electrodes attached to your skin, and you can expect discomfort in the middle of your chest where it was opened and in your leg (if that's where the vein for the bypass graft came from).

It's possible that you will also use a breathing tube and a urinary catheter inserted into your body after surgery, but this will not last long. Generally, most people bounce back. Your stay in the CCU may last 12 to 24 hours. That's when your recovery really begins. Once your doctor has determined that your body is working well on its own and you no longer need on-line monitoring, you may be moved to a cardiac unit or floor where you will learn that recovery loves company. My roommates were very talkative, exchanging tips about the food and introducing their families. It was reassuring.

You will also find that cardiac units have highly skilled nurses who bear the majority of the care for patients after surgery. While you will be able to sit up, eat solid food customized to your dietary needs (e.g., low-fat food for diabetes), you are not going to feel like playing 18 holes of golf or even taking a walk down the hall, which the nurse will want you to do.

This is where you have to find motivation. Your nurse will suggest that you walk, and it will involve getting up and lugging your oxygen unit with you. When you're in bed, you'll get oxygen support through an uncomfortable tube with little plastic prongs in your nose. A pulse oximeter attached to your finger painlessly measures the concentration of oxygen in your bloodstream. If you get up and walk around, the exercise will help strengthen your lungs. That knowledge got me up and walking, pulling my tank on its little cart up and down the hall. I wanted to go home. Your motivation in the period after surgery is up to you, but as you do get stronger and you feel better, you'll be glad you took the first step.

The First Days of the Rest of Your Life

When you get home, usually in five or six days after surgery, you will certainly feel better, but you will still be tired and weak. You will also have a unique souvenir from your surgery. Down the center of your chest will be a scar that most bypass patients call their "zipper" and, possibly, also a scar on the inside of your leg extending from above your ankle to your thigh, where the saphenous vein has been harvested for use in the bypass. (Frequently, an artery called the internal mammary from inside the chest is used.) This may be the first time you realize exactly what has happened to you: Someone opened your chest, stopped your heart, repaired it, and restarted it. This can be a very intense moment, much different from the realization that you have heart disease.

Beyond the emotional issue, you also will have to take care of that scar. Not only has your chest been split open, but it's been put back together, sometimes with special internal medical wires that will remain forever. (They will not set off an airport alarm.) Taking care of the chest and leg incisions requires basic hygiene, using mild soap and water. Your nurse or doctor will instruct you, indicating when it is safe to have any bandages removed.

Report any excessive tenderness or swelling around your incisions. Do not ever hesitate to call your doctor or surgeon about your concerns. They will not mind because the last thing they want is a negative outcome for you. *It cannot be overstated that in the aftermath of bypass surgery, you should remain in contact with your doctor.* If you have trouble breathing, dizziness, or feel angina-like chest pain, make that call!

You will be allowed to take a bath or shower; however, they should be quick and, if possible, keep the shower spray from hitting your chest incision directly.

A few things that you may expect include the following:

○ Soreness and muscular pain (a result of your body's recovering from the surgery)

○ Tightness in the chest around your scar

○ Swelling in the legs from where the vein was harvested (in many cases, you will be told to keep it raised), which should resolve over time

○ Keeping your legs stretched out to ensure easy blood flow

○ No driving for at least 30 to 60 days to protect your chest while it heals (which made me very frustrated, since I hate to rely on others, but it is far better than ending up back in the hospital)

○ No bike riding or lifting of heavy objects

○ Diminished appetite or change in taste

○ Interrupted sleep or trouble getting back to sleep once awakened

○ Gastric problems, such as constipation

Be Aware of Your Feelings

There are a few other things that are specific to recovery after bypass surgery. Primary among them is the potential for the depression described earlier. You may have mood swings throughout the day. While these periods are very common, you should be aware of their severity. If, for example, you find yourself not just "down" or "blue," but in despair or having suicidal thoughts, get help. Some reports attribute this to fear of the future regarding your health, or you may be worried that your health is now compromised and your old life is gone. Virtually anything can set off depression after bypass, but *it must not be taken lightly*. Be forthright with your doctor. Get professional help.

Bypass patients also report something that I found both curious and disquieting. You may be unable to remember certain things, have problems with short-term memory, or not feel as "with it" as before the operation. For months I was convinced that something had happened during the surgery and that my family wasn't telling me about it.

As it turns out, some cognitive changes can be attributed to the enormous stress on your body that goes along with this surgery. It is thought that having your heart stopped while your brain and circulation are maintained on the heart-lung machine contributes to this phenomenon. Fortunately, these are generally mild, temporary changes.

Is it scary? Sure, but it goes away with time. Within a few weeks, certainly by the time you go back to work, you may only notice it occasionally. However, if you continue to suffer from any sort of unusual psychological stress, talk with someone as soon as you can. Keep in mind that open heart surgery is an exceptional event. Despite the high success rate of this surgery, you must pay attention to what your body tells you as you heal.

Your Sex Life

There is no reason your bypass operation should prevent you from having a normal sex life and some good old-fashioned TLC. Intimacy, warmth, and comfort from your partner or spouse work wonders.

One rule of thumb I often hear is that "sex requires as much energy as walking up a flight of stairs. When you can do that, you are good to go." While this may be accurate, a better standard is the one your doctor sets for you.

Pay attention to your doctor's advice about the use of **erectile dysfunction** medications because they can't be taken with some heart medications, such as nitrates (see **Month Eight**).

Exercise Guidelines

○ Stop any exercise if you experience shortness of breath, dizziness, leg cramping, unusual fatigue, and/or chest pain (angina). Notify your doctor if these symptoms persist.
○ If your post-exercise pulse rate is more than 30 beats faster than your resting pulse rate, or if your rate of perceived exertion is over 13, you have exercised too hard. In order to correct these conditions, you will need to modify your next exercise session.

Pulse Assessment

Monitoring your pulse rate helps you to keep your activities within a safe heart rate range. To take your pulse, place your index and middle fingers on the lower part of your thumb, then slide your fingers down to your wrist or place them at the carotid artery in your neck. (Do not use your thumb, as it has a noticeable pulse that will confuse your count.) If you do not feel the pulse, try moving your fingers over a little bit in the

When to Resume Usual Activities

Weeks 1–6

Light housekeeping:
-Dusting
-Setting the table
-Washing dishes
-Folding clothes

Light gardening:
-Potting plants
-Trimming flowers

Needlework

Reading

Cooking meals

Climbing stairs

Small mechanical jobs

Shopping

Restaurants

Movies

Church

Attending sports events

Riding in a car

Walking

Using the treadmill

Stationary biking

Shampooing hair

Playing cards/games

After 6 weeks

Continue activities of weeks 1–6 (you may be able to tolerate a more intense level)

Return to work part-time (if your job does not require lifting and if returning is approved by your surgeon)

Heavy housework:
-Vacuuming
-Sweeping
-Laundry
-Ironing

Heavy gardening:
-Mowing the lawn
-Raking leaves

Business or recreational travel

Fishing

Light aerobics (no weights)

Walking the dog on a leash

Driving a car or small truck

Boating

After 3 months

Continue activities of 1–3 months (but you may be able to tolerate more)

Heavy housework:
-Scrubbing floors

Heavy gardening:
-Shoveling snow
-Digging

Football/Soccer

Softball/Baseball

Tennis

Bowling

Hunting

Jogging

Bicycling

Golfing

Weight lifting

Motorcycle riding

Push-ups

Swimming

Water skiing

Skydiving

* Keep in mind that all of these activities need to be within or under the 10-pound weight limit until six weeks after surgery.

** Visitors: Limit your visitors for the first couple of weeks. If you become tired, excuse yourself and lie down. Your visitors will understand.

This chart was developed by the Barnes-Jewish Hospital and Washington University School of Medicine cardiothoracic-surgery performance-improvement team. Reprinted by permission.

same area. Once you can feel the pulse, count it for 15 seconds and multiply by 4. This will tell you how many times your heart is beating in one minute. Your doctor or her or his nurse can help you to find the pulse in your wrist if you have difficulty.

(Reprinted by permission from the Barnes-Jewish Hospital CABG discharge instructions.)

IN A SENTENCE:

> *Coronary bypass recovery, similar to recovery from a heart attack, involves overcoming both emotional and physical issues and dedicating yourself to reversing your **negative health behaviors**.*

DAY **7**

What to Expect Emotionally

HEART DISEASE is a family disease. Obviously, the level of your illness, its progression, and the restrictions on your life may define the impact on everyone in your home. Heart disease is also a chronic illness. However, unlike a stroke victim who may require many levels of care, you *may* be able to manage without a caretaker. Still, heart disease presents many daily challenges such as these:

- ❍ Are you on a new diet?
- ❍ How mobile are you?
- ❍ Can you take care of yourself?
- ❍ Are you taking a confusing array of medications?
- ❍ Do you have more than one medical problem?
- ❍ Will your recovery be long?
- ❍ When can you go back to work?
- ❍ Do you need home nursing care?

These are only a few of many *practical issues* that you and your family will have to cope with when you are being treated for any sort of heart disease. However, heart disease can, and usually does, have an emotional impact that can be obvious or, as it did in my case, it may sneak up on you without warning. Heart disease can do all of the following to you:

○ provoke depression
○ affect intimacy
○ diminish self-esteem
○ create a constant state of anxiety
○ cause resentment of other, healthy family members
○ affect communications between family members
○ cause embarrassment
○ create denial, slowing your recovery

Whether you've been told you are at risk for heart disease, diagnosed with a congenital heart malformation, or are in recovery for a heart attack, you are faced with significant lifestyle changes. In most cases, it's not simply giving up trans-fatty foods or something more difficult, like smoking or that daily six-pack. It's time to decide whether you want to live or die. You're going to have to deal with problems like these and, possibly, many more.

Keep in mind that these steps back to a normal life come in stages, and, thankfully, do not occur all at once. Yet, the question of motivation and how you attain your recovery goals is not answered easily. It's absurd to think that anyone can do this alone. Add to the list of things you have to consider in your life: what sort of help you need and where you are going to get it.

My Story

Over more than a decade from the time of my first MI to this very day, I have experienced and overcome every one of the emotions and problems mentioned previously. That does not mean they have come and gone and will not reappear. If there is one thing that influenced my positive behavior and the desire to survive, it was finding reasons to do so.

When you find yourself facing this moment, every cliché in the book will be thrown at you: Do it for your kids. Don't you want to walk your daughter down the aisle? You're still young; you have so much to live for and accomplish. Then there's my favorite: Consider the alternative.

As much as these were nice, rational reasons to make an effort to change 40 years of ingrained negative health behavior, they simply weren't working for me. Like most people after a heart attack, I'd been given a set of therapeutic directives that included attendance at a cardio-rehab program, exercise, and nutritional counseling. There is no question that anyone who is recovering from heart surgery or who is diagnosed with some other cardiac issue should be in a cardio-rehab program. I went to all of the classes after my MI and again, five years later, after my bypass surgery. I listened to my internist's lectures on my cholesterol and blood-sugar levels. Unfortunately, then I went off to the store for bags of cookies and stopped at the video store so that I could hit the couch, kick back, inhale the cookies, and watch a movie while the cholesterol and pounds added up.

During those periods, I had plenty to live for: two great children in college and the career I'd always dreamed about. These should be important motivators, and they were hardly superficial, but by themselves, they didn't do the trick. Here is the key: I can't emphasize enough that a serious, chronic illness provokes emotional issues that have to be coped with as quickly as possible. Like me, you may not recognize that this is the problem. Looking back, my emotional battle with heart disease also matched my medical battle, dividing it into "before bypass" and "after bypass" phases. The first phase was definitely a losing battle, and the second has gotten me to where I am now—the healthiest I've been in a decade plus.

From the period of my heart attack until I was faced with the undeniable opinions of *four* cardiologists that I needed quadruple bypass, I went through several years marked by depression, mood swings, despair, and loneliness. Yet I went to work every day, spending $1\frac{1}{2}$ hours commuting to the office on a New Jersey transit train and two subways. I had two high-stress executive jobs that meant business lunches without a single heart-healthy dish on the menu. Occasionally, the thought that fried shrimp, french fries, and a caesar salad drenched in creamy dressing was not going to help my already clogged arteries passed my mind, but not before the food passed my lips.

I have since learned that my story, post-MI, is not all that unusual, but with one strong exception. While I was increasing my risk factors, somehow I managed not to have another, perhaps fatal, heart attack. This is where the first step after any sort of heart disorder recovery really begins. You have to realize that you are not just living for others; you're working to prevent going through what you have just been through!

There are multiple step-by-step recovery and risk-reduction programs for each heart disorder. These include exercise, diet, medication compliance, dealing with insurance companies, and the mechanics of recovery. They begin in **Month Two.** These rehabilitation programs will involve your own group of people, but as you will learn, this group is not a permanent team, as many books suggest.

Your cardiologist or surgeon will set up a formal program for you, but you'll face several potential challenges that require more than advice from recovery and treatment specialists. These are the challenges that test your medical and emotional recovery, and your response will help you over the long term.

Depression: The Sneak Attack

Depression has long been associated with heart disease, both as a precursor and an after effect. According to research by the National Institute of Mental Health (NIMH) and other studies, depression is so prevalent among people who develop heart disease that it could almost be categorized as a risk factor. Persons who are depressed are between 1.5 to 4 times as likely to develop heart disease as are those who are not depressed.

Looking at this from the post-program side, if you have survived a heart attack, the NIMH says, you are far more likely to become depressed. While about one in 20 American adults experiences major depression in a given year, the number goes to about one in three for people who have survived a heart attack. In addition, if you develop depression after a heart attack, you have a greater risk of death.

You can't underestimate what a bout of depression can cause in your recovery, especially if you have some concomitant illness. In stroke victims, 40 percent to 50 percent suffer from depression. Not surprisingly, diabetic men with depression have a higher level of erectile dysfunction, although this can also be related to other conditions, such as high

---

Watch for These Symptoms of Depression

○ Persistent sad, anxious, or "empty" mood
○ Feelings of hopelessness, pessimism
○ Feelings of guilt, worthlessness, or helplessness
○ Loss of interest or pleasure in hobbies and activities that once were enjoyed, including sex
○ Decreased energy, fatigue, feeling "slowed down"
○ Difficulty concentrating, remembering, making decisions
○ Insomnia, early-morning awakening, or oversleeping
○ Appetite or weight changes
○ Thoughts of death or suicide, or suicide attempts
○ Restlessness or irritability

If five or more of these symptoms are present every day for at least two weeks and interfere with routine daily activities, such as work, self-care, child-care, or social life, seek an evaluation for depression. (**Source: National Institute of Mental Health**)

---

blood pressure, elevated cholesterol, smoking, and medications including insulin.

Of all the emotional disorders, constant or occasional depression is enormously crippling. The textbook symptoms are well known: feeling anxious, empty, worthless, hopeless, pessimistic, or helpless. The textbook hardly tells the story, as anyone who has been through this will tell you. Depression can wreak havoc with your cardiovascular system, which is one reason depression is also a risk factor for stroke. Any anxiety disorder can upset your heart rhythms, shoot up your blood pressure, and affect your blood-clotting ability and cholesterol levels. Depression, which provokes stress, can trigger metabolic changes that cause the release of stress hormones like cortisol or adrenaline that weaken your ability to recover.

It's likely you'll be told to expect some form of post-surgical depression. According to the American Heart Association, "Depression (during recovery from a heart attack) is normal, and in 85 percent of the cases, it goes away in three months." To be honest, I, like many, had suffered some periods of anxiety and depression that had sent me into counseling and, ultimately, into treatment with medication for several years. How-

> ### Depression
>
> Anyone can be struck by depression. Almost 10 percent of American adults—19 million people above age 18—suffer depression every year. About 80 percent of people who are treated get better, but only about 50 percent of the people with depression get help. (NIMH)

ever, nothing could have prepared me for what happened after my quadruple bypass surgery.

Not surprisingly, after five days in recovery (**Day Six**), I wanted to get out of the hospital. I was finally given extensive marching orders and was sent home to begin my formal and personal rehab. In Day Six, you can read about the formal program, but I had a goal and began my comeback with a determined attitude. My goal? To get back to work as quickly as I could, of course. I wanted to be at a photo shoot in Mississippi in 30 days, and my cardiologist told me that if I passed a stress test in 28 days, I could go.

That energized me. My friend Dr. Solomon in Boston told me that the secret "was to do everything they told me to do twice." It worked. Within two weeks, I was walking all the way around the courtyard at my apartment complex. I had enough energy to work from home for several hours each day, and I'd made it to all my physical rehab classes.

About two weeks after my surgery, I was working and listening to a soundtrack from a cult movie, ironically titled *Still Crazy*, about a group of musicians looking back on their lives. The cut was called, "What Might Have Been." The message, wrapped in a beautiful melody, is pretty straightforward, but for some reason, the lyrics rocked me in my gut:

What might have been/
What might have been—a portrait of my life. . .

I'd heard this song many times, but this time as I listened, the tears started to flow. I began to cry harder than I'd ever cried before. My body shook for half an hour. I couldn't move, and pretty much didn't move for the next few days, during which I was wracked by a wide range of negative emotions. The song had triggered years of bottled emotions, according to my counselor, and I was suffering from depression. It was different from other bouts of depression related to an inherited brain-chemistry imbalance or a divorce or a death in the family.

I had been hit by a train unexpectedly, which is exactly what I'd been warned about. This type of depression is often triggered by stress or a life-threatening experience. Worse, it also threatened to dislodge my newly discovered will to make a healthy comeback. Fortunately, I had a good support system, although I lived alone. My friends and family refused to let me wallow, and I realized that my goal—the trip—was at risk if I didn't get back on track. This time, unlike many times in the past, I got out of bed and got back on my way.

Intimacy

After depression, intimacy is one of the trickiest parts of emotional recovery. First, the term "intimacy" means so many things. Are we talking about sexual intercourse, or do we simply mean nice moments, snuggling, hugging? Many emotions can surface, ranging from fear of another heart attack to fear about your ability to perform if you are male.

Ironically, if you are suffering some transient depression (the "blues") the warmth of a good hug or just waking up every morning with someone to hold can become anxiety provoking to anyone who has suffered a cardiac event.

Everyone experiences "recovery" in this area differently. To present this issue properly, an entire section of this book—**Week Two**—has been devoted to it, covering both the emotional and chemical (medication) issues.

More Steps Back to the Real World

While overcoming the two "biggies"—emotional distress and/or depression—a return to intimacy during your recovery may seem like a lot to cope with. But there are more problems that might strike unexpectedly or may simply come and go.

Low self-esteem. You might find that you have a sense of diminished self-esteem after a significant bout with heart disease. Generally, it goes along with depression, so you should consider it a possible early warning sign.

For a heart patient, failing self-esteem may be something that only another patient can describe. For many of us, our level of heart disease is a direct result of failing to do something to prevent it from getting worse. You are determined, as I was, to get back on that treadmill and stick with the program. Most of all, you want to get back to work for a variety of reasons. The biggest of these is to regain your sense of self-worth.

This may seem trivial, in that you are happy to be alive, but this issue can sneak up on you. First, you may feel that the old days of physical activities—sports or ballroom dancing or many other things—are over. Second, you may be reluctant to push yourself the way you did before at work, yet your colleagues still are working 80-hour weeks. Third, you now have to watch your diet, too. This means that when the boss or your friends take you out to lunch to welcome you back to work, you have to watch what you eat, and this might make you uncomfortable.

Here's the answer. If you reduce your stress, if you take it slow in resuming activity, and if you learn to eat properly, your risk for another heart attack or more advanced cardiovascular disease will be reduced. You will be in top shape. You'll be able to look in the mirror and see a healthy person. The best way to deal with issues of self-esteem is to work at becoming healthy.

Embarrassment. Some people feel that asking for help is an imposition. Horribly scaring someone who loves you when you collapse on the kitchen floor or in a pick-up game at the park really is an imposition. Trust me on this one. They are much happier that you are alive. You can overcome all of your fears of embarrassment by getting as healthy as you can. Embarrassment is a valid emotion, but it does not last.

Anxiety. This may be another constant when you are beginning to recover. To be honest, I put on a great show of bravado when I came home from the hospital after my bypass, but I was terrified to go to bed. I lived alone, and despite having close friends and neighbors to call on, I still relied on anti-anxiety medication for quite some time. When I was busy working or keeping occupied with a movie and some popcorn, I was fine. I rarely, if ever, took a pill during the day.

Finally, I hit on the perfect solution, and I recognize that this is not a universal answer: I got a cat. I took my daughter to the animal rescue and found my new best friend. Today, seven years later, Mr. Sneakers, a

black-and-white tuxedo cat, is lying on the table next to my desk, waiting for some reassuring petting whenever I need it.

Everybody has to find his or her own solution to the natural feelings
that come out when you are recovering from cardiac surgery, changing a
lifestyle to prevent further damage, or simply coping with a new self-
image as a "sick person." Often, people turn to their faith, which I found
helpful. I also sought counseling. However, there is one thing I can tell
you, something my father used to say to me, and he was always right:
"This, too, will pass."

Resentment. I have heard versions of this true story many times.
John, an active 77-year-old, has passed away after a six-year battle
with heart disease. During that period, he had two major heart attacks. After the first one, his wife, Maria, was told to call her family
because he was not going to live, but, somehow, he did. The ensuing
years were difficult for John and Maria. He wanted to pursue his only
passion, golf, and Maria watched him like a hawk. What did he eat
and when did he eat it? Why did he have to work eight hours? He
could cut back now. Much worse, the doctor wouldn't let him back
onto the golf course.

John's final heart attack came shortly after his 77th birthday. John
and Maria had been married 51 years. They owned a small jewelry business that they had built over the years that secured their lives and put
three children through college. When John died, the couple had seven
grandchildren and two great-grandchildren.

A few years later, Maria followed several of her widowed friends to a
retirement area in Asheville, NC, that she and John had picked out
many years before. Within a few years, Maria had adjusted, begun a new
life, and moved on, including meeting a new man, Frank, who reawak-
ened some emotions that she thought she had buried with John. As
many people with aging, widowed parents know, there are many couples
or live-ins in our senior-citizen communities.

Maria and her new friend became so close that they came to family
events together, and the relationship was quickly accepted by her children, who decided to let Mom know that if she and Frank wanted to get
married or live together, they would have no objections.

Her response was direct and surprising: "Are you serious? I'll never
take care of a sick man again!"

The family was shocked, never once having suspected that Maria resented taking care of their dad. You may have heard stories like this, or you may even sense it within your own support group. You also may resent healthier members of your own family who can eat what they want or hit the links every weekend. Resentment sometimes goes hand-in-hand with embarrassment, and it is one of the more insidious emotional reactions to heart disease that you have to watch for.

Resolving resentment from both sides requires effective communication among family members and as much education about heart disease as possible.

Denial. This problem can slow your recovery as much as or more than anything else.

Several things may cause denial, but two are common. One, ironically, is that reasonably soon after your treatment you may feel much better than you did. After all, you may have spent years with creeping CAD that slowly hampered your ability to even walk up the stairs. Now your bypass has given your heart fresh, oxygen-rich blood to draw on each day. You may be back on the golf course several weeks after surgery when your doctor has cleared you.

Your denial may not be intentional, but you may believe, as I did for a time, now that you have been treated, your underlying health problems, risk factors, or failure to comply with diet and exercise programs aren't that important.

The other reason that denial occurs is the obvious one. It's understandable that you may simply want to avoid many of the emotional problems, such as embarrassment, lack of self-esteem, or resentment, and the possible unpleasant side effects of medication you may not want to take (**Month Eight**).

IN A SENTENCE:

> *As you recover from heart disease, there are many practical issues you have to face, and the emotional ones can sneak up on you; however, if you are prepared and build a support system, these issues need not be devastating.*

The Family Impact

CONSIDERING WHAT you may encounter emotionally as a heart patient, does this mean you will become a burden for your family members, spouse, friends, or caregivers? Recovery from and living with any chronic disease is not easy. That is a simple truth, and it is likely that your family and you will have to make changes in many areas, depending on the severity of your condition. Care is not the only critical issue—preventing progression of the disease is equally important.

It's hard to emphasize how much you need other people in your life to help you when you have heart disease. Unfortunately, few resources have considered this aspect of heart disease in any depth. "Family" and "heart" are more often classified under risk factors, or, more recently, the effect on family if the patient is female and household functions are dependent on her health.

Embracing help during your recovery is very important. Your recovery and long-term prospects will be easier if you don't try to go it alone. As you read on, keep in mind that you and your caregivers are only human. You may not be able to do all the things suggested in your first year of recovery, but most of us don't live the "white picket fence" life. Keep trying! It will take time, but you and your family can do this—together.

Getting with the Program

Overall, the most important thing that has to be in place is a medically supervised program, one that everyone understands. The American Heart Association makes the salient point that "the long-term success of any secondary prevention program is directly related to patient compliance. Evidence suggests that . . . diet, exercise, and drug therapy benefits patients. And those who quit smoking significantly reduce their risks of another heart attack, sudden death, stroke, and total mortality compared with those who continue to smoke."

This can be a tall order for someone who has not only had to deal with a life-changing health event, but who is now coping with the concomitant processes of physical and emotional recovery. Unfortunately, the major focus is on the patient, and the family members may feel that they are expected to get with the program and alter their lives to become caregivers. That can be overwhelming.

Underlying the recovery period will be myriad changing emotions: fear, uncertainty, frustration, distress. It is a good reason to consider counseling as a first step and throughout the recovery period. Try to understand what it's like to be in the shoes of your caregivers. If you are joined by family members in counseling or in the meetings with your physician and/or members of the rehab team, you will all have the same, unfiltered information.

Here are just a few general areas that are going to be a lot easier to cope with when you have the help and understanding of a supportive family or other group.

Forming a Support Team

Your medical support group is pretty straightforward, and usually is dictated by your cardiologist and surgeon. These will include nurses with the physical and occupational rehab programs, a social worker to help you with insurance and other family issues, a trusted and capable pharmacist, special programs, like weight loss or smoking cessation, and perhaps your clergyman or -woman.

Your personal recovery team is as important, if not more so. Unfortunately, like parenting skills, we are not born with the innate sense of what we have to do to take care of someone who is sick or recovering from a serious illness. Some of the more complex aspects of caring for a heart patient on their road to recovery are discussed below. The reality is that you are going to find some people in your family who are more helpful to you than others. However, this is not a negative because you want someone who is not only willing to help, but can handle the emotional process.

I was more dependent on outside help than most people. I found my driver, my medication helper, my friend to call in the middle of the night, someone to exercise with, and, eventually, one person who came into my life and, understanding my need to be independent, helped me only when it was clear that the next step back would be a big one.

We all have different lives before and after our heart disease is identified. You can't make people who were around you change simply because you have. You can, however, be aware of how they may feel now and work to share your emotions and theirs to help you come back to a life that is better than ever.

Are You on a New Diet?

Certainly if you've had a heart attack, if you suffer from cardiovascular disease, high cholesterol, or other lipid problems, *and* if you have concomitant disorders such as diabetes and hypertension, french fries, rich desserts, and baked potatoes loaded with butter and sour cream may be things of the past. You may not only have to make a radical change in your diet to protect your heart directly, but you may also need to lose the weight that is adding stress to your system.

Dietary modifications, even extensive ones, do not have to be a battleground, as they often are, even though this is one of the hardest parts of your life to change. The knee-jerk reaction that I've experienced and have witnessed often follows when a nutritionist or a physician puts together a diet and orders you to follow it. Since diet is one of the major risk factors for cardiovascular disease, it's logical that someone who loves you and cares about your future will focus on it. After all, it's one thing they can have some input into and, perhaps, even control.

How do you avoid this?

First, it's important to realize and *believe* that the changes you are making are not simply to treat a disease. A healthy diet and lifestyle are something everyone should follow. Keep in mind that no one expects everyone in an entire household to change their lives immediately. It would be naive to expect that you or your family members can turn their lives around on a dime. Recovery is a marathon, not a sprint.

Here are a few basic ideas for a program to help keep peace in the home as you make dietary changes:

- ○ Do not treat this as a "recovery plan." This is a diet and lifestyle change for everyone in the family for now and in the future.
- ○ Make it positive and goal-oriented. For example, introduce a healthy vegetable into your meals regularly.
- ○ Make it educational for everyone. Learn about heart disease.
- ○ Involve the whole family. One goal is to reduce risk in your children, too.
- ○ Do not obsess. If you have to go to a business lunch or a party once you are back to work and the only food is not on your diet plan, it's OK.
- ○ Do things that are active. Even if it's not a sport or exercise, keep your brain and everyone else's stimulated with games, museums, mini-vacations, a club, or a charity activity.
- ○ Don't make or even suggest changes in diet or treatment unless your physician approves them. If you read an article or find something on the Internet, or your aunt in Florida swears that her son-in-law's uncle was saved by the bark of a Peruvian tree, ask the doctor before you try it.
- ○ Plan heart-healthy menus together one or two weeks ahead.

Are You Still Smoking?

If you smoke and you have survived a heart attack or stroke, you are very lucky. Thousands of indisputable studies link smoking to increased risk of cardiovascular disease, stroke, and cancer.

None of this is news to you. If you or a member of your family support team smokes, you've heard about it from your doctor, and you've read about it every day. You are virtually a pariah in the workplace, and you are excluded from restaurants and public spaces where smoking is increasingly banned. It is very likely that you agree with what you read and are told: Smoking will shorten your life.

Similarly, if you live with a smoker (you both may be smokers), then you also are facing a major challenge, one much more difficult than altering diet or sedentary lifestyle. To use addiction terms, you are an enabler, and you'll have to reach a solution to this problem. Smoking cessation programs are outlined in depth in **Month Three**, but the reality is that you (and your spouse, perhaps) are trapped in nicotine addiction, one of the most difficult addictions to kick. How and what you do to undo this addiction is up to you; however, substance-abuse experts will tell you that you need motivation and support.

How Mobile Are You?

Of all the aspects of recovery from my bypass surgery, being "grounded," forbidden to drive a car, was the worst for me. This dictum is consistent for all bypass patients, who are told not to drive for four to six weeks to ensure that in case of an accident, the chest incision is not harmed. For the first few weeks, I realized that driving was not a good idea and that I probably would have endangered everyone else on the road. Since I lived alone at the time, with no family near, I had to rely on friends to drive me to the market, cardio rehab, the video store, and elsewhere.

Part of my disease was my self-imposed stress that only increased when riding in a car driven by someone else. Two weeks after surgery, I felt much, much better and could see no reason why I couldn't drive. I called the doctor, who emphasized that if anything happened, I'd find myself back in the hospital in much worse peril. So, miserably, I admitted my powerlessness, accepted help from my family and friends, and concentrated on walking more laps around the courtyard until my cardiologist cleared me. The blessing here was that all the extra work did strengthen me and I passed the 30-day stress test and was back on the road.

The general rules on mobility are dictated by your doctor; however, in general, the rule should be to take it easy and take advantage of this time. The family and your support group are on the same emotional roller coaster as you are, and the best thing you can do is to open lines of communication. You are going to want to get up and about, and this is what experts recommend now. Lying in bed is not the norm; you need cardiovascular fitness that comes with any sort of light exercise in the beginning.

Family members have a tendency to walk on eggshells, but if you get them to join you in your daily walk or other exercise, they will understand that you are improving each day and back off.

Can You Take Care of Yourself?

This is a loaded question. From your point of view, the answer may be simple. Of course you can take care of yourself! The answer from your family may be simple, also: "Hey, if you can take care of yourself, how'd you get yourself into such trouble?"

To your family, this may seem like a fair question; however, it's really not. Of course you may have increased your risk factors, or your problem may have been congenital and your DNA is responsible for your problem. You may be, as many are, doctor-phobic, and your problem could have been diagnosed during a regular physical. Regardless, you are now a person who has had a bypass, a heart attack, heart failure, vascular disease, angina, or another cardiac condition. That is you now, and you need some level of care as you get back to your new and improved life.

See this as an opportunity. Don't see it as a weakness. You are going to be adjusting and changing each day. Your emotions are going to be riding a roller coaster and there is no reason not to ask for help. Time is going to be your best friend. You and your support groups are both going to have to reach accommodation. Here are some recommendations.

Are You Taking a Confusing Array of Medications?

Taking your medications as directed cannot be overemphasized, and it is a situation in which a family member or significant other can make a difference. It is likely that you will be on multiple medications (**Month Eight**) that include not only prescriptions for your heart, but also for other conditions, such as diabetes or high blood pressure. It is not uncommon to find someone taking five to ten different pills a day.

Multiple medications present a wide-ranging set of problems, including side effects, potential interactions, and general confusion about timing and conditions. Do you take this pill on an empty stomach? Should this pill make you nauseous? Why do things taste odd after you take a certain pill? Worse, does this medication reduce libido and cause other unpleasant sexual side effects? Essentially, medication is in the neutral zone. Your doctor has prescribed the pills, and the side effects are what they are. The fact that you have to take pills raises multiple issues that can be discussed, such as reluctance to follow a diet and medical plan because of the drugs, problems with intimacy, and even depression.

Here are a few tips that can help:

○ Involve your family in developing a daily routine for taking your medication, rather than seeing their reminders as nagging.
○ Go to any pharmacy and pick up some inexpensive pill holders that allow you to divide your medications over one or two weeks at a time.
○ Ask your spouse or someone else to help you separate the pills.
○ Carefully review the patient information from the pharmacist and ask others who are helping you to read it so they will understand it and can recognize when a side effect emerges.
○ Learn the basics of each medication; for example, what you should do if you discover that you've missed a dose.
○ Most important, ensure that everyone knows what to do in an emergency that might result from an unexpected drug interaction.

Do You Have More Than One Medical Problem?

If you are very fortunate and have not been diagnosed with any other medical problem, it is likely that you may develop one in the future. The odds are not in your favor unless you are able to prevent your risk factors from increasing. This is yet another reason why you need a good support system. Recovering from a heart attack is difficult enough, but, as you've seen, integrating diet, exercise, and emotional issues into the rehabilitation program are also not going to be easy. If you can't lower your risk—in any area—you may find yourself in more trouble.

Exact data on the number of heart patients who have another disorder are hard to pin down, possibly because the frequency of different disorders occurring differs between sexes, among various ethnic groups, and at different ages. However, there are statistics that overlap that can give you an idea of how one disease can create risk for another.

According to the American Diabetes Association, "two of three women with diabetes die from heart disease or stroke." In general, those with diabetes have a risk two to four times higher than others of developing heart disease if their diabetes is not controlled.

The famous Framingham Heart Study that has followed 5,000 people since 1948, conducted by the National Institutes of Health, also has reported parallel risks. "Excess body weight is strongly and independently associated with increased risk of heart failure. This risk, which increases continuously with increasing degrees of body weight is 34% higher for *overweight individuals* and 104% higher for *obese persons*."

In addition, the CDC reports that nearly one-third of us has two or more of the six top risk factors for heart disease. These include high blood pressure, high cholesterol, diabetes, smoking, obesity, and inactivity.

If you do have more than one medical problem, then what you have to do is simple: Strive for risk reduction and be sure you are in compliance with your doctor's orders. The indisputable statements given here clearly spell out what will happen if you do not stick with the plan. The same answer applies if you are a victim of more than one disease. In this situation, however, you still have a very good chance of recovering your health because the solutions are the same.

Will Your Recovery Be Long?

You will probably ask your doctor these questions, and perhaps, you'll get answers that are not particularly satisfying. Everyone has a different recovery/rehab plan. Again, this is where your support group can be helpful. Sit down with your doctor or rehab team and set out a plan with specific goals for return to work. Get answers to questions such as

○ When will you be able to return to work full-time?
○ Will you need some sort of vocational counseling?

○ What level of work is appropriate at different points along the way?
○ Can you travel?
○ What safety measures do you need to take when traveling?

IN A SENTENCE:

> It's very difficult to recover from heart disease without having family and other people in your life to help, but it's important to realize that it can be difficult for them because of the changes that everyone may have to make, from diet to lifestyle to simple concern for your future health.

FIRST WEEK MILESTONES

○ You have learned what heart disease is, why you have it, and the first steps to take

○ You have learned how doctors confirm their diagnosis

○ You know the first steps to take to assess your risks

○ You have overcome denial, which got you into this trouble

○ You have begun to take the first steps to recovery

○ You have learned how to choose a cardiologist and get a second opinion

○ You understand the emotional impact on you and your family

Returning to Sex and Intimacy

SEXUALITY AND intimacy play different roles in everyone's life, and for heart patients, it's no different. While there is a great deal of commonality in medical issues among patients, no one, beyond self-appointed relationship experts, can really tell you what is right and wrong. I am no different, except in one respect. Having gone through both a heart attack and a heart bypass, years apart, I've faced the questions about sexuality and intimacy more than once at different stages in life. When I was younger and had a heart attack, regaining sexuality was first among my priorities. Several years later, intimacy was what I needed most. All I can offer is my own experience, lessons I've learned, and some suggestions that have worked for me.

For many patients, sex and intimacy can be the proverbial 800-pound elephant weighing down your recovery. When you've come through the post-crisis period of your diagnosis or cardiac event and your life is beginning to seem more normal, is great sex next?

I've talked with cardiologists, psychologists, social workers, and patients about the most intimate details of heart surgery ("Now, here's where we put the catheter!"), but sexuality didn't come up voluntarily or often. If you think about it, how frequently did it come up before your heart disease became apparent? Difficulty in broaching the subject should be expected, but it does not have to stop your progress.

The intimacy question for a heart patient has two other parts: What was your sex life like before your diagnosis? What are your expectations of sex in the future? Upon examining your levels of intimacy before you became sick it may become clear that stress and a workaholic lifestyle were part of your crash and that intimacy or sex was not part of your life then, either. Similarly, too often, heart disease patients have unrealistic expectations for future sex that can provoke guilt and fear. Intimacy after any chronic-disease diagnosis or surgical procedure— breast cancer, a crippling accident—is going to have to be out on the table and discussed honestly with your partner, spouse, and your doctor or counselor.

When I had my heart attack, I was in the middle of a very stressful time, but I was not living alone. Several years later when I had my bypass, however, I was living alone and had no serious significant other in my life. I was fortunate (blessed) that someone later came into my life who provides love and emotional support for me. However, the first year of loneliness and bouts of depression and sadness after the bypass were hard to handle.

While having a heart attack or some other form of heart disease may slow you down, you might eventually return to the old behavior that got you into trouble, as I did. If intimacy and sex were not part of your past lifestyle, that's probably not going to change now. But changing that situation is something that you should have as a goal in your recovery because there will be many times when you really do need that hug.

Where Do You Start?

The most important aspect of your first step back to intimacy and sexuality is to *start with restoring intimacy, not having sex, as a goal*. This means redefining intimacy as holding hands on a walk if you like that, hugs when you feel down, watching a movie together, cooking dinner, or talking about the day before you turn off the lights and go to sleep.

Don't forget that at this time, when you may want to begin sexual relations, other things are going on in your recovery that can affect your desires. Your body is adjusting to new medications, you are back at work after several weeks away, and you may bear scars from surgery and some embarrassment.

These psychological land mines may affect your ability to have sexual relations and may provoke other problems, like erectile dysfunction (ED) or loss of desire. In some ways, sexual problems caused by heart disease may be similar to those caused by aging for men and women, but with some new twists. High blood pressure, diabetes medications, fluid-reducing pills, antidepressants, pain meds, and drugs for irregular heartbeats can cause erectile dysfunction and problems achieving ejaculation. In women, these meds may reduce vaginal fluid, causing painful intercourse and loss of desire, and an OB/GYN should be consulted as soon as possible.

Could Sex Cause Another Heart Attack?

Will sex harm you or cause another heart attack? Even if you have talked to your doctor about this, you *must* discuss this with your partner in your initial period of intimacy. First, sex is on your mind, even if you deny it. I've been there, and as good as I am at denying major health issues, anxiety about sex and a heart attack took a long time to resolve in my mind. The same question is also on your partner's mind. After all, how would your partner feel if something happened while you were making love?

Along with fear that you or your spouse might have a heart attack during sex is the tendency to be overprotective. You will make each other crazy. Even worse is the tendency to buy into some of the common myths that surround sex and heart disease, such as the belief that any sort of chest pain during sex means you will never have sex again. This is totally untrue unless the pain is severe and mimics the symptoms of a heart attack.

Another myth is that having a few drinks will relax and protect you. Booze can actually hurt your performance and might interact with your medications. You must talk to your doctor about the things you hear from well-meaning friends or read on the Internet.

One guideline used by many doctors regarding the point at which you can progress from intimacy to sexual relations is that sex does not place extreme demands on your heart. It is more like walking up a few flights of stairs at a regular pace. So if you can make it from the basement recreation room to the second-floor bedroom, you are good to go, but check first with your doctor!

Resuming Intimacy

Returning to intimacy is often thought of as a "male issue," perhaps because the media today is so focused on the physical issues associated with male sexuality. Men are, unfortunately, concerned with function more than women are; women are more likely to see the issue from an emotional point of view. The main rule for both sexes is "go slowly." As you read earlier in this book, whether you are a man or a woman, you have just been through a terrible psychological and physical ordeal, and it's normal to experience wild mood swings afterward. Take your reentry into the bedroom as gradually as you need to.

Generally, cardiologists and recovery specialists suggest that common sense should govern your actions unless your physical condition is truly severe, such as the following:

○ Unless there is a sound medical reason, don't turn your house into a hospital room. You can sleep in your own bed, which is often a quicker route to comfort and normalcy.

○ There is no rule relating to when you can resume having intercourse, regardless of what you read on the Internet or in self-help books. *Your physician must be your main decision maker.* Sometimes timing is related to the healing of your chest incision or your condition before surgery because those in better health tend to bounce back faster.

○ Once you are cleared by your physician *and* sexual desire returns, the first move is obvious: Talk to your partner. Conventional wisdom says that most people are reluctant to talk about sex. It's hard to believe that in a time of information saturation by erectile dysfunction TV commercials, you and your significant other can't or don't talk about sex.

○ If you don't normally talk about sex, this is a good time to start, and you should not be reluctant to seek professional assistance, either alone or as a couple. Stereotypes suggest that women will talk to a friend, while men won't. This might be true, but returning to sexual relations is something that can have long-term effects. Talk to someone who has professional counseling experience. Your cardiovascular-rehab team will be happy to direct you to a good counselor.

○ Some attitudes about sex may be cultural or gender- or age-related, but they all boil down to the same issue: Even though my doctor says it is safe, what does that mean?

○ You may have concerns about your or your partner's expectations, as well as concerns about the energy requirements and safety of sex, regardless of the doctor's OK.

○ It would be dishonest to say that a cardiac event is not a unique life crisis. There are very little data that predict how you will relate to each other and whether or not you will each respond sexually, and the problems you might have had before you became ill may be magnified.

○ There are also reams of "how-to" advice relating to safe positions, concerns about your physical appearance (the incision), and even sexy lingerie. Again, the message is the same: Talk to each other, and talk to your doctor.

○ You and your doctor must talk candidly about your prior sex life and what is appropriate now. In general, when the doctor tells you that you will be able to resume sex, take it easy before trying anything too strenuous—you will get there eventually. Check in with your doctor after you've begun and report how you felt, such as whether you experienced angina or chest pain during intercourse. It is likely that after a few months, you will be back to normal.

The American Heart Association has some general guidelines for couples resuming sex that make sense and that can probably work for almost everyone:

○ Choose a time for sex when you're rested, relaxed, and free from the stresses brought on by the day's activities.

○ Wait one to three hours after eating a full meal to allow time for digestion.

○ Select a familiar, peaceful setting, free from interruptions.
○ If prescribed by your doctor, take your medications before having sexual relations.

IN A SENTENCE:

Returning to intimacy and sexuality during your recovery from heart disease, surgery, or a heart attack should be a slow and gentle process that enables you to take up where you left off or even to improve your relationship.

ED Medications: Are They for You or Your Partner?

WHAT ABOUT those erectile dysfunction (ED) pills—sildenafil (Viagra), tadalafil (Cialis), and vardenafil (Levitra)—and others that may come along in the future?

To say that this is a growing business is a vast understatement. According to the Food and Drug Administration, the number of men *diagnosed* with ED has risen by 250 percent. Clearly, this does not indicate that we have had an epidemic; rather, we have had an outbreak of men seeking a solution to a problem that few of us have been willing or able to talk about.

In the not-too-recent past, this has been beyond a hot topic for a lot of men. When Viagra hit the market in 1998, the little blue pill changed both the culture and the dialog. Erectile dysfunction came out of the bedroom and into the mainstream for most people. The market has grown with the introduction of the other two medications that claim superiority to each other by time of onset or duration of action.

The Internet and online advertising contain millions of hits and pages that mention ED drugs. One website claims, "The name recognition of Viagra is so good that nearly every

---

Do ED Pills Really Work?

I am one of those millions of men who have tried and regularly use them (and no, I'm not going to do a product endorsement beyond saying that I've tried them all and they pretty much work the same). How well do they work? My medication-induced erectile dysfunction has reversed.

The reason why I decided to try them is obvious, but I did not make the decision alone. I discussed it with not only my partner (first, guys!) but also my cardiologist. He demanded one health condition, and that was significant weight loss, so for all of you baby boomers out there looking for motivation to slim down, this is it.

The most important thing I learned from using ED meds is why they work. There are clear biological functions they correct, but it all starts with a signal given off in the brain.

The other thing that is also interesting is that as I've lost weight and my diet and lifestyle have helped my biological function that is required and described below. You may find as I did that you need lower doses, less frequently.

---

adult in America has heard of the drug and can tell you what it does." Another manufacturer claims that 300 million tablets are dispensed each year.

Despite some restrictions, most heart patients can use ED meds. However, it's important to remember that erectile dysfunction is *not* the same as loss of libido, which can be a side effect of medication or which can be caused by emotional problems like those mentioned in the previous section. This is why, with all drug treatments, you always should discuss use with your doctor first.

How ED Meds Work

Erectile dysfunction has more to do with anatomy than with desire. Most people with cardiovascular disease suffer from impaired blood flow throughout their vascular and arterial systems. Vascular blockages are only part of the problem preventing you from having an erection. It's likely that you did not simply wake up one day and discover that your potency had diminished. You've probably suspected something has been wrong for a while.

What has been happening is a slow change in the brain-penis connection that is similar to the connection that your brain uses when it sends orders to certain muscles in your body, such as when your brain tells your arm to move or your leg to kick a ball.

Normally, when your brain becomes sexually aroused, a complex chain of chemical events leads to an erection. When you feel aroused, you can almost feel the blood flow into your penis through the arteries. At the same time, the veins in the penis constrict and keep the blood from flowing out. This is why the term "engorged" is often applied to an erection. What happens is that whenever your brain wants something to happen in your body, it generates a signal through your nervous system, and many of these signals are quite specific.

For an erection to occur, the signal goes to specific nerve cells, which, in turn, release nitric oxide. This provokes an enzyme that produces further chemical reactions and release of a chemical called cyclic guanosine monophosphate (cGMP) that causes the smooth muscles in the penis to relax and allows blood flow to expand the penis.

If you have reduced blood flow in your vascular system, you are going to be at higher risk for ED, but this does not mean that ED drugs increase the amount of blood in your body. Where ED drugs come into the picture is that the brain also produces a chemical called phosphodiesterase–5 (PDE–5), which can halt production of cGMP. PDE is naturally produced—there are 11 different variations of this chemical in the body—but only PDE–5 can prevent cGMP from allowing enough blood flow for an erection. In normal arteries, this is not a problem. But in a compromised system, not enough cGMP is produced, resulting in ED.

The ED drugs (PDE–5 inhibitors) simply stop or reduce the amount of PDE–5 in the system, which allows cGMP to accumulate and increase blood flow into the spongelike muscles in the penis, the corpora cavernosa, which cause the penis to become erect. This particular ability of the active ingredient of ED drugs is the breakthrough that many men were waiting for.

However, ED drugs have side effects that can be harmful to anyone and potentially deadly in cardiac patients. These are prescription drugs for a reason, so *do not take them without clearance from your doctor.* (See **Month Eight** for a list of heart drugs and their side effects.)

Anyone who is taking a nitrate medication such as nitroglycerin should not take an ED drug because one of the principal actions of this class of drugs is to increase nitric oxide, which opens your arteries.

Because ED is such a widespread problem, a subculture of "cures" from the worlds of alternative medicine and "illegal" sales has emerged. There are two reasons. Legitimate, FDA-approved ED medication is absurdly expensive, usually costing $10 a pill (with insurance). Further, most insurance plans limit the number of pills you can get per month. Often the drive to acquire this medication outweighs the health considerations. You may be tempted to order from sources that pop up on your e-mail and at websites that are likely to be bogus. This is simply endangering yourself for no reason. Try to keep in mind that ED medications influence only one part of sex and intimacy.

Another source of these medications are the snake-oil salespeople who sell "natural" supplements, creams, and cures that promise to even surpass legitimate ED meds in effectiveness and duration. *Stay away from these because many contain the same medications that are found in approved ED meds and can interact with nitrate heart medication you may be taking!* Buying any medication for anything—especially for ED—without talking to and getting approval from your cardiologist is a very dangerous thing to do. In fact, it can be deadly!

Some new ED drugs are in development that promise to do more then restore your erection. According to the Center for Sexual Health in Albany, NY, a new medication, hMaxi-K, uses a form of gene therapy called "naked DNA" that "transmits a human genetic code into target cells." When the cell reads this code, it makes a protein that tells smooth muscles to relax. Many studies will be necessary before this therapy is ready for FDA review and approval, but if hMaxi-K is approved, it will revolutionize ED treatment.

ED is really not a laughing matter, and the reality is that for millions of people like me, PDE–5 inhibitors have removed one more area of stress from life. These drugs have made intimacy easier for me because I am more relaxed, and it may do the same for you and your partner. However, you can never forget that no one with heart disease should ever use one of these drugs without a doctor's approval. They are only safe to use when your doctor says so.

IN A SENTENCE:

Medications for erectile dysfunction have helped millions of men overcome the sexual problems caused by side effects of many heart, high blood pressure, and diabetes medications; however, they should not be taken by heart patients who are on any nitrate drugs and should only be taken if you have your doctor's approval.

living

Women and Heart Disease

ACCORDING TO the American Heart Association:

○ In 2003, almost twice as many women died from cardiovascular disease than from cancer.
○ More women (38 percent) than men (25 percent) will die from heart disease within a single year.
○ The death rate associated with heart disease among minorities, especially African American women, is significantly higher than among Caucasian women.
○ More women are hospitalized in a given year for heart disease than for any other disorder.

Today, we know that women are at just as much risk for heart disease as men are, and that at least one in four women will die from some form of cardiovascular disorder. In fact, each year 349,000 women will die from heart disease. The problem does not threaten only older women. Coronary heart disease is the number-one killer of women over age 25. According to the American Heart Association (AHA), 64 percent of women who died suddenly of heart disease had no previous symptoms. One in 2.6 female deaths is from heart disease, compared to one in 30 from breast cancer. Finally, heart disease in women claims more lives than do the next four most common causes of death combined!

Is there any good news? Yes. The National Institutes of Health announced in February 2007 that new data show a definite reduction in the number of women who die from heart disease per year. The one-in-four figure mentioned above was one-in-three deaths in 2003.

For many cardiologists, OB/GYNs, and other doctors who might have large female populations in their practice, these numbers are not surprising. However, until a few years ago, they were about the only medical professionals who discussed heart risk with their patients. It has only been in the last decade that the enormous effect of heart disease on women has been widely understood and has been backed by scientific studies. Despite the grim, well-documented statistics, the threat of heart disease in women is still not universally understood, but the word is spreading rapidly.

Fortunately, in 2004, organizations like the AHA and grass-roots groups joined to create and promote a universal understanding of the high risk of heart disease women face. This program, known as "Go Red For Women" (celebrated every February), is dedicated to "taking action to fight heart disease" and to "teaching women to improve their heart health." This program is helping combat the reality that women have been left out of the heart disease risk-reduction equation for a long time.

All too frequently, women don't have the information they need at an early enough time to reduce medical risk. Fortunately, awareness is increasing. Here are the facts that you need to know about how heart disease affects women.

Why Weren't We Made Aware of the Risk of Heart Attack or Another Coronary Disorder in Women until Recently?

The answer to this question is not simple; however, it is becoming clearer with each year. For the past 50 years, the medical profession has struggled to get heart disease under control. This battle has been fought on medical, educational, and direct risk-modification fronts. The problem for you, as a female, is that it's largely been a battle fought within and through the male gender. Some studies have shown that, even today, less than 20 percent of physicians recognize that more women than men die of heart disease. One reason is that only 25 percent of participants in all heart-related research have been women. This has been labeled "cultural gender bias" by some groups who point to the fact that heart disease rates have dropped more dramatically for men but have stayed about the same for women over the past few decades.

There is no doubt that one reason a gender bias has been created is that doctors have used the traditional list of risk factors when assessing both men and women, not recognizing that this can automatically create a decided difference in the diagnosis. Since "being male" is on virtually every list of default heart disease risk, the factor "being a woman" does not automatically ring a bell for some doctors, although we now know that "being male" skews the diagnosis incorrectly. The reality today is that being a woman, a child, or an adolescent should be a default risk, too. *Everyone is at risk.* Over many decades, this lack of attention to sex differences has created the myth that most men die from heart attacks, and most women succumb from breast cancer. Today's evidence shows this is untrue.

Risk of cardiovascular disease is often first identified by your family or primary physician, and, based on what they find they may refer you to a cardiologist. They, too, may be looking at the traditional male risk factors, including gender, family history, and age, along with others, including smoking, weight, lifestyle, and elevated blood pressure when you see them for a check-up or with a specific symptom. It's very possible that you may have none of these risk factors and may still be at risk for heart disease—and you may not be referred to a cardiologist.

How Do Cardiac Symptoms Differ Between Women and Men?

Perhaps the most significant and overlooked difference between women and men is that there actually are several different cardiovascular symptoms and risk factors for each gender. *Your primary physician may not ask you about those or recognize them as important although they have been known for some time. Unless your doctor is a cardiologist or OB/GYN, he or she may not be as familiar with issues that affect only women with heart disease.*

In 1996, the National Institutes of Health initiated the **Women's Ischemia Syndrome Evaluation Study (WISE),** one of the most important studies of women and heart disease. Their goal was to understand how heart disease develops in women, and to evaluate the influence of hormones. What they discovered was quite surprising:

"In as many as 3 million U.S. women with coronary heart disease, cholesterol plaque may not build up into major blockages, but instead spreads evenly throughout the artery wall. As a result, diagnostic coronary angiography reveals that these women have 'clear' arteries—no blockages—incorrectly indicating low risk. Despite this, many of these women have a high risk for heart attack." This condition was labeled "coronary microvascular syndrome," and is a prime example of why risk for women is often missed. In this case, according to the NIH, "plaque accumulates in very small arteries of the heart, causing narrowing, reduced oxygen flow to the heart, and pain that can be similar to that of people with blocked arteries, but the plaque does not show up when physicians use standard tests."

WISE investigators found that the majority of women with "clear" angiography who are not diagnosed will continue to have symptoms, a declining quality of life, and repeated hospitalizations and tests.

"When a diagnosis of this condition is missed, women are not treated for their angina and high cholesterol, and they remain at high risk for having a heart attack," says National Heart, Lung, and Blood Institute (NHLBI) director Elizabeth G. Nabel, M.D. "This study and the high prevalence of coronary microvascular dysfunction demonstrate that we must think out of the box when it comes to the evaluation and diagnosis of heart disease in women."

Estrogen and Heart Disease

However, over the past decade, cardiovascular disease in women has been widely and correctly studied in relation to the general biological differences between men and women. Chief among these is the connection between heart disease and **estrogen,** a naturally occurring hormone in women that is produced by the ovaries and that affects the menstrual cycle and development of secondary sexual characteristics, such as breasts. Ongoing studies indicate that estrogen may affect many organ systems in women. These effects range from increased incidence of blood clot formation to lowered blood pressure. These responses may be negative, influencing clot formation, but at the same time, they may have a positive effect on blood pressure.

The presence of estrogen is partially responsible for another myth about women and heart disease: that women have special protection because of their anatomy and biology (also called "sex protection"). This concept comes from data that show that women have lower risk at the age when men's symptoms of heart disease begin to appear. It's thought that estrogen is the reason that women have usually developed heart disease at a later age than men do. There is evidence that this is partly true. In fact, women's risk for heart disease, in general, is lower prior to the onset of menopause.

Estrogen has a positive effect on the good cholesterol, HDL, and a lowering effect on LDL, the bad cholesterol, in pre-menopausal women. Even with elevated total cholesterol, estrogen still offers some lowered risk to women. When estrogen levels are reduced at menopause, statistically, the risk levels of heart disease rise for females until, at age 65, men and women have the same risk on the basis of the three basic risk factors mentioned previously.

In addition, most women undergo menopause in their early 50s. Unfortunately, along with the rising risk of heart disease, there are many uncomfortable symptoms of menopause, such as hot flashes. The solution for many women seemed to be a medication that not only would diminish menopause symptoms, but that might extend the sex protection. This solution set off controversy when hormone replacement therapy (HRT) using synthetic estrogen and the drug progestin was widely prescribed in the early 1990s. While HRT seemed to relieve menopause symptoms, several large studies linked increased risk of heart attack with HRT.

One large study, HERS (Heart and Estrogen-progestin Replacement Study), conducted in 1998 and published in the *Journal of the American Medical Association,* revealed that women who had had a previous heart attack and who were on HRT for one year had a 50 percent higher risk for stroke and heart attack. Yet, after another year on the same treatment, it appeared that the women's heart attack risk had dropped. This puzzled researchers, so another look was taken after three years. One conclusion, now accepted widely, is that after a certain period of time,

HRT might help protect certain women against stroke and heart attack; however, this protection did not extend to women who had already had a heart attack or stroke.

About the same time that the HERS was reported, a second large study was initiated worldwide. Called the Women's Health Initiative (WHI), it looked at a larger range of HRT effects. It ultimately revealed that estrogen made matters worse, increasing risk for stroke and providing very little protection from heart attack. The results of these studies and a second HERS (HERSII) review initially caused a severe decrease in the use of HRT. By late 2004, some conclusions were finally reached about the use of HRT among post-menopausal women and how it relates to heart and stroke risk.

The American Heart Association and the Food and Drug Administration have published official guidelines that indicate the following:

○ HRT is not for heart attack prevention. It does not replace the natural estrogen that protects younger women.
○ At times, HRT has been prescribed for other uses, such as prevention of bone disease; however, the benefits and the risks are not proven.
○ Anyone currently at risk for heart disease or with heart disease should not use HRT without a physician's specific approval.
○ HRT is a good method of reducing post-menopausal symptoms over a short period.
○ HRT does not prevent heart disease with long-term use.

An important point to remember when considering the controversy is that hundreds of thousands of women use HRT every day, and have done so for years. Clearly, this is a decision between you and your physician; however, there seems to be very little question that once you hit menopause, the natural biological advantage of reduced risk of heart disease that you have as a woman is no longer present.

Specific Cardiovascular Risk Symptoms in Women

Overall, one of the most important and positive events that has surfaced over the past decade of studies of women and heart disease is our understanding of the difference between the symptoms that men and women experience when heart disease is present.

Among the most prominent difference is that women may experience shortness of breath without chest pain. This is similar to the symptoms that diabetics experience when they have angina. It is also a common symptom of other conditions, such as anxiety.

Other symptoms include those that may be common to other conditions, such as chills, cold sweats, nausea, lightheadedness, and palpitations—basically, feeling like you have the flu (see **Day Five**). This is why your doctor and you should be aware of your risk factors. Given that these symptoms can be signs of either a common ailment or a life-threatening event, you cannot afford to ignore any illness. You cannot say, "I'll tough it out." Many men choose to do so, but these ambiguous symptoms in women can mask a heart attack and can lead to your death.

Women suffer from the same heart attack symptoms as men (see **Week Three**), including chest pain, angina, severe chest pressure that comes and goes, pain up and down the left arm, and pain in the neck or jaw. The pain may feel like severe indigestion or heartburn (mine did), and you may experience sudden exhaustion.

Oral contraceptives, which contain estrogen, have been shown to increase risk through a link to C-reactive protein (CRP). Produced in the liver to reduce inflammation, high CRP has been linked to heart disease. Meanwhile, inflammation can cause atherosclerosis. This, in turn, suggests that higher levels of estrogen can produce inflammation and can promote coronary artery disease.

Studies of a link between the pill and heart disease have shown that when used by smokers or by women with high blood pressure, there is a significant risk. However, for women under age 35 who do not smoke and who use low-estrogen pills, the risk is minimal. Researchers point out that oral contraceptives are usually used by younger women whose risk of heart disease is lower anyway. If you add smoking, obesity, and poor diet to oral contraceptives, you significantly increase your risk. According to the Mayo Clinic, "Concurrent use of birth control pills and smoking boosts the risk of heart attack 39 times" when compared to non-smoking oral contraceptive users.

Should you become pregnant if you have heart disease or some other heart risk? In theory, there is no reason why you cannot; however, this is a subject that can only be settled between you and your doctor. The American Heart Association has issued specific recommendations in this area. Women who are at the top of the risk list are those who have a heart defect that can increase the risk of birth defects in the child. In these cases, close monitoring with fetal ultrasound or other tests should be considered.

Just being pregnant places stress on the body; however, this can be counterbalanced through good diet, never smoking or drinking, and making sure that you take all medications as directed. *Remember, take no medication that is not explicitly prescribed by your doctor*.

As most women who have been pregnant know, other problems can occur. One is a **heart murmur** (a measured volume of blood flowing through the heart), which can be a normal occurrence, but also must be carefully monitored. Some women develop arrhythmias (irregular heartbeats). *It's very important that you report any heartbeat sensation that seems to be faster, then slower*.

About 8 percent of pregnant women develop high blood pressure (hypertension). It's important to make sure your blood pressure is stable by having it checked frequently and by not taking any medication without your doctor's knowledge and consent. Should you gain weight quickly, develop swollen legs and ankles, and have protein detected in your urine, you are at risk for **toxemia** or pre-eclampsia. In each of these cases, blood flow to the fetus is limited and can reduce its viability.

Pregnancy in and of itself does not create heart risk; however, heart risk, either prior to pregnancy or during pregnancy, can threaten both the mother and the baby. Reducing the effect of normal heart risk through diet, exercise, eliminating smoking and drinking, and good prenatal care can significantly reduce heart attack risk.

What Are the Common Risk Factors Shared by Women and Men?

Beyond such problems as coronary microvascular syndrome and the benefits of estrogen that create different age risks for women with heart disease, common risk factors with men are just as crucial.

Denial. One common risk factor that can be identified across the gender line is personal attitude, which appears two ways. Many cardiologists report that denial is one of the most common problems they encounter in any patient.

Related to denial is the response many women have to symptoms of heart disease: "I don't have time to be sick" or "I'll be fine." While there is no question that men also have this attitude, it appears more common among women. My mother ignored her own heart problems, claiming that she had to be there for my ailing father. Some data suggest that women are more likely to die from a heart attack than men, possibly because of anatomical issues—smaller and more easily damaged coronary arteries—or because women don't seek or receive treatment as soon as men.

Smoking is a risk factor for virtually everything that can go wrong in your body, and it is not an exclusive heart risk factor for women. No one will be surprised by the fact that smoking is the single most preventable cause of death in the U.S. There is some evidence that more than half of heart attacks in women are related to smoking.

Smoking and oral contraceptives together increase risk even more. Simply put, smoking is about as self-destructive as you can get. Virtually every medical specialty sees the effects of smoking on the vascular system. For example, an orthopedist told me, "Smoking is extremely destructive. It increases the likelihood of osteoporosis and it clearly impedes healing, since blood flow is required to heal the bones, and smoking harms circulation."

In **Month Three,** you will find information on different effective methods of smoking cessation. Today, virtually every hospital and every doctor can direct you to a program, and many have started clinics that are low-cost or free. Keep in mind that even if you are still smoking, once you stop, your heart risk lowers by 50 percent after one year and by 66 percent in two years.

We also live in a society that emphasizes achievement, and that often causes stress. An "overstuffed" lifestyle full of saturated fats and too little exercise adds up to a heart attack set-up. For many women, the common risk factors can add up faster because more may be expected of them in the workplace with the added responsibilities of taking care of a home and family.

If you have any of the following risk factors, common for women and men, then you should be seeing a cardiologist or discussing them with your primary care physician:

○ **Family history.** Your internist, OB/GYN, and even your dentist should know about your family history of heart disease.

○ **Total cholesterol and other lipids.** High HDL, LDL, and triglycerides are risk factors and symptoms. Diet is only one way to control elevated lipids. Many effective, proven medications can help (see **Month Eight**) to bring high cholesterol under control quickly.

○ **High blood pressure (hypertension)** and **diabetes** often accompany heart disease and raise risk. Both can be controlled through medication, diet, and exercise. Add to these **obesity** or simply being **overweight**, and you have a perfect trifecta for heart disease risk.

○ **Stress, depression, and other emotional factors** are frequently listed as risk factors for heart attack and heart disease. We often hear the phrase "broken heart" to describe the cause of a heart attack.

While not a typical risk factor, aspirin use, which is widely endorsed for use after a heart attack and with high success potential, may not have the same effect for women.

In 2005, a study published in the *New England Journal of Medicine* took a look at the risk and benefits of aspirin as a preventive measure among women. The results showed that the benefit was not as clear as the benefit seen in males. In this case, more than 40,000 healthy women, age 45 and older, took either 100 mg of aspirin or a placebo. The results showed that there was virtually no difference in the risk for heart attack. There was, however, a 17 percent reduction in stroke risk. When the study was analyzed further, it was determined that women over age 65 did benefit significantly from aspirin use, not just in heart attack prevention, but also for stroke and other heart disorders. The main issue with aspirin use is that it can cause stomach upset and, in some cases, stomach bleeding.

The bottom line on aspirin is that your doctor should decide with you, balancing all of your risk factors when it comes to preventing a first event. Since there is clear evidence that aspirin does help prevent a second heart attack in both men and women, you will probably be told to consider it. There is evidence that some people do suffer from aspirin resistance, which prevents clotting, so ask your doctor about this when considering aspirin use.

Treating Heart Disease in Women

Beyond the issues of hormone replacement therapy, treatment of women for heart disease may differ from treatment of men because in general, women are built on a smaller scale than men. The heart is smaller, and so are the arteries, which can make angioplasty more difficult. Several other factors may enter into treatment for women; however, the same arsenal of behavior modification, medication, surgery, and risk reduction are still the front-line defense.

As we learn more about the different gender risks, treatment will improve. For example, an important key to good heart health is weight loss. According to the Society for Women's Health Research, "weight gain and fat deposition differ between women and men. Research into these differences can generate tremendous information about the development and progression of disease." As this group reports, it's well known that fat distribution and body shape between men and women are different. Adipose tissue, present in men and women, stores fat and is drawn upon when you need energy. However, distribution of adipose fat is different between men and women, which may play a role in cardiovascular risk.

What Is the Medical Community Doing to Reduce Women's Cardiovascular Risk?

The past decade has seen a decided sea change in the understanding of clinical issues relating to women and heart disease and, with the initiation of Go Red For Women, a leap forward in the public consciousness.

"Through WISE, we have made tremendous progress toward better understanding of heart disease in women. Too often, women are tested again and again, go untreated, and still have high risk for heart attacks," says George Sopko, M.D., NHLBI project officer for WISE.

This new focus on women was highlighted in February 2007, when the AHA issued further important recommendations for women ages 20

Recommendations from WISE Investigators

○ *Identifying Candidates for Exercise Stress Testing*: Using the evaluative tool Duke Activity Status Index (DASI) in women with heart disease symptoms prior to stress testing can help determine who would be eligible for an exercise stress test versus a stress test using intravenous medications to increase the heart load instead of exercise. Current guidelines offer physicians little guidance on how to identify women who would not be able to sufficiently complete the exercise test. The DASI previously has been validated as a useful tool for determining functional capacity.

○ *Low Coronary Flow and Scores on Function Test Indicate Poor Outcomes*: Women who have low DASI scores also have lower coronary flow velocity, a combination that may explain the poor outcomes seen for women with heart disease but no blocked arteries.

○ *Role of Pre-menopausal Hypertension in Disease Risk*: Women who have high blood pressure before menopause, especially high systolic blood pressure, should be considered at a higher risk and treated accordingly.

---

and over. In "Guidelines for Preventing Cardiovascular Disease in Women," important issues, such as aspirin use, mineral supplements, hormone therapy, and stroke prevention were announced. These are reflected in the information above.

"The updated guidelines emphasize the lifetime risk of women, not just the more short-term focus of the 2004 guidelines," said Lori Mosca, M.D., Ph.D., director of preventive cardiology at New York–Presbyterian Hospital and chair of the American Heart Association expert panel that wrote the guidelines. "We took a long-term view of heart disease prevention because the lifetime risk of dying of cardiovascular disease (CVD) is nearly one in three for women. This underscores the importance of healthy lifestyles in women of all ages to reduce the long-term risk of heart and blood vessel diseases."

Go Red For Women is the beginning of a movement that emphasizes to women that "your heart is in your hands." The program urges women to understand that they can and should control their risk factors, such as high blood pressure, smoking, elevated cholesterol levels, and obesity, themselves.

Highlights of the AHA Recommendations

○ Lifestyle changes to help manage blood pressure include weight control, increased physical activity, alcohol moderation, sodium restriction, and an emphasis on eating fresh fruits, vegetables, and low-fat dairy products.

○ In addition to advising women to quit smoking, the 2007 guidelines recommend counseling, nicotine replacement, or other forms of smoking-cessation therapy.

○ Physical activity recommendations for women who need to lose weight or sustain weight loss have been added: a minimum of 60 to 90 minutes of moderate-intensity activity (e.g., brisk walking) on most, and preferably all, days of the week.

○ The guidelines now encourage all women to reduce saturated-fat intake to less than 7 percent of calories, if possible.

○ Specific guidance on omega–3 fatty-acid intake and supplementation suggests eating oily fish at least twice a week and taking a capsule supplement of 850 to 1000 mg of eicosapentaenoic acid (EPA) and docosahexaenoic acid (DHA) in women with heart disease, 2 to 4 g for women with high triglycerides.

○ Hormone replacement therapy and selective estrogen receptor modulators (SERMs) are not recommended for preventing heart disease in women.

○ Antioxidant supplements, such as vitamins E, C, and beta carotene, should not be used for primary or secondary prevention of CVD.

○ Folic acid should not be used to prevent CVD, a change from the 2004 guidelines that did recommend it be considered for use in certain high-risk women.

○ Routine low-dose aspirin therapy may be considered in women age 65 or older, regardless of CVD risk status, if benefits are likely to outweigh other risks. (Previous guidelines did not recommend aspirin in lower-risk or healthy women.)

○ The upper dosage of aspirin for high-risk women increases to 325 mg per day, rather than 162 mg. This brings the women's guidelines up to date with other recently published guidelines.

○ Consider reducing LDL cholesterol to less than 70 mg/dL in very high-risk women with heart disease, which may require a combination of cholesterol-lowering drugs.

With this elevated visibility, it is likely that not only will we learn more about heart disease and the differences between women and men, but we will also dispel the many myths that have prevented many women from receiving early diagnosis.

IN A SENTENCE:

> *Despite the widespread incidence of heart disease and coronary fatalities among women, new efforts at education and awareness have begun to show success, and the rise of cardiac disease has slowed.*

Pregnancy and Heart Disease

IF YOU'RE a woman of childbearing age and have a heart condition, be sure to talk with your cardiologist if you intend to become pregnant. However, even if unplanned pregnancies occur, it does not mean that you should panic or that you or your child are automatically at great risk. The growth of specialized prenatal care and more specialists in the pediatric world have improved the health of mothers and children. However, two cardiovascular risks that can occur during pregnancy include a congenital heart defect risk to the fetus and risks to the mother who may have an existing heart condition.

A range of heart problems can appear during pregnancy, whether existing heart problems are present or not. These include the following:

- O **Rapid** or **irregular heartbeats** (**arrhythmias**) sometimes appear during pregnancy; however, they may have been present prior to pregnancy but not detected. Your doctor may pick up an arrhythmia in a regular exam, or you may feel faint, have palpitations or dizziness, or feel lightheaded. You may be asked to wear certain devices, like a Holter monitor, or to undergo tests such as an ECG or echocardiogram.

○ **High blood pressure** can be very serious during pregnancy, especially in women who were hypertensive before pregnancy. It's estimated that 8 of 100 women will have high blood pressure beginning in the latter part of the second trimester (at 20 weeks). You must be very careful about what sort of medication you take, such as angiotensin-converting enzyme (ACE) inhibitors, which are used to treat a number of heart problems, such as congestive heart failure and high blood pressure. These drugs may cause birth defects or kidney problems in the second and third trimester. High blood pressure also can lead to a stroke, and, coupled with such high risks as smoking and obesity, increases danger to you and your fetus.

○ **Stroke** can be fatal. Symptoms may include extremity numbness, pain, vision problems, and serious headaches.

○ The most significant problem caused by high blood pressure during pregnancy is **pre-eclampsia (toxemia of pregnancy)**. If you notice rapid weight gain and swelling in the ankles and your doctor discovers protein in your urine, you may have this disorder. Blood flow through the arteries, kidneys, liver, and brain can be affected, leading to decreased blood flow to the fetus. It's also possible that the pregnancy can fail at this point because the uterus is not able to grow steadily, or toxemia can lead to premature birth. Pre-eclampsia is the leading cause of pre-term birth in the U.S.

○ A **heart murmur** is another common finding that can arise during pregnancy. It is often completely normal and reflects a measured volume of blood flow during the pregnant state. While heart murmurs are common, they can also mean that your heart valves may not be working properly. In general, heart murmurs are not life-threatening and should not cause great concern.

What Other Non-heart Problems Should Heart Patients Be Aware Of?

○ **Type 2 diabetes** (also known as gestational diabetes) can appear in non-diabetic women who are pregnant. Fortunately, it usually is resolved after birth; however, it is another condition that has to be properly monitored. Gestational diabetes may reappear in subsequent pregnancies.

○ **Varicose veins** are unpleasant, unsightly bluish veins that stand out on your legs and may make their first appearance during or after pregnancy. During pregnancy, your body has a greater than normal amount of blood running through it, which causes blood vessels to bulge or swell. There is not much that you can do about it, and having a family history of varicose veins or being over-weight may increase your odds. Elevating your legs may help.

○ **Blood clots** are the number-one cause of death in pregnant women. They can appear in either the veins close to the surface or in deeper veins (superficial vein thrombosis and deep vein thrombosis). A clot may break off the wall of the vein and travel through the blood vessel, clogging it and causing either a pulmonary embolism in the lungs or a stroke. Anticoagulants may be given to the mother to reduce the risk. Another very rare potential embolism is the **amniotic fluid embolism,** which can occur if the placenta ruptures, sending amniotic fluid to the lungs and causing sudden cardiac arrest. Fortunately, these occurrences are infrequent.

What Are the Risks for the Mother Who Has a Congenital Heart Condition?

Along with stress, every pregnancy has certain risks that are more challenging in women with heart disease or heart defects. If you have a congenital heart condition, you should talk with your doctor because you need to take certain precautions.

○ Make sure pregnancy is safe. If it is not, institute appropriate family-planning measures.

○ Your child has a greater chance of a heart defect. It is likely that you will need more careful prenatal monitoring through tests such as ultrasounds.

○ Focus on a healthy lifestyle. Talk to a nutrition specialist to plan a diet that takes into account the health problems you have and to address the needs of your baby and yourself to ensure a successful pregnancy.

○ Don't drink, don't smoke, and make sure your medications are safe to use during pregnancy. As a rule, always ask your pharmacist.

There are dozens of books on pregnancy. Anyone who has a heart problem and who is considering getting pregnant or becomes pregnant *must* get as much information as possible to ensure a healthy pregnancy and a healthy baby.

IN A SENTENCE:

> *In the past, it was considered dangerous for a woman with heart disease to become pregnant; however, the growth of specialized prenatal care and more pediatric heart specialists have enabled many women with congenital heart disorders to safely experience a successful pregnancy.*

living

Congenital and Acquired Heart Disease

IT IS heartbreaking to think of a child with heart problems. Growth and other areas of physical or social development can be impaired and, in some cases, the child may not survive. However, the medical profession has become far more adept at diagnosis and treatment of these diseases. It's common now for doctors to suggest genetic testing for diseases that run in various populations to detect anomalies that may develop.

Heart disease in children comes in two categories: congenital disorders, which you are born with, and acquired disorders, which you might pick up while you are growing. It is also not an uncommon occurrence. According to the American Heart Association, today almost twice as many children in the U.S. die from congenital heart problems than will die from all cancers combined.

Congenital disorders are actually a birth defect and, of all birth defects, heart defects are the leading cause of death. More than 90,000 lives are lost to congenital heart defects, 40,000 new cases occur annually, and estimates indicate that at least 1 million people, young and old, are living with some sort of congenital heart problem, according to the March of Dimes. If you are a heart patient and you have young children or grandchildren, you should be aware of how heart disease can affect them.

Note: Heart problems in children and teenagers can often be a result of obesity, a rapidly spreading crisis in our nation. A complete discussion of this problem and other dietary issues that complicate heart disease is found in **Month Four.**

What Causes Congenital Heart Defects?

A congenital heart defect occurs when something—and researchers are not completely sure what it is—goes wrong at the time of conception. Heart defects can be so slight that your child may look, act, and remain healthy for many years before symptoms appear.

These problems also can manifest after birth in children who have other problems, such as Down's syndrome or Turner's syndrome (which can affect height). It's known that some environmental factors, such as German measles early in pregnancy, some viral infections, industrial chemicals, and alcohol, increase the risk of congenital defects.

Certain chronic diseases in the parent increase the risk of heart defects in children. Diabetes can increase risk. Any diabetic who is pregnant should be closely monitored.

Dietary factors also can increase risk. A diet designed for you by your OB/GYN and cardiologist is a good idea for ensuring a healthy baby and a healthy mother.

The March of Dimes reports, "Scientists are making progress in understanding the genetics of heart defects. Since the 1990s, they have identified several gene mutations (changes) that can cause heart defects." For example, a March of Dimes–funded scientist discovered a series of genetic steps that appears to contribute to a common, important group of malformations affecting the heart's outflow tract. He also identified a gene that can cause a heart defect called an atrial septal defect (a hole between the upper chambers of the heart) and one that may contribute to hypoplastic left heart syndrome (underdevelopment of the heart's main pumping chamber).

"Heart defects also are common in children with a variety of inherited disorders, including Noonan (short stature, learning disabilities), velocardiofacial (craniofacial defects and immune deficiencies), and Holt-Oram (limb defects) syndromes," according to the organization.

What Are the Most Common Congenital Heart Defects?

While more than 40,000 children are born each year with one of the heart defects described below, parents should not blame themselves. Fortunately, today there are special pediatric facilities that offer sophisticated medical or surgical solutions to most of these defects.

These are some of the most common congenital defects:

○ **Patent ductus arteriosus.** Before birth, a large artery (ductus arteriosus) lets the blood bypass the lungs because the fetus gets its oxygen through the placenta. The ductus normally closes soon after birth so that blood can travel to the lungs and pick up oxygen. If it doesn't close, the baby may develop heart failure. This problem occurs most frequently in premature babies. Drug treatment, catheter-based closure devices, or surgery can close the ductus.

○ **Septal defect.** This is a hole in the wall (septum) that divides the right and left sides of the heart. A hole in the wall between the heart's two upper chambers is called an atrial septal defect, while a hole between the lower chambers is called a ventricular septal defect. These defects can cause the blood to circulate improperly, so the heart has to work too hard. A surgeon can close the hole by sewing or patching it. Small holes may heal by themselves or may not need repair at all.

○ **Coarctation of the aorta.** Part of the aorta, the large artery that sends blood from the heart to the rest of the body, may be too narrow for the blood to flow evenly. A surgeon can cut away the narrow part and sew the open ends together, replace the constricted section with manmade material, or patch it with part of a blood vessel taken from elsewhere in the body. Sometimes this narrowed area can be widened by inflating a balloon on the tip of a catheter (tube) inserted through an artery.

○ **Heart valve abnormalities.** Some babies are born with heart valves that do not close normally or that are narrowed or blocked so blood can't flow smoothly. Surgeons usually can repair the valves or replace them with manmade ones. Balloons on catheters also are frequently used to fix faulty valves.

○ **Tetralogy of Fallot.** This combination of four heart defects reduces the amount of blood reaching the lungs. As a result, the blood that is pumped to the body may not have enough oxygen to satisfy the needs of the body. Affected babies have episodes of **cyanosis**, which is a bluish or grey tint of the skin or lips, and may demonstrate slow growth. This defect is usually surgically repaired at approximately three to six months of age. Most affected children live normal or near-normal lives.

○ **Transposition of the great arteries.** Transposition occurs when the positions of the two major arteries leaving the heart are reversed, so that each arises from the wrong pumping chamber. Affected newborns suffer from severe cyanosis due to a lack of oxygen in the blood. Recent surgical advances make it possible to correct this otherwise lethal newborn defect.

○ **Hypoplastic left heart syndrome.** This combination of defects results in a left ventricle (the heart's main pumping chamber) that is too small to support life. This defect is the most common cause of death from **congenital heart disease**. However, over the past 20 years, survival rates have dramatically improved with new surgical procedures and, less frequently, heart transplants. The long-term outlook for children with this heart defect remains uncertain.

(Adapted from and used by permission of The March of Dimes.)

What about Acquired Heart Disease in Children?

While less common, acquired heart disease in children can be just as life threatening. Most acquired childhood heart disorders appear or develop during childhood. The two best known are rheumatic fever and Kawasaki disease.

Rheumatic fever (RF) is not seen frequently in the more developed nations today. It is often seen in children and adolescents in regions that lack good hygiene or sanitary conditions. According to The World Heart Federation, 15.6 million people worldwide suffer from rheumatic fever and die from the consequences of the disease each year. There is a larger incidence of rheumatic fever in Polynesian populations, and women appear to experience more severe disease.

Initially RF often mimics a cold or a strep throat caused by the streptococcus bacterium. In some children who have reduced immune protection, the virus spreads to the heart valves and creates damage that may not be noticed. Symptoms include red, swollen, painful, hot joints; sore throat and fever; tiredness; and shortness of breath, pain, and cyanosis on exertion. People tend to recover—at first—but the damage to the heart valves progresses over decades until symptoms actually appear. By that time, surgery is typically indicated and can ameliorate the symptoms.

Antibiotics and early detection can reduce the incidence of RF. Penicillin given monthly for a period of time, can prevent the strep bacteria from spreading and damaging the heart.

Kawasaki disease is another acquired heart disease that usually appears in very young children under the age of five. Not much is known about this disorder, but when it's detected early, it can be treated successfully. While relatively uncommon (19 in 100,000 U.S. children), it occurs most often in children of Asian origin.

Since early detection is the best defense in Kawasaki disease, children with a fever lasting longer than five days who have a full body rash, red eyes, and chapped lips should be seen by a doctor immediately. Other symptoms can include swollen lymph nodes, swelling in the palms and soles of the feet, and a swollen tongue with a white coating or red bumps. Unfortunately, if you are unable to take the child to a doctor as soon as the symptoms appear or if it's not diagnosed correctly, then heart complications can develop. After a week or more, **vasculitis** (inflamed blood vessels) can harm the coronary arteries, affecting blood flow to the heart. Once this occurs, the heart muscle can become involved and the heart valves can begin to fail because the natural rhythms of the heart are disrupted.

One of the problems with Kawasaki disease is that it can mimic Rocky Mountain Spotted Fever, scarlet fever, a drug allergy, juvenile rheumatoid arthritis, and several other conditions, so they have to be simultaneously considered and ruled out. This can entail blood tests and heart-function tests, such as an echocardiogram. Treatment is usually through a high dose of intravenous gamma globulin that boost the immune system and help defend against the infection.

What Other Childhood Heart Problems Should You Know About?

Children, like adults, can suffer heart failure, a term that actually refers to improper function, rather than a total breakdown. In fact, people of all ages suffer from heart failure, although adults usually experience heart failure as a result of other disease states, such as coronary artery disease, high blood pressure, or diabetes, which aren't common in very small children. In children, heart failure is usually a result of overcirculation failure (sometimes called pump failure).

Overcirculation only appears in about 1 percent of all births, and is a result of a structural heart defect, usually a hole between the chambers of the heart. Blood from the arteries and from the veins flows together, which leads to an inefficient overflow of blood and can create problems with heart-muscle functions and overload the heart muscle, rendering it weakened and fatigued.

A viral infection can lead to pump failure in a child, just as it does in an adult, harming the heart muscle. If the coronary arteries are also affected by any sort of virus, the same problem will occur, preventing blood flow to the heart and weakening it. Virtually any sort of congenital defect, such as an electrical malfunction that affects heartbeat or even a side effect of other medical problems, can create heart failure.

Children suffering from heart failure can have a range of symptoms, including troubled breathing, poor appetite, fevers, delayed growth, sweating and lethargy. Watch for these symptoms and contact your pediatrician if you see any of them. Your pediatrician should refer you to a pediatric cardiologist. These conditions can be treated by both medication and surgery. Treat this decision as you would any adult medical decision about the procedure and choice of a pediatric cardiologist. In **Day Four**, there is a complete guide to making this sort of decision.

Are There Any Other Congenital Disorders?

One of the main goals of the March of Dimes and many other research institutes has been the search for a genetic link to pediatric heart problems. A single gene, if identified, says the March of Dimes, would help us learn what factors affect the molecular pathways responsible for fetal development. In the past few years, studies have pointed to a mutation in the GAT4A gene, which seems to be responsible for the normal separation of the heart into right and left chambers.

Other known genetic disorders can cause heart malformations, although they are not specifically heart disease. Among those are DiGeorge and velocardiofacial syndromes. For further information on these and other birth defects, contact your local state office or the national March of Dimes office (www.marchofdimes.com).

IN A SENTENCE:

> *Heart disease in children can either be congenital or acquired later in life, and together, these account for the most deadly threats to young children today, but thanks to early diagnosis and treatment and the advent of genetic testing, many more children with heart disease go on to lead long, healthy lives.*

Gaining a Global Perspective

DESPITE THE fact that we live in a country with so much excess that our risk factors practically guarantee you can eat, drink, or loaf yourself into heart disease, diabetes, and high blood pressure, significant levels of heart disease are not limited to the U.S. You are not alone. Almost one-third of all deaths around the world—more than 16 million—are caused by cardiovascular disease. Eight percent of these deaths occur in low- or middle-income countries, and half occur in women. Here's another real shocker: Heart disease takes five times more lives than does HIV/AIDS in these countries.

The international spread of heart disease is certainly not limited to third world or underdeveloped countries. More than 19 million people die from cardiovascular disease in the European Union (E.U.) alone. This accounts for almost half of all deaths in most E.U. countries. In Canada, another land of plenty, someone dies of heart disease and stroke every seven minutes! The cost to the Canadian economy is over $18.4 billion per year.

As you know, heart disease kills more men and women in the United States than does any other disease. While the overall death rate has slowed among U.S. men, it continues to grow among women. Globally, the gap between men and

Heart Disease Is a Worldwide Threat

Heart attack, though, is not the only form of heart disease that is spreading. Rheumatic heart disease (rheumatic fever), a valvular disease (see **Day Two**), is relatively uncommon in the U.S. today. According to the AHA, there have been "few outbreaks" in the past three decades; however, it is serious and has a mortality rate of 2 to 5 percent. Twelve million people worldwide are affected by rheumatic fever, two-thirds of them are children, and about 300,000 people die from it annually. Of this group, 3 million have ended up in the hospital, and many will require surgery at some point.

women also is closing. According to the World Health Organization (WHO), in 2005, 53 percent of men and 47 percent of women died from coronary heart disease around the world.

Fortunately, the global problems caused by heart disease, especially strain on medical resources and the economy, are now being understood. Literally hundreds of new studies and data have described the socioeconomic impact of heart disease in virtually every country in the world.

If you grew up in the era where at dinner you had to be a member of the "clean plate club" because "children were starving in China," you have much less to worry about. The number of obese Chinese men and women has actually caught up to that of American men and women. From 1980 to the late 1990s, the rate of overweight men and women in China grew by 135 percent and 95 percent, respectively. Now, however, there are more obese Chinese women (40 percent) than Chinese men (37 percent). Those children in many parts of China may not be starving anymore; instead, they may have eaten themselves into a high risk for heart disease (see **Week Four**).

Joining China is India, which also has become a cardiac disease disaster site. WHO reports that "60 percent of the world's cardiac patients will be Indian within the next 3 years."

The future global spread of chronic disease, according to WHO, is likely to continue unless measures to reduce risk factors are taken. "It is clear," WHO says, "that the chronic disease problem is far from being limited to developed regions of the world."

"It's clear that the earlier labeling of chronic diseases as 'diseases of affluence' is an increasing misnomer, as they emerge both in poorer countries and population groups." WHO reports that not only is this tak-

ing place faster than it did during the spread of disease in the industrialized countries 100 years ago, but the threat to overall world health is
greater due to population density. Not only will chronic disease account
for 71 percent of all deaths worldwide by 2020, but 71 percent of those
deaths will be from chronic heart disease.

Why Is Heart Disease So Common Worldwide?

As I have mentioned, heart disease and other forms of coronary artery disorders are largely a result of increased risk factors, and there is no
question that this is at the root of the global problem. One area that is
widely recognized by groups like WHO and American medical organizations is family history, which is harder to track because it requires medical histories taken directly from each patient. This information may not
be as easy to gather as statistical information drawn from patient records
is. While family history may play a part in developed countries like the
U.S. and Europe, our other risk factors, such as high blood pressure, tobacco use, and diet, are common among all countries.

Some emerging studies suggest a genetic relationship between heart
disease and certain ethnic groups. In some studies of Asians, there is a
possible underlying relationship to genetics; however, one expert notes
that in India, for example, diet excess was balanced by "physical demands of life that were high. Now the pendulum has swung in the opposite direction, and we refuse to do anything. If we could drive to the
bathroom, then we would do that. People simply refuse to move."

If there is one overriding reason for the worldwide epidemic of heart
disease outside the United States, it would be smoking. In 2005, there
were still over 1.3 billion smokers (multiple packs per day) worldwide,
an estimate that will continue to rise to 1.7 billion soon.

But the news is not all bad. Anyone who has been abroad recently
knows that the non-smoking trend that is catching on here is being du-
plicated in many places. Among the countries that have some sort of
smoking bans are Australia, Belgium, Bhutan (the first!), Canada, Czech
Republic, Denmark, Finland, France (in most public spaces), Hong
Kong, Iceland, Ireland, Italy, Lithuania, New Zealand, Norway, Portugal,
Sweden, and Uruguay. Even China has some bans under consideration.
While education and strong warnings from federal government agencies

---

The "Thrifty Gene" Theory

A number of hypothetical theories regarding heart disease in certain ethnic populations have been advanced, including the "thrifty gene" theory. Studies of some Asian groups in Canada suggest that because this population suffered from famine over many generations, their bodies adjusted to the deprived conditions needed to survive. Thus, they had a "thrifty gene."

Now that food is plentiful, their bodies have difficulty absorbing the food and they develop obesity or diabetes because their bodies are still trying to retain much of the surplus food for future use. It's estimated that it might take a few generations for their genetic make-up to adjust.

---

have helped reduce smoking here, around the world it is a major risk factor driving many of the statistics above.

Perhaps the worst environment in the world for a non-smoker is Asia, especially Japan. Surveys conducted by the Japanese tobacco industry itself report that an astonishing 62 percent of men in their 30s and 24 percent of women in their 30s are heavy smokers. In the U.S., the smoker is relegated to small rooms, outside the office, or banned totally. In Japan, if you are a non-smoker, you'll be lucky to find anyplace where smoking is banned. Despite laws that ban sales to people under age 20, cigarettes are easily available in vending machines everywhere. Some progress has been made in recent years with a single no-smoking car on commuter trains and a government-sponsored education program; however, tobacco is a $33.8 billion-per-year business in Japan, and major curbs are not likely in the near future.

Among the estimates of damage from smoking are the following statistics:

- ○ A 50-year study by the British Heart Foundation reported that deaths among daily smokers were 60 percent higher than among non-smokers and 80 percent higher in heavy, multi-pack smokers.
- ○ WHO says, "tobacco is the single greatest cause of death and disability worldwide, accounting for 10 million deaths a year."

○ Adults are not the only victims. Underage smoking and second-hand smoke will kill 250 million children and adolescents, about one-third of whom are in developing countries. (Think of where most of this tobacco is coming from.)

○ More than 60 percent of men in China smoke.

It's hardly surprising that, in addition to smoking, many of the other traditional risk factors for cardiovascular disease around the world are the same ones you face. However, many of these are a result of lifestyle excess that has not traditionally been present in other countries. For example, a recent story in *Time* profiled the residents of Okinawa, one of the islands of Japan that is known for residents who lived lengthy, healthy lives throughout many generations. Until recently, their diet was about as healthy as it gets: fish, rice, vegetables, and no saturated fats. In 1976, Okinawans got a present from their American friends: their first McDonald's.

Today, there are 44 McDonald's restaurants on Okinawa, and by the mid-1990s, Okinawans had fallen from the healthiest population to 26th of 40 Japanese districts studied. Almost half of all men in Okinawa aged 26 to 60 now are obese.

In countries like Japan, China, India, and Vietnam, where the main cause of death was traditionally infectious disease or malnutrition, the tables have been turned. American-style fast food and tobacco have created a far greater impact on the lives and deaths of people there.

In addition, the traditional risk factors for heart disease also are spreading worldwide. The AHA reports:

○ 66 percent of men and women worldwide have high cholesterol levels

○ 44 percent of men and 35 percent of women worldwide are overweight

○ Obesity rates among men in the U.K. have tripled in the past two decades, catching them up to the female population

○ The proportion of people in India who are overweight will increase from 9 percent in 1995 to 25 percent in 2025

○ The proportion of obese men in countries in the E.U. (not including the U.K.) is higher than the U.S.

Statistics may give us a snapshot of how our cultural lifestyle has spread, but what else do they really mean? The AHA draws this conclusion: "Obesity in the developing world can no longer be considered a disease of groups of higher socioeconomic status. The burden of obesity in a particular developing country tends to shift toward the groups of socioeconomic status as the country's gross national product increases. The shift of obesity apparently occurs at earlier stages of development among women than among men."

Even in the U.S., people who are poorer have less access to good health care, do not have insurance, and are not health-literate. In other countries, where access ranges from universal health care to very little care, risk factors and negative health behavior seem to be spreading among both men and women. Already we see consequences beyond cardiovascular disease. For example, the number of adults with diabetes worldwide is well over 170 million. Estimates for China and India show an increase in diabetes as well.

What's Your Risk as Part of an Ethnic Population in the U.S.?

Two things specifically increase heart disease risk in the U.S. within the various ethnic or racial populations, and these factors are similar to those of other poor countries. First is the level of risk we assume by our lifestyle. The other, which is much too common, is lack of access to proper health care and proper nutritional education. Added to these are non-modifiable and modifiable risk factors discussed earlier in this book (see **Day One**).

Today, heart disease is the leading cause of death among U.S. ethnic groups each year.

- O Hispanics: 130,000
- O African Americans: 206,000
- O Native Americans: 80,000
- O Asian and Pacific Islanders: 78,000
- O Caucasians: 259,000

Along racial lines, African Americans are far more likely to suffer from heart disease; however, the numbers have not dropped as they have in the general population. Almost 50 percent of African American women and 45 percent of African American men are likely to develop heart disease at a younger age and with more severe symptoms than any other racial population. The reason more African Americans are more likely to end up hospitalized and at greater risk seems to be widespread hypertension and diabetes within this group. High blood pressure has been increasing rapidly in younger African Americans of both sexes.

Heart disease is also widespread in Hispanics, but they are much less likely than African Americans to die from heart attacks. Still, heart disease and stroke are the number-one killers of Latinos and Hispanic Americans. This group is also prone to high blood pressure but is less likely to have it than Caucasians and African Americans are. Excess weight and obesity also are a problem for Hispanics, Latinos, and African Americans.

Statistics about different populations around the world and within the racial or ethnic groups in our country give us one strong message: We have a big problem that will not subside, according to many experts, including the National Institutes of Health, until the frequency of health care increases among minority groups. For example, only 50 percent of American Indians/Alaskan Natives, 44 percent of Asian Americans, and 38 percent of Mexican Americans have had cholesterol reviews or counseling in the last two years.

A study conducted by the Henry J. Kaiser Family Foundation in 2002 indicated that "African Americans were less likely than whites to receive diagnostic procedures, revascularization procedures, and thrombolytic therapy for heart disease." More startling, says the report, "Hispanics are less likely to receive aspirin and beta-blockers when hospitalized for heart attack than whites."

The U.S. Department of Health and Human Services cites two other factors that can also deprive someone from achieving good heart health. One is education. Those with less education are less likely to have high blood pressure identified, monitored regularly, and treated when necessary. The same situation is true in individuals with low income.

Sadly, no matter how much data are collected, studies conducted, and population groups examined, the problems caused by heart disease are clear. From Asia to the U.K., and in every ethnic or racial group in the U.S., the risk for heart diseases increases daily. Large segments of the population do not have adequate (or any) medical insurance. In countries where health care is available, people embrace the worst risk factor possible: smoking.

It's often said that we live in a shrinking world. Technology, communications, and travel have contributed to rapid information transfer. One byproduct is how much we know about the health-care crisis around the world. Many efforts are under way to bring health education to high-risk populations, largely through training foreign doctors and medical personnel in the U.S. Unfortunately, the crisis may be outrunning the solution, especially since even underdeveloped nations are showing growing risk of heart disease. Poverty, malnutrition, infectious disease, and lack of regular medical care are prevalent in many places where resources are scarce.

What can you do? The best place for us to start is at home and in our communities, especially since we know first-hand what heart disease can do. Supporting school-based education programs and food banks to get healthful food into the hands of those who cannot afford it is an excellent starting place.

IN A SENTENCE:

> *Looking at the global picture, you can see how the risk factors of smoking, poor nutrition, lack of exercise, and poor medical care easily can put entire populations at risk—yet, while you can't change the world, you can change your life.*

FIRST MONTH **MILESTONES**

○ YOU HAVE LEARNED THE STEPS INVOLVED IN RECOVERY FROM A HEART ATTACK.

○ YOU HAVE LEARNED HOW HEART DISEASE AFFECTS WOMEN DIFFERENTLY.

○ YOU HAVE LEARNED ABOUT SEXUALITY AND INTIMACY WITH HEART DISEASE.

○ YOU HAVE LEARNED HOW HEART DISEASE AFFECTS OTHER POPULATIONS IN THE WORLD.

living

Getting Control: Taking Inventory

UNLIKE MANY other people, you have the chance of a lifetime: an opportunity to clear the past and open a new way for the future. You have an opportunity to rebuild, regroup, and readjust. You are still alive. As the old joke goes, if you are reading this, you have made it through a heart attack, or perhaps congestive heart failure, angina, congenital heart disorder, cardiomyopathy, arrhythmias, rheumatic heart disease, valve problems, and other problems, such as diabetes or hypertension.

In **Month Two**, you will see how easy it can be to create a goal-based plan to get your health back, a process comparable to starting a new business with you as the product. The strategy shows you how to set goals and markers for assessing your progress. However, you need one thing before this plan can be created that is essential to any new product development: raw materials. You have to have some basic assets to create an inventory that you can draw on as you need.

In your case, the process is slightly different because you are going to both acquire raw materials and discard some intrinsic behaviors that have held you back. It begins with an inventory.

Your Health Inventory

Over the past weeks, as you've learned more about heart disease, you should have learned to recognize your risk factors for heart disease. Start by putting this knowledge to good use.

First, list your current top-ten risk factors.

For example (in no particular order):

1. Family history: mother and grandmother
2. Heart attack (year, severity)
3. High cholesterol
4. Diabetes
5. 20 pounds overweight
6. Smoking (packs per day)
7. Gender and age
8. Junk-food junkie
9. Have never exercised regularly
10. Major denial

With the exception of smoking, I can plead guilty to all the items above. They are my risk-factor inventory. Keep in mind that this is not a medical assessment test that leads to a score. This is a look at the impediments to your personal rebuilding, identifying them and helping you to create a whole new inventory to draw on.

Take the next step. What are the top ten worst risk factors in your present inventory?

1. _____
2. _____
3. _____
4. _____
5. _____
6. _____
7. _____
8. _____

9. _____

10. _____

Assess Your Inventory

Not a day goes by that I don't think about what I did to accumulate such a messy life that led to heart attack, bypass surgery, and years of recovery. Had I really focused on the things I could have changed or influenced and attacked each one, many things in my life would have been different. You can avoid that trap now. With your list, now you can become proactive.

For example, finally controlling two risk factors that I had at the time of my MI were keys to my recovery. I was diagnosed with diabetes years before I developed heart disease. Two in three people with diabetes die from heart disease. That was significant, but no one told me that diabetes can affect blood chemistry, promoting and accelerating atherosclerosis or hardening of the arteries, a major coronary risk factor. I also had high cholesterol. High triglycerides and low HDL are often present in diabetics, a particularly concerning combination, creating increased heart attack risk.

Further, my elevated lipids indicated that my diet was not great. It was filled with fats and other unhealthy food, and loaded with sugar going right into my bloodstream because my diabetic body was not generating enough insulin to absorb it. This cycle is only a quick example. You simply can't see this as a simple, one-time effort to eradicate a risk factor. If you cut out all sweets and fried food, you have begun to apply brakes, but you've already harmed the central machine—you have heart disease—and you need to initiate widespread recovery.

The first step is to sit down with your doctor and your risk-factor list and understand the medical treatment options in the context of your family history, damage to the heart, and your current physical condition. Ask your doctor these questions:

1. Do I need medication?
2. Do I need angioplasty?
3. Do I need surgery?
4. Do I need all three treatments?
5. Have I omitted any risk factors, and what are the priorities in managing my risk?

Discuss with your doctor your goals. Do the same with a therapist or counselor and a nutritionist.

Replace Your Risk Factors

Reversing or eliminating most of your risk factors is a good start. More important, you want to *replace* these risk factors with positive behaviors that will enable you to reach your goals, *especially the long-term goals you noted in the last section.* In the next sections, we'll look at ways to reduce your risk factors. Here's another exercise: Using your list of top-ten risk factors, begin examining your risk factors and swap each for something that can help you move forward.

For example:

1. **Family history: mother and grandmother.** There is not a lot you can do with the cards you've been dealt—or can you? My mother died from heart disease at age 75 after a second bypass. I am now 15 years younger than she was, and I've had an MI and a quadruple bypass. I have set my mother's ultimate longevity—75 years—as a minimal goal, and have looked at the elements of her lifestyle that I can avoid. I have discussed with my children my mother's heart disease and mine as examples of what ignoring DNA-related risk factors can do.

2. **Heart attack (year, severity).** I have made learning about my heart attack and heart disease an integral aspect of my life. I subscribe to several online newsletters that go beyond covering heart disease because recovery, in my case, applies to several problems. I am proactive in my own care and education. If I have a question, other than a medical emergency, I do as much research as I can, starting with the Internet. You can go from link to link, picking up information for later on. Chat rooms and similar sites work well, but I also find links from the American Heart Association and professional journals interesting.

3. **High cholesterol.** There are many ways to attack this problem and they are described in depth in **Month Three**; however, one of the most important things you can do is to ask your doctor to refer you to a lipid clinic. Lipid clinics have been instrumental in bringing my blood values into the normal range. Through regular monitoring and medication adjustment, they also have been a great motivator.

4. Diabetes. Information about this subject, including a top-notch book in this *First Year* series, is everywhere, and self-education is certainly a vital part of diabetes treatment. Diabetes is one of the few conditions in which the patient has a large role in the success of the treatment. Everything, from a determination to take medication that can have unpleasant side effects to self-administered insulin injections, tracking sugar levels, and dietary control, rests on your shoulders. Simply getting past this part of your duel with diabetes is a great start.

5. 20 pounds overweight. I was only a few pounds overweight when I had my first MI. Several years later, when I had my CABG, I had gained more than 40 pounds. For the next several years after surgery, I tried to have a more active life, primarily defined by golf and a few sessions per week on the treadmill. Naturally, my weight crept up until complications like backaches and breathlessness set in. When I came finally under the care of Dr. Rimmerman at the Cleveland Clinic, he created a series of challenges for me, similar to goal setting. Then I discovered a weight-loss program that worked for me (see **Month Four**)— Weight Watchers—and over 15 months I have lost and kept off 20 pounds, with more still to go.

6. Smoking (packs per day). I would not be alive today if I had smoked. If there is one single risk factor that any doctor or medical professional will tell you must be stopped, it is smoking. This includes pipes, chewing tobacco, and the like. Smoking is an equal-opportunity killer, and it's just a matter of time that determines whether you'll develop lung cancer, vascular and heart disease, emphysema, or heart failure. If you smoke, put this on the top of your list of health issues as something you absolutely must deal with. It will not be easy, but stopping smoking will save your life.

7. Sex and age. These won't be easy to change. You are what you are in this case, but you can be aware of what these factors mean for your risk levels. As you've seen previously, heart disease affects men and women differently. Keep this in mind as you continue your day-to-day research and also discuss with your doctor any new information available on the topic.

Age is unfortunately not reversible, but we do seem to be living in an age when your age truly is a number. As several of my landmark birthdays approached, I couldn't decide whether I should celebrate or get into bed and pull the covers over my head for a few days. But I did not hide, and I am healthier for that positive attitude. Now I do not think about my age except in the concept of how good I feel!

8. **Junk-food junkie (JFJ).** I was capable of eating an entire pack of cookies at once. I lived on candy, and loved french fries. This addiction—the sugar and caffeine rushes—is hard to kick, especially if the habit began in childhood, as mine did. My parents were JFJs and they were my enablers. Today, I've changed my diet and I really don't miss the junk food as much as I had expected (see **Month Four**).

9. **Have never exercised regularly.** Perhaps you are athletic and you don't particularly like the exercise machine/gym scene. That's totally understandable. I skied, played tennis, and played softball for more than 20 years as an adult. I loved each season and never thought I'd have to give it up. Before I was 50, my MI forced me to the bench, and then into retirement. My skis, racket, and mitt went into storage, and that was it. I tried the exercise programs and joined the YMCA, but always found something "more important" to do. Yet I found a way to change that. You can find out how to set up a regular exercise program that you'll want to stick with in **Month Five.**

10. **Major denial.** Of all my risk factors, denial was probably the one that held me back the most from making a rapid recovery. In fact, denial is the ultimate catch-22 because you don't really know you are in denial if you are actually in denial. Looking back at my lengthy period of denial that extended through my heart attack and even through my CABG, I can easily see all the signs that manifest themselves in the risk factors I've listed here. However, the denial was ultimately broken because I developed a game plan to return to health. If you follow it, you will be on the right path.

Your doctor can be a great help when it comes to guiding you through the rest of the process of taking control of your recovery.

From a Doctor's Side of the Fence

Marty Kanovsky, M.D., has seen it all as a suburban cardiologist in his offices near Washington, DC. His patient population varies widely; however, it tends to be on the older side. "Sometimes," Dr. Kanovsky jokes, "there are so many walkers in my waiting room, I can barely get through."

Beyond treating his patients medically, Dr. Kanovsky finds that motivating each patient is a major part of his work. "I want to put a positive spin on what I tell them," he says, "but I also want scare them just enough to make them do the right thing."

In general, Dr. Kanovsky finds that there are very specific patterns among his patients.

"I see several types. One typical group, I call the *deniers*. These are the people who search the Internet to find something that supports what they want to do," he explains. For example, if they don't want to take their statins (LDL-lowering medications), they will keep looking until they find something that supports their feeling that there are potential risks with statins.

"These are also the patients who I know aren't telling me the truth. We'll be sitting in the office discussing diet or exercise, and while the patient is talking, the spouse is sitting off to the side, shaking her head. I usually find that the men are the biggest deniers, while the wife wants them to be doing the right things."

"Some patients are trying, but they simply are not getting it right," Dr. Kanovsky says. "For example, I asked a patient what he was having for lunch, and he said a ham-and-cheese sandwich with a glass of milk. They think they are following the diet and telling you the truth, but they aren't. In the same vein, I will see people who are very careful about their medications and take them correctly, but do nothing else that they are supposed to do."

On the brighter side, he sees fewer smokers now than in the past. "While smoking is going down, the bad part is that obesity is definitely increasing, much more than ever before," Dr. Kanovsky says. He emphasizes reducing cholesterol and looking at not only total cholesterol, but also HDL, LDL, triglycerides, and other important markers beyond genetic risk factors.

Putting people on the right diet track and motivating them to lose weight requires tapping into the right motivator, which, in many cases, is the spouse, who can provide positive reinforcement, according to Dr. Kanovsky. Beyond providing plenty of directed patient information, he encourages all of his patients to go beyond simple cardio-rehab exercise programs.

"The people who go to complete cardio-rehab programs that include classes and supervised exercise do much, much better," he says. "One reason is that many hospitals have every possible sort of exercise equipment with very active, enthusiastic, and positive trainers to help you. The classes are also very helpful because they not only help you learn, but you meet other people like you and others who are at different stages. Many people make friendships in these classes and exchange information about what has worked for them.

"Patients also have a tendency to have a real letdown after surgery or a heart attack, simply because they have had so many other worries. All of a sudden, they start to think about what has happened. A rehab class can also help with the psychological issues," Dr. Kanovsky adds.

Another reason that the rehab classes are important, Dr. Kanovsky points out, is that "most of my patients have something else wrong with them: diabetes, hypertension, and high cholesterol."

As for motivation, his observation has been that human nature tends to be a major factor. For example, Dr. Kanovsky explains, "if you like your job, you are probably going to be more motivated to get back to work than someone who doesn't want to go back so quickly. Of course, a patient whose problem is discovered early can have a lower-risk operation and will recover quickly."

IN A SENTENCE:

You have an opportunity to rebuild, regroup, and readjust, having made it through a heart attack, or perhaps other coronary disease, and the place to begin is by identifying and assessing your risk factors.

Getting Control: Making a Game Plan

AFTER LEARNING that you have heart disease or multiple risk factors for significant consequences, such as a heart attack or open heart surgery, you now know that something about your life is just not right. You may, as I did, finally admit that it is time to get it together, get past the denial, and decide what you'd *like* your future to be. Now that you have some understanding of the basics of heart disease, you do have the knowledge to put a plan together to restore your health. You know that recovery can be an emotional roller coaster, but you also know that you can overcome this particularly difficult challenge.

Getting control of your life when you've recently been diagnosed with heart disease requires more than just fear of more illness. You need a game plan for life that will help you to

- ○ continue increasing your knowledge of your condition
- ○ understand what your treatment options really are
- ○ develop close and open communication with your medical team, especially your physician
- ○ develop family support and other support systems
- ○ create a game plan for specific risk reduction
- ○ develop a plan to rebuild your body

○ develop a plan to rebuild your mind-set
○ determine life changes that can help your recovery
○ make changes at work that can help your recovery
○ create specific motivators to keep you on track

Any sort of game plan for sports, education, or business usually requires two components: a strategy and a goal. Overcoming a medical illness, especially heart disease, requires a third component. Call it intestinal fortitude, guts, or any other term, but it boils down to *how much you want to recover.*

Develop a Strategy: The Profit Is Your New Life

Start thinking about getting control by developing a personal strategy for recovery soon after you are diagnosed. If you include the elements listed previously, you will have a better path to renewed health and health behavior. Begin by seeing your recovery as a new business you are starting. You are the product, and the new, improved model you develop as you recover can be a smash hit.

If you've ever run a business or worked in a management position, the term "strategic thinking" is probably familiar. For years, when I ran my own company or when I was an executive in high-stress corporate settings, this was a daily, almost unconscious method we used to increase profits. Essentially, strategic thinking is a process that begins by examining what you have to do or what you need to have on hand to reach a specific goal. It sounds simple, but it's not, especially if you apply the idea of thinking strategically as a way to get healthy.

The first thing to do is to develop goals with your doctor and rehab team. One thing to note is that although you may have identified what you need to fill in your strategic plan, you can't count on the conditions remaining stable. For example, you may decide you are going to walk outside 30 minutes each day, but what happens when it rains every day for two weeks? You have to include in your plan creative and flexible contingencies.

One other thing you may want to keep in mind as you develop your strategy: Since strategic plans are influenced by outside factors, you also must keep up with what is happening in heart disease treatment. One of the best things you can do for yourself is to become as educated as possible (which you will read more about here), but the point is to use that information to update your plan.

Set a Goal

What *should* your goals be after your recent diagnosis? Certainly, there are several important ones that your doctor will set, such as compliance with your medications, attending cardio-rehab, setting a return-to-work date, and making changes in your diet and lifestyle. Simple. No problem. No stress, right?

This is why you need a plan of your own that enables you to comply with what your doctor wants, but that does not make you feel as though all you are doing is treading water and trying to not drown. You want to be able to clear the debris clogging the stream taking you toward your goal. Put more simply, you don't want a second heart attack, or to make any other condition worse, which would turn the odds against your profitability or, in real terms, your survival.

Goal setting can be a tricky thing. We often set goals that are either too high or too low. You may want to consider another trick. Look at your whole recovery plan and break it into small, reachable goals that will lead to your ultimate destination.

Try filling in some of your goals below (copy this or write it out on a pad).

List four short-range goals (Examples: Walk around the block once, then twice, be able to drive again, start an exercise and cardio rehab program)

1. _____
2. _____
3. _____
4. _____

List four medium-range goals (Examples: Go back to work, play golf every weekend, go back to school, go to Paris)

1. _____
2. _____

3. _____
4. _____

List the four most important long-range goals you have (Examples: See your children graduate from college, have grandchildren)

1. _____
2. _____
3. _____
4. _____

Once you have completed this exercise, you will have two things you didn't have before you started:

○ Concrete, positive reasons to continue rebuilding your health or achieving your goals
○ A plan that can be implemented by choosing the methods to construct the platforms you need to keep going

Implement the Plan

If you continue with this rebuilding model, you now have to acquire the tools for reaching the goals you've set. This includes the short-, medium-, and long-range goals you've listed above, and don't forget to consider how you are going to measure your progress.

List Your Two Most Important Short-Range Goals

1. _____
2. _____

Answer These Questions

What do I have to do to reach the goals I've listed above? How can I do this safely and given the reality of my condition? (Examples: Find the right cardio-rehab class, regain my independence, stop smoking, begin a proper diet)

_____

_____

_____

_____

_____

Now List Your Two Most Important Medium-Range Goals

_____

_____

_____

_____

_____

Answer These Questions

Where do I stand now? How have I done? Have I accomplished my first set of goals?

_____

_____

_____

_____

_____

_____

What do I have to do to build on my accomplishments to get to my two most important medium-range goals? Am I ready to do this? (Can I go back to work? Am I ready to travel?)

_____

_____

_____

_____

_____

You're Back in Business

After you have reached your short- and medium-range goals, your life may be returning to normal, or, more specifically, to a new and improved normal, the great product you've been working so hard to become. You have followed your strategic plan by setting and reaching or exceeding your goals. You are back in business, going to work, hitting the links over the weekend, taking a vacation, and doing the things you used to take for granted, like shopping for a new pair of shoes.

Let's go back to the original concept of rebuilding your life through a strategic plan. By this time, you've used many of the suggestions in the list at the start of this section to help you reach your goals, and the result is very positive. However, remember that you really are just starting out. You'll want to keep your investment solid, and not get in too far over your head. For example, just because you can walk several miles on the treadmill doesn't mean you are ready for the 5K. Like a business, you want to build slowly.

Another thing you'll want to do at this point is to take a look back and see how well you have done. If you are back at work, feeling well, and your doctor has told you, "See me in a few months," you should be smiling. The question to ask yourself next as a part of your strategic plan is, "Where do we go from here?"

This is important because your next move will determine how well you do on your way to those long-range goals.

What about the Long-Range Goals?

The secret to achieving your long-range goals is to integrate the things you've used to get you this far along in your recovery into every part of your life. Yet that's not enough. To really reach your long-range goals, you have to embrace the third element I mentioned earlier: the intestinal fortitude to make it happen. In other words, how much do you want to see your children graduate from college or to hold your grandchildren?

It's one thing to develop the motivation to recover enough to go back to work. After all, you need to pay the mortgage and meet your other responsibilities. You have gone to cardio-rehab and rebuilt your strength so that you will feel better and will be able to do some of the recreational activities you've enjoyed.

To reach this long-range goal, you have to make a commitment to really change your life. This means that the behaviors that led to the de-

> ### **True Story**
>
> Early after my first myocardial infarction, I was back at work, standing on the train platform, sipping my coffee. I noticed a friend who had had a severe heart attack about a year before while shoveling snow. He was the first of our group of middle-aged guys to have an MI. We hadn't seen each other recently, so I walked over to see how he was doing and exchange war stories.
>
> To my enormous shock, he was puffing away on a cigarette, and I knew he'd been a heavy smoker. After exchanging family news and medical updates, I asked him, "Are those (cigarettes) prescribed by your doctor?" He laughed and kept on smoking.
>
> We lost contact when I moved, but I read in the newspaper that his daughter had become a highly recruited tennis player. I hoped he was still healthy and able to see her play in college.

velopment of your primary risk factors (**Day One**) have to change permanently. You'll have to change certain aspects of your lifestyle. Before your heart attack, you may have thought you were living the good life, but obviously, you weren't. Now you have the chance to live the good and healthy life.

Everything you may have done in the past that your doctor has told you to change not only will have to change, but you'll have to find the strength to do it. Much of this will have to come from deep inside.

To do this, you are going to have to develop a series of motivators that enable you to make changes to ingrained behaviors. For example, I was one of the worst junk-food eaters on the planet, capable of eating entire bags of cookies in a single sitting. I had never read a food label. Today, I go into supermarkets and I don't even see the junk food that lines 90 percent of the shelves. I have become so used to a healthy diet that if I taste anything that's not low-sodium or fat-free, it tastes awful. You can do this, too (see **Month Five**)!

This didn't happen overnight. In fact, it took me over a year to just get to this point, but each day gets easier.

How do you find or create these motivators? When I complained about my situation and the difficulty of overcoming it, friends said to me over and over, "Sure, but what's the alternative?" As well-meaning as my friends were, this drove me crazy. I needed motivation, and this comment suggested that just avoiding death was a good motivator.

You've just had a profound wake-up call from your diagnosis. You do not need negative motivators, even if your friends did not intend it in that way.

IN A SENTENCE:

> *You have a second chance to rebuild your life and body, and to begin you must take inventory of the risk factors and negative behavior to begin creating a plan.*

Quitting Smoking

IN THE next few sections, you will find information to help you focus on reducing or eliminating the toughest cardiovascular risk factors. You already know that just getting to this point in your recovery, where your heart health has improved considerably, has not been easy. I know it was not easy for me. It has taken motivation, overcoming fear, regaining lost self-esteem, and adapting to a new lifestyle that includes both diet and exercise.

Your life has been turned over, and you've tumbled down a steep, boulder-strewn hill. Now it's time to dust yourself off and climb back up, but this time, you have to make some very specific, long-term changes that will help you scale the slope to good health.

Regaining your overall health requires long-term behavior modification, a classic technique that is supposed to make you change your behavior by giving you a positive reinforcement/reward when you do something good or that will deliver a negative reinforcement (punishment) if your behavior is not up to snuff. You will have to find new motivation to make changes in your daily life and activities, but the motivation for change has to be intrinsic.

As you reach this stage, you will have to reward yourself and tailor the methods of modifying past unhealthy behavior to your daily needs. Certainly, you should seek and get help in this effort. However, regaining your overall health has to be an ongoing personal process, not just a series of single attempts. In previous sections, some methods of gaining control of your risk factors have been suggested. Now is a good time to build your knowledge bank of certain behaviors to help you climb to lifelong heart health.

According to the American Heart Association

> Cigarette smoking is the most important preventable cause of premature death in the U.S. It accounts for nearly 440,000 of the more than 2.4 million annual deaths. Cigarette smokers have a higher risk of developing several chronic disorders. These include fatty buildups in arteries, several types of cancer and chronic obstructive pulmonary disease (lung problems). Atherosclerosis (buildup of fatty substances in the arteries) is a chief contributor to the high number of deaths from smoking. Many studies detail the evidence that cigarette smoking is a major cause of coronary heart disease, which leads to heart attack.

Smoking: Personal Health Enemy No. 1

Second only to having a family history of cardiovascular disease, smoking is as dangerous to your heart and just about every other organ as it gets. With every puff, you inhale 400 different toxins and 43 known carcinogens. These chemicals circulate in your body, continually putting you at long-term risk. Thousands of studies have proven this (as well as tacit, if grudging, admission by the tobacco industry). Former U.S. surgeon general Richard Carmona, M.D., referred to these studies as "massive and conclusive."

More than $4 billion is spent on cigarettes each year in the U.S. alone. Where heart risk is concerned, more than 440,000 people die each year because of smoking and 135,000 additional deaths are linked to the effects of cigarettes on the cardiovascular system. Smokers are two to three times more likely to die of cardiovascular disease than are non-smokers, according to the American Heart Association.

Is the Threat from Secondhand Smoke Real, Too?

Just to ice the cake, environmental or secondhand smoke is just as deadly. Up to 60 percent of non-smokers have "biological evidence of

Smoking Stats

In the U.S., an estimated 25.1 million men (23.4 percent) and 20.9 million women (18.5 percent) are smokers. These people are at higher risk of heart attack and stroke. The latest estimates for persons age 18 and older show the following data:

○ Among Caucasians, 25 percent of men and 21 percent of women smoke.

○ Among high-school students of all races, 29 percent of boys and 28 percent of girls smoke.

○ Among non-Hispanic blacks, 23.9 percent of men and 17.2 percent of women smoke.

○ Among Hispanics, 18.9 percent of men and 10.9 percent of women smoke.

○ Among Asians (only), 17.8 percent of men and 4.8 percent of women smoke.

○ Among Native Americans/Alaska Natives, 37.3 percent of men and 28.5 percent of women smoke.

○ Studies show that smoking prevalence is higher among those who have earned a GED diploma (39.6 percent) and among those with nine to 11 years of education (34.0 percent) compared with those with more than 16 years of education (8.0 percent). Smoking is highest among persons living below the poverty level (29.1 percent).

National Health Interview Survey (NHIS), 2004; National Center for Health Statistics and NHLBI; and American Lung Association, 2002.

exposure," according to the surgeon general's report. Fortunately, this is beginning to change as a result of smoking bans in many states and countries. Smoking rates in most groups, except for teenage females, are dropping. Unfortunately, many potentially harmful substances, like alcohol and tobacco, have been around for hundreds of years and are part of our culture. As a result, they are not easy to remove from our lives.

American Heart Association data indicate that "the link between second-hand smoke (also called environmental tobacco smoke) and disease is well known, and the connection to cardiovascular-related disability and death is also clear. About 37,000 to 40,000 people die from heart and blood vessel disease caused by other people's smoke each year. Of these, about 35,000 nonsmokers die from coronary heart disease, which includes heart attack."

European specialists are beginning to study secondhand smoke seriously. In 2007, Greek researchers studied more than 200 patients who had been admitted to hospitals for a heart attack or unstable angina. The scientists discovered that 46 percent reported being exposed to secondhand smoke at home and on the job. Two other disturbing facts were found: Exposure to secondhand smoke on the job was more dangerous than was exposure to smoke at home, and secondhand smoke was a directly contributing factor to the patients' heart disease and angina.

Smoking is most often associated with cancer; however, its effect on the cardiovascular system is both quiet and deadly. The more you smoke, the greater are the chances of atherosclerosis, which results in blocked arteries and reduced blood flow to your heart. If other health behaviors—diet and exercise—are already bad, smoking multiplies the risk, leading to angina and coronary artery disease. In smokers, the peripheral arteries that carry blood to the arms and legs are also at increased risk for blockages and can result in symptoms of intermittent claudication; central artery blockages can also occur and result in increased stroke risk.

According to the Cleveland Clinic's Heart and Vascular Institute, "A person's risk of heart attack greatly increases with the number of cigarettes he or she smokes. There is no safe amount of smoking. Smokers continue to increase their risk of heart attack the longer they smoke. People who smoke a pack of cigarettes a day have more than twice the risk of heart attack than nonsmokers."

Oral Contraceptives

The Cleveland Clinic also cautions that "women who smoke and also use oral contraceptives (birth control pills) increase several times their risk of coronary and peripheral artery diseases, heart attack and stroke compared with nonsmoking women who use oral contraceptives."

Why Is Quitting Smoking So Difficult?

Why do people continue to smoke, knowing what we know about its effects on health? The short answer is simple: The active ingredient in tobacco, nicotine, is just about the most addictive compound in the world. According to the National Institute on Drug Abuse (NIDA), a division of NIH, "Nicotine's 'kick' is caused in part by the drug's stimulation of the **adrenal glands** and resulting discharge of epinephrine (adrenaline).

"The rush of adrenaline stimulates the body and causes a sudden release of glucose, as well as an increase in blood pressure, respiration, and heart rate. Nicotine also suppresses insulin output from the pancreas, which means that smokers are always slightly hyperglycemic (i.e., they have elevated blood sugar levels). The calming effect of nicotine reported by many users is usually associated with a decline in withdrawal effects, rather than direct effects of nicotine."

Other substances in tobacco smoke are associated with the release of other naturally occurring substances in our brains, such as the neurotransmitter dopamine, which affect pleasure and pain. Dopamine makes you feel good, but when you stop smoking, you feel miserable, which our body interprets as withdrawal pains.

It may be hard for you to stop smoking for another, more insidious reason. A study released by the Harvard University School of Public Health in January 2007 confirmed a similar study by the Massachusetts Department of Public Health that found that nicotine levels in cigarettes increased by 11 percent between 1997 and 2005. Further, studies by the University of Pittsburgh School of Medicine published in *Public Health Reports* show that there may be increased smoking in both African American and Hispanic populations due to targeted advertising by tobacco companies.

"Cigarettes are finely tuned drug delivery devices, designed to perpetuate a tobacco pandemic," Howard Koh, associate dean for public health at Harvard, told the Associated Press. "Yet, precise information about these products remains shrouded in secrecy, hidden from the public." Tobacco companies disputed the initial report from the Massachusetts Department of Public Health, but the data were confirmed by researchers at Harvard.

How Do You Get Addicted?

Nicotine causes addiction, a term that is widely misunderstood. Addition is *not* caused by an addictive personality. Further, all the stereotypes of why people smoke, such as to look cool or to be one of the gang, are reasons why someone might start smoking or experiment with smoking, but they are not reasons for why you can't quit. Biologically, addiction is caused by your body's exposure to something that makes it feel good. However, when you take a second dose, the effect is not quite as strong, so, you have to increase the dose to equal the effect of the first dose. Over time, you need more and more just to feel "normal."

That's not all of the process, however. Once your body has decided it likes what you are putting into it—and this can also apply to things like chocolate or coffee—you develop a specific need that makes it hard to turn down another dose. That is dependency. That's where the increasing dose comes in: Your body adapts to the level or the dose. In the case of smoking, the nicotine makes you feel good, calm, and alert, while, at the same time, your body wants more of the nicotine and adjusts to whatever you give it. That's *tolerance*.

Finally, addiction also is characterized by the decision to continue consuming the substance, despite knowing that the substance causes you harm. Drinking and driving makes no sense, but people do it. Do you know anyone with a drinking problem who gets into a car and says, "I'm going out on the highway to cause a 10-car pile-up"? Of course not.

Nicotine is almost the perfect drug when it comes to keeping people hooked and forcing them to increase their daily dose. Addiction experts will tell you that relapse is also part of the definition of the disease. It takes more than one effort for most people to stop smoking. This is good news because it means that the more you try to stop, the better the odds are that you will eventually make it.

What about Psychological Addiction?

Some experts believe that there is a difference between physical and psychological addiction. Does a psychological addiction imply that you are a damaged person who can't help yourself? Psychological addiction is supposed to be a precursor to physical addiction or an excuse for not stopping the behavior. There is some evidence that you might be a risk taker who tries potentially harmful activities, but that is a different issue. Regardless, once you start using something that gets you high or makes you feel good, pretty soon you'll need more and more to get that buzz. For heart patients, it really doesn't matter. It's all bad.

Addiction specialists point out that the process of becoming addicted can be subtle. One theory is that all drugs that cause addiction are gateway drugs. This means that one substance leads the person to addiction or to multi-drug use. To go along with that concept, some experts suggest that many drugs lead to a crossover effect. This is controversial because it suggests that smoking cigarettes leads to smoking marijuana, which leads to heroin use or other multi-drug-use scenarios. The data supporting this theory are inconclusive and anecdotal where heart patients are concerned. You have to stop, no matter how you got started or why you are continuing to use tobacco in any form—cigarettes, chewing, sniffing, pipes, or hookahs!

How Do I Stop?

For decades, the office of the surgeon general of the U.S. has led the battle to reduce smoking, educate the public, and make inroads on the problem of teen smoking, which remains widespread. Two websites, www.surgeongeneral.gov/tobacco/ and www.smokefree.gov, are good places to gather information on nicotine addiction and to find hotlines and contact information to immediately begin the process of quitting smoking.

Contacting a website for information is a great first step; however, it is only the opening round in overcoming a very serious physical addiction. You have options open to you:

○ Join a smoking-cessation program
○ Use nicotine replacement/medication
○ Quit "cold turkey"

Before you choose the approach you want to take to stop smoking, prepare yourself to succeed. *I cannot emphasize how important it is to set yourself up for success.* The Centers for Disease Control and Prevention, the office of the surgeon general, and the federal Department of Health and Human Services recommend five actions (the first words of which form the acronym **START**). The entire excellent program can be downloaded as a manual at www.smokefree.gov/pubs/clearing_the_air.pdf. START stands for

S = **Set** a quit date.

T = **Tell** family, friends, and co-workers that you are quitting.

A = **Anticipate** and plan for the challenges you'll face while quitting.

R = **Remove** cigarettes and other tobacco products from your home, car, and workplace.

T = **Talk** to your doctor about getting help to quit.

Here's one more bit of motivation: According to the National Institute of Drug Abuse, "Within 24 hours of quitting, blood pressure and chances of a heart attack decrease. A 35-year-old man who quits smoking will, on average, increase his life expectancy by 5.1 years."

Join a Group

It has been my experience in every aspect of recovery from heart disease that participating in a group has been exceptionally helpful. Whether the group is led by a professional or by a facilitator or member, discussing common problems and exchanging experiences has always helped me.

You will pick up behavior-modification tips that have worked for others that might fit into your lifestyle, such as making lists that remind you of why you want and need to stop smoking, or keeping a journal that helps you record times (triggers) when you needed a cigarette so badly you broke out into a sweat. It will also demonstrate to you that there are others who are facing the same challenges. Feeling part of a team can be comforting and, in my estimation, leads to greater chances of a successful outcome.

Use Medication

Many medical treatments for smoking cessation are based on nicotine replacement. The most common are the transdermal nicotine patch, nicotine gum, and nicotine nasal inhalers. The concept of these products is that they reduce the withdrawal symptoms that occur when you stop smoking. The nicotine they give off counterbalances the nicotine you crave, but does not give you the buzz, and your heart and body are spared the dozens of deadly chemicals delivered every time you inhale. While originally available by prescription only, both the gum and patches are available over-the-counter. There are also lozenges and any number of alternative products, from potions to fake cigarettes, to help break your oral fixation on cigarettes.

For some time, there has been a search for a "magic pill" to break the tobacco habit. For the last few decades, an antidepressant, bupropion (Zyban), has been found to provide the same effect as the replacement devices do in releasing small amounts of dopamine in the brain. The latest and most controversial similar medication is the highly promoted varenicline (Chantix), which became available in 2006. It releases dopamine in the brain, but it also is supposed to block the sites (receptors) in your brain where nicotine activates those positive feelings. Chantix is expensive, but it certainly costs less than cigarettes, although it is unclear how well it works. In addition, numerous side effects, mostly gastric, have been reported.

The Mayo Clinic's opinion about Chantix is straightforward: "For your best chance at quitting smoking with Chantix, you must be committed to your goal. Chantix and other stop smoking aids may increase the likelihood that you'll quit smoking, but they don't make quitting easy. Most smokers try many times to quit. Most try many different medications and strategies, such as counseling, to stop smoking before they finally succeed. Quitting smoking is very difficult and requires planning and persistence, but it can be done.

"Talk to your doctor about your many options for quitting smoking, including counseling. Together, you can decide what stop smoking medication or strategy might be best for you."

As with all smoking-cessation products, you can improve your chances of success by participating in some form of counseling.

Going Cold Turkey

Going "cold turkey" is a slang term for simply stopping smoking suddenly and completely. You have probably talked to or met people who have simply stopped smoking and have been successful—for at least a time. It is not an urban myth that cold turkey doesn't work because you relapse. Remember that you are fighting an addiction and that addiction specialists also consider *relapse as part of the definition of recovery.*

Fighting an addiction is often so difficult that you can be successful at quitting smoking for a period, then you start smoking all over again, then you quit again. Remember that the day you stop, you begin to recover health. So the day you stop again, you start recovering again. Be aware of websites filled with "quit cold turkey" devices. They can be traps for people desperate to quit smoking.

There is no reason not to want to go cold turkey; however, again, the final decision about what will work for you should be made by your doctor and you.

What About Weight Gain?

By far the most common excuse for refusing to stop smoking is that it leads to weight gain. The reality, say the experts at the Cleveland Clinic, is that not all people pack on pounds when they stop smoking. Of those who do, most only gain six to eight pounds. Only 10 percent of people who quit gain more than 30 pounds. So while most smokers weigh about four to ten pounds less than non-smokers, weight gain after quitting smoking generally levels off within six months.

Most people gain weight after smoking because smoking increases your metabolic rate, which burns more calories. In addition, quitting may be an excuse to fill the void with candy, alcohol, and sugar-filled soft drinks and foods. The reason is simple: Sugar and carbohydrates have a similar effect on the brain's pleasure centers. In fact, all foods have the same effect, and most of the food we eat also provides needed vitamins, calories, and nutrients. Snacking is fine, but limit it.

Losing weight after ceasing smoking is not quite the same as simply going on a diet because years of smoking may have damaged your heart and lungs. Adding weight rapidly may do further damage, leading to diabetes or more stress on your cardiovascular system. You may feel massive cravings as your system withdraws from nicotine. Weight-loss plans begun after quitting smoking should be cleared with your doctor. A great tool to answer many questions about weight control after quitting smoking is at www.smokefree.gov/pubs/FFree3.pdf. This document was created by the H. Lee Moffitt Cancer Center & Research Institute at the University of South Florida.

Pregnancy

It's absurdly redundant to point out that if smoking is so deadly for people, then smoking while pregnant is simply asking for trouble. According to the National Institute of Drug Abuse, "In the U.S., it is estimated that 18 percent of pregnant women smoke during their pregnancies." Deadly substances given off by tobacco, like carbon monoxide and nicotine, can reduce blood supply to your baby. Worse, "nicotine also readily crosses the placenta with concentrations to the fetus as much as 15 percent higher than levels in the mothers." The data show that nicotine is found in breast milk and in the amniotic fluid.

If you smoke during pregnancy, your baby will be harmed. Women who smoke more than a pack a day during pregnancy nearly double the risk that the child will become addicted to tobacco if she smokes later in life. Every bit of scientific evidence about smoking and pregnancy screams, "If you care for your baby, don't smoke!"

Children and Cigarettes

It's hard to believe that any parent would want a child or adolescent to smoke. Yet by growing up in a house with smokers puffing away in every room, children are already feeling the effects of secondhand smoke. Parents have a tremendous amount of influence over children who may be tempted to use any substance of abuse, so parents who smoke are sending a terrible message, and the message is, unfortunately, getting through to their children.

The National Institute of Drug Abuse reports that

- 4 million adolescents used a tobacco product during the past month (2004);
- 90 percent of smokers begin before age 18; and
- more than 6 million adolescent smokers will die prematurely from smoking-related diseases.

Besides the "I look cool with a cigarette" attitude that many teens have, there is also evidence from animal studies that indicates that teenagers may have an actual sensitivity to cigarette smoke that can increase their dependency on cigarettes.

The bottom line on smoking is simple. Don't smoke around your children. Talk to your children about peer pressure and how to handle it. Stop together—make it a family event! Educate children about the health and economic issues surrounding cigarette use. Excellent information is available from a local smoking-cessation program or government resources.

IN A SENTENCE:

> *To stop smoking, you will have to seek every resource and source of inner strength you have, but it's worth it to save your heart and your life.*

Lowering Your Cholesterol

THERE IS a single battle that I have waged to reduce my heart disease risk that has been more difficult for me than any other. That is to bring my cholesterol and other lipid levels down to a normal range. One reason it has been so hard is that I was born with a family history of high cholesterol. Another is that, for many years, I did not practice the sort of dietary and health behavior that would bring about change. There is no question that my predisposition for **hypercholesterolemia** (high cholesterol) was handed down genetically from family members who had serious and ultimately fatal heart disease.

Cholesterol and other lipid levels in your blood correlate directly with your odds of a heart attack, angina, and other coronary artery diseases. Pile bad diet, obesity, and a sedentary life on top and you might as well check into the coronary care unit now because you could end up there at some point. My wake-up call came when I was being discharged from the hospital after my quadruple bypass. Along with a set of cardiac-rehab instructions, there was a set of target goals for my cholesterol levels and my current blood tests. I realized that my chances of beating the odds without some intervention were not great.

What Is Cholesterol?

Cholesterol is a waxy, white, odorless, tasteless substance that forms part of every cell in your body. Cholesterol circulates constantly through your body, and it is an essential part of every organ. It is not a fat, as many people think. The body needs certain levels of cholesterol. We also need certain kinds of fat to keep the body energized. Generally, we acquire this fat through dietary cholesterol, but if we eat foods that are rich in cholesterol, it can be harmful to us. When we eat foods that are lower in cholesterol, our risk decreases.

For most people, cholesterol's effect as a heart disease risk factor is largely a product of lifestyle; however, some people are born with a heightened level of harmful cholesterol in their bodies, a condition called hyperlipidemia.

Good Cholesterol, Bad Cholesterol— What Does It Mean?

Until recently, I had always found the "good" and "bad" cholesterol discussions confusing, and you may feel the same. Think of it this way: HDL stands for "highly desirable levels"; LDL stands for "less-desirable levels" of cholesterol.

HDL ("good cholesterol") and LDL ("bad cholesterol") have different but equally legitimate functions in the overall health picture. LDL helps our bodies with cell membrane growth. However, because that can involve the structure of the arterial walls, too much LDL in the bloodstream builds blockages. HDL cholesterol is high in protein, and it is removed by the body through the liver, lowering the possibility of arterial blockages.

How Do Cholesterol Levels Affect Heart Disease?

Blockages caused by high LDL levels lead to atherosclerosis, a buildup of plaque and other substances on the inner wall of the arteries that narrows them. Narrowed arteries reduce the normal flow of blood that carries oxygen to the heart. Without oxygen, stresses on the heart increase, making it pump under duress to maintain normal function.

This reduction in blood flow can lead to chest pain, known as angina, and, ultimately, a heart attack.

In addition, triglycerides, which store fat as an energy source for metabolic activity, also have to be carefully watched. As triglyceride levels increase, so do atherosclerotic obstructions.

Managing your cholesterol and other harmful substances in your bloodstream is one of the most important ways to control heart disease risk. Cholesterol and other lipids (the body's fat substances, including triglycerides) are needed by our body to create internal energy. They are the essential building blocks of body tissues and organs.

There are other ways of measuring heart health, but because our cholesterol levels are correlative to whether or not we are developing dangerous blockages in our arteries, it can be a good measure of our risk. As you remember, modifying risk factors is key to recovery from heart disease. Cholesterol is an important risk factor to keep under control. Further, it is not easy to do this, but it is one thing that you can do with some effort and discipline.

To be successful in reducing or managing heart disease risk, make sure you receive your LDL and HDL levels from the doctor and make sure you get the patient information handout from your pharmacist with your prescriptions. These are important tools.

It is likely that your cardiologist will want to treat all of your lipids. When you talk to your cardiologist, ask about joining a lipid clinic. Most top-notch cardiology practices have a physician-led program that is staffed by nurse practitioners, physician's assistants, or other clinical associates who will see you regularly and keep track of your progress.

Staying on top of your cholesterol levels can also be a complicated process involving a combination of diet and multiple medications. It's important to note that beyond family history, age and gender can affect cholesterol levels. With age, both men's and women's cholesterol levels rise, especially in women after menopause (see **Week Three**). Smoking and high blood pressure also can promote higher levels of cholesterol.

What Are the Right Cholesterol Levels?

Over the past three decades, the effects of cholesterol have been studied extensively, and there is a general agreement within the medical profession about its effects and how much of it indicates a serious risk factor. While cardiologists do sometimes disagree about which cholesterol value (or number) is more important, they agree that the main goal is to get all of these values into line.

Unless you've had a heart attack or you suffer from angina, you may never know that your cholesterol levels are not in balance. In general, having high cholesterol levels does not produce symptoms. You may only know that these levels are elevated when it's too late, which is another reason to make sure that your regular exams include what is called a blood lipid panel, which produces a **lipid profile**.

Cholesterol levels are measured through a simple blood test that should be done after you have had no food for 12 hours. This fasting test will measure your total cholesterol and levels of HDL, LDL, and triglycerides. The actual measurement is the amount of cholesterol in your bloodstream expressed in a numerical value. This test will show how many milligrams of cholesterol your body has per deciliter of circulating blood (expressed as mg/dL).

The numerical value is measured against a scientifically accepted range that indicates your risk potential.

According to the American Heart Association, these values are as follows:

Total cholesterol:

- ○ Below 200 mg/dL lowers your heart disease risk
- ○ 200–239 mg/dL is borderline high risk
- ○ 240 mg/dL and above is high risk

LDL cholesterol:

- ○ Below 70 mg/dL would be the best goal for patients with established atherosclerosis (coronary artery disease)
- ○ Below 100 mg/dL is ideal
- ○ 100–129 mg/dL is good, but not optimal
- ○ 130–159 mg/dL is borderline high
- ○ 160–189 mg/dL is high
- ○ 190 mg/dL is very high

HDL cholesterol:

- ○ Below 40 mg/dL increases risk for heart disease
- ○ 40–59 mg/dL is good
- ○ Above 60 mg/dL is excellent

Triglycerides:

- ○ Below 150 mg/dL is ideal
- ○ 150–199 mg/dL is borderline
- ○ 200–499 mg/dL is high
- ○ 500 mg/dL is dangerously high

None of the above should be seen as absolutes. Age and other factors can affect triglycerides, and different forms of cholesterol at different levels have individual effects. It is up to your cardiologist or primary care physician to interpret the results of your lipid profile with you to set a treatment plan.

Your doctor may point out that your total-cholesterol-to-HDL ratio is out of whack. This ratio is represented by a number derived from dividing your total cholesterol by your HDL number. In the best case, you would want this ratio to be less than 4 and certainly not above 5. The higher the ratio, the greater your risk for a heart attack. You may also see ratios of LDL/HDL; however, the former method is more common.

Managing Cholesterol

The standard American diet is largely composed of animal-based foods, such as eggs, red meat, some shellfish, and products from whole milk. These and other typical, high-fat choices introduce LDL into the body. In addition, a host of factors, such as smoking, your weight, family history, and age can affect your levels of LDL.

Eliminating cholesterol totally is not the goal because we need some food to stoke the body's energy centers for growth and daily activities. Reducing the amount of certain types of fats is the objective.

Trans Fats

Another dietary product, trans fatty acids, are found in many foods, including vegetable shortening, french fries, most candies, and similar foods. In the early 1900s, trans fats were commercially produced when it was discovered that they were a by-product of partial hydrogenation of plant oil, a method used to create products like Crisco. These products became popular because they had a high melting point, giving them a long shelf life.

While saturated fats, mostly found in meats, increase LDL, trans fats are even more damaging to your health. Studies conducted over the past three decades suggest that trans fats are linked to 30,000 heart disease fatalities each year.

In 2003, the Food and Drug Administration (FDA) required levels of trans fats to be included on all nutrition labels. Recently, cities and restaurants have made headlines by removing trans fats.

These are

- ○ **Saturated fats,** which are found in animal products such as beef, liver, butter, whole milk, eggs, and cheese, and palm and coconut oils, increase LDL levels.
- ○ **Monounsaturated fats** are found in olive and peanut oils and have little effect on cholesterol levels.
- ○ **Polyunsaturated fats** are found in safflower, sesame, cottonseed, sunflower, and soybean oils, and can actually reduce the level of LDL cholesterol in the bloodstream.

The National Heart, Lung, and Blood Institute promotes a dietary program for lowering cholesterol, called the **TLC Diet (Therapeutic Lifestyle Changes)**. It can be found at www.nhlbi.nih.gov.

Reducing the amount of saturated fat–filled foods and replacing them with monounsaturated and polyunsaturated fats that are less damaging should be a daily goal. Mono- and polyunsaturated fats usually are found in some seafoods and most vegetables, and can help to lower the level of LDL and increase the level of HDL in your body. The more HDL you have in your system, the more you lower your heart health risk. Maintain a diet rich in vitamins and nutrients, fruits, vegetables, and whole grains, and stay away from sodium, saturated fats, and refined sugar products.

Cholesterol Medication

It seems as if you can't turn on the TV or read a newspaper or a magazine without finding an article about a cholesterol-lowering breakthrough or yet another advertisement for another medication you "should talk to your doctor about." Medications designed to raise, lower, stabilize, or modify cholesterol come on the market every day, and their value, popularity, cost, and recall change just as quickly. For example, there seems to be some controversy over which is more important: raising HDL or lowering LDL. Different studies have been published, but there is a lack of medical consensus, except that having all your lipid values in the proper range is the best.

Here are some of the more widely used medications for cholesterol regulation:

Fibrates
gemfibrozil (Lopid)
This drug raises HDL cholesterol levels and lowers triglyceride levels.

Resins
Resins are also called bile acid–binding medications. They work in the intestines by promoting increased disposal of cholesterol. According to the University of Pennsylvania Health System, "when used with dietary control, bile acid resins can reduce LDL levels by 15 to 20 percent. When bile acid resins are combined with nicotinic acid, LDL levels can drop as much as 40 to 60 percent."

Some of these drugs include cholestyramine (Questran, Prevalite, Lo-Cholest), colestipol (Colestid), colesevelam (WelChol), and clofibrate (Atromid-S).

Statins
Statins are effective for lowering LDL cholesterol levels and have few immediate short-term side effects. They interrupt the formation of cholesterol in circulating blood. Commonly prescribed statins include

○ atorvastatin (Lipitor)
○ fluvastatin (Lescol)

○ lovastatin (Mevacor)
○ pravastatin (Pravachol)
○ rosuvastatin calcium (Crestor)
○ simvastatin (Zocor)

Niacin (nicotinic acid) comes in prescription form and as a dietary supplement. Dietary-supplement niacin is not regulated by the U.S. Food and Drug Administration (FDA), as prescription niacin is. It may contain variable amounts of niacin, and the amount of niacin may even vary from lot to lot within the same brand. Dietary-supplement niacin must **not** be used as a substitute for prescription niacin. It should **not** be used for lowering cholesterol because of potential side effects. Also, if you are taking any of the medications discussed here, it is important that you do not stop taking them without consulting your doctor.

IN A SENTENCE:

> *Normalizing your cholesterol levels requires diet, exercise, and a wide range of medications that your doctor will tailor to your specific situation, but you must take them as prescribed for the greatest effectiveness.*

Obesity

OBESITY IS a major problem worldwide. Each year, more than 400,000 Americans die as a result of obesity. We are actually heading toward a point when obesity is a greater health risk than starvation is. Of the 6 billion people worldwide, 1 billion are overweight, compared to 800 million who lack enough food, according to the World Health Organization (WHO).

Obesity and weight loss have been prominent topics in conversations with heart patients in my recovery group, and with experienced cardio-rehab specialists. Being overweight is also one of the toughest risk factors to get under control. Losing weight and maintaining that weight loss is not easy, and anyone who tells you that it is isn't telling the truth. My own battle with my weight has been critical to regaining my health. If I can overcome the obstacles that lead to restored health, especially losing weight, you can, too!

Are You Obese?

Defining obesity is not hard. Accepting that you are obese *is* hard. Yet there is a wide range of solutions, from counseling to surgery, so don't give up.

The simple definition of obesity, according to the American Heart Association (AHA) is "too much body fat." According to the National Heart, Lung, and Blood Institute, obesity is expressed as a ratio of your height and weight. This provides your Body Mass Index (BMI) value, which is generally accepted as a measure of excess weight and your heart risk.

To Calculate Your BMI:

Multiply your weight (in pounds) x 704.5. Divide that number by your height (in inches), then divide that number by your height again. This gives you a BMI number that you can round off.

An example:

187 pounds x 704.5 = 131741.5. Divided by 67 (inches) = 1966.29 divided again by 67 (inches) = 29.34. This is the BMI number.

(Note: This is a formula used by NIH. There is some small variation in the multiplier used by other groups; however, the difference is negligible.)

Another way to find your BMI is to use the chart on the following page.

To find a BMI Calculator for children from the Centers for Disease Control log on to http://apps.nccd.cdc.gov/dnpabmi/Calculator.aspx.

What Does Your BMI Mean for You?

If you have a BMI of 30 or above, you are technically obese. However, if the number is below 30, you still are not in the clear. You still may be **overweight**. Multiple groups, such as WHO, define "overweight" as a BMI of 25 or higher. One of the problems with using the BMI scale is that many people who are fit and trim have a high BMI because their bodies are muscular. (Still, a pound of muscle weighs the same as a pound of fat.) On the other hand, a person might have a low BMI but be malnourished and unhealthy.

BMI is a good general measure because it is a simple reference point that you can use as a personal benchmark. The point is that *if you have a high BMI, it is likely that you have a seriously increased risk for heart disease, high blood pressure, and diabetes.*

Body Mass Index Table

To use the table, find the appropriate height in the left-hand column. Move across to a given weight. The number at the top of the column is the BMI for that height and weight. Pounds have been rounded off.

BMI	19	20	21	22	23	24	25	26	27	28	29	30	31	32	33	34	35
Height (in.)							**Body Weight (pounds)**										
58	91	96	100	105	110	115	119	124	129	134	138	143	148	153	158	162	167
59	94	99	104	109	114	119	124	128	133	138	143	148	153	158	163	168	173
60	97	102	107	112	118	123	128	133	138	143	148	153	158	163	168	174	179
61	100	106	111	116	122	127	132	137	143	148	153	158	164	169	174	180	185
62	104	109	115	120	126	131	136	142	147	153	158	164	169	175	180	186	191
63	107	113	118	124	130	135	141	146	152	158	163	169	175	180	186	191	197
64	110	116	122	128	134	140	145	151	157	163	169	174	180	186	192	197	204
65	114	120	126	132	138	144	150	156	162	168	174	180	186	192	198	204	210
66	118	124	130	136	142	148	155	161	167	173	179	186	192	198	204	210	216
67	121	127	134	140	146	153	159	166	172	178	185	191	198	204	211	217	223
68	125	131	138	144	151	158	164	171	177	184	190	197	203	210	216	223	230
69	128	135	142	149	155	162	169	176	182	189	196	203	209	216	223	230	236
70	132	139	146	153	160	167	174	181	188	195	202	209	216	222	229	236	243
71	136	143	150	157	165	172	179	186	193	200	208	215	222	229	236	243	250
72	140	147	154	162	169	177	184	191	199	206	213	221	228	235	242	250	258
73	144	151	159	166	174	182	189	197	204	212	219	227	235	242	250	257	265
74	148	155	163	171	179	186	194	202	210	218	225	233	241	249	256	264	272
75	152	160	168	176	184	192	200	208	216	224	232	240	248	256	264	272	279
76	156	164	172	180	189	197	205	213	221	230	238	246	254	263	271	279	287

BMI	36	37	38	39	40	41	42	43	44	45	46	47	48	49	50	51	52	53	54
Height (in.)									**Body Weight (pounds)**										
58	172	177	181	186	191	196	201	205	210	215	220	224	229	234	239	244	248	253	258
59	178	183	188	193	198	203	208	212	217	222	227	232	237	242	247	252	257	262	267
60	184	189	194	199	204	209	215	220	225	230	235	240	245	250	255	261	266	271	276
61	190	195	201	206	211	217	222	227	232	238	243	248	254	259	264	269	275	280	285
62	196	202	207	213	218	224	229	235	240	246	251	256	262	267	273	278	284	289	295
63	203	208	214	220	225	231	237	242	248	254	259	265	270	278	282	287	293	299	304
64	209	215	221	227	232	238	244	250	256	262	267	273	279	285	291	296	302	308	314
65	216	222	228	234	240	246	252	258	264	270	276	282	288	294	300	306	312	318	324
66	223	229	235	241	247	253	260	266	272	278	284	291	297	303	309	315	322	328	334
67	230	236	242	249	255	261	268	274	280	287	293	299	306	312	319	325	331	338	344
68	236	243	249	256	262	269	276	282	289	295	302	308	315	322	328	335	341	348	354
69	243	250	257	263	270	277	284	291	297	304	311	318	324	331	338	345	351	358	365
70	250	257	264	271	278	285	292	299	306	313	320	327	334	341	348	355	362	369	376
71	257	265	272	279	286	293	301	308	315	322	329	338	343	351	358	365	372	379	386
72	265	272	279	287	294	302	309	316	324	331	338	346	353	361	368	375	383	390	397
73	272	280	288	295	302	310	318	325	333	340	348	355	363	371	378	386	393	401	408
74	280	287	295	303	311	319	326	334	342	350	358	365	373	381	389	396	404	412	420
75	287	295	303	311	319	327	335	343	351	359	367	375	383	391	399	407	415	423	431
76	295	304	312	320	328	336	344	353	361	369	377	385	394	402	410	418	426	435	443

To find a BMI Calculator for children from the Centers for Disease Control log on to http://apps.nccd.cdc.gov/dnpabmi/Calculator.aspx

You are not alone if you are obese. According to researchers

○ one in three Americans is obese.

○ 81.6 percent of African American women and 75 percent of Mexican American women are overweight or obese.

○ 69 percent of African American men and 76 percent of Mexican American men are either obese or overweight.

○ 20 percent of the population in certain urban areas of China are overweight or obese.

○ 23 percent of people in the U.K. and 12 percent of German citizens are obese.

○ compared to 3.6 million a decade ago, 5.9 million people in France today are obese.

What Causes Obesity?

It's hardly surprising that fat causes obesity, but not the fat you see when you're in the dressing room trying on a new pair of tight jeans or a new bathing suit. That is what we usually call "flab," but it's actually cutaneous fat. The fat that is at the root of obesity is called visceral fat, and the amount of it found in your body is indicative of your heart risk. You look heavy because the cutaneous fat lies near the skin and piles up, while the visceral fat is deep in your body, wrapped around your liver, heart, and other organs and accumulating in your abdomen. This is why it is sometimes called "organ fat," and it's fat that will kill you.

Visceral fat metabolizes in the liver, producing circulating blood cholesterol, creating the plaque that keeps oxygenated blood from the heart. Not surprisingly, visceral fat also comes from consuming certain foods that contain certain saturated fat: butter, fried foods, fatty meats, and the like.

A sedentary lifestyle can increase visceral fat. One study (*Science Daily*, 2003) carried out at Duke University Medical Center matched a group with high levels of exercise against a group who had lower amounts of exercise and found that the more active group had significant decreases in visceral fat over a fairly short period of time.

One sure sign that you are accumulating visceral fat is the growth of your paunch. The Duke researchers "were surprised by how rapidly fat accumulated deep in the abdomens of participants who did not exercise." The less you exercise, the quicker your life can go downhill. A simple way to think of this is that if you continue to take in more calories than you burn, you automatically increase your weight and add strain to your system, including your heart (see **Month Six**).

Are You an Apple or a Pear?

Your body shape, especially when you are overweight, seems to have a connection to your heart risk. The "pear" shape indicates that you have a great deal of cutaneous fat; the "apple" shape equates with greater risk because it indicates a greater proportion of visceral fat. While both shapes indicate excess weight, heart risk is greater for those with the "apple" shape.

Some researchers think that a high waist-to-hip ratio—your waist and hip circumferences are close—also is a strong risk factor for heart attack. A large study published in *The Lancet* (November 2005) reinforced this point when it reported that BMI measurements indicated a clear risk for a heart attack—and so can your waist size. This study also included both men and women and cut across multiple ethnic groups in several countries.

What Does Obesity Lead To?

There is very little disagreement about the risk of heart disease and other conditions caused by obesity. Add to that smoking, family history, and high cholesterol levels, and you are a walking time bomb. Eventually, if you do not do something, you'll explode, as I did.

As you add pounds, you immediately begin to increase your blood pressure. With continual stress on your cardiovascular system, soon you will have high blood pressure, or **hypertension.** High blood pressure is a silent, asymptomatic disorder that leads to stroke. The older you are, the higher the risk of stroke. According to the Centers for Disease Control and Prevention, *half of Americans between ages 55 and 64 have high blood pressure!*

Obesity clogs your arteries with more LDL than HDL, which leaves you at enormous risk for a heart attack.

For people who have a family history of diabetes, obesity can increase or create risk in those with no history by creating insulin resistance. Insulin is a naturally occurring substance secreted by the pancreas and carried in the blood. It is vital to regulating the level of energy our cells produce. However, high amounts of visceral fat eventually prevent the insulin from reaching the proper cells, causing the pancreas to produce more and more insulin until it eventually wears down glucose levels, resulting in atherosclerosis and type 2 diabetes.

Multiple studies in men and women have shown that obesity increases the risk of coronary artery disease by three to four, leading to a heart attack. Obesity is also linked to congestive heart failure, possibly some cancers, gallstones, osteoarthritis, and sleep disorders.

The Risk Has Already Spread to Your Children

It's hardly news that children around the world are heavier than they were in previous generations. It's almost a self-fulfilling prophecy, given that our kids spend so much time in sedentary pursuits. Previous generations of kids had little choice but to be active because we were told to go out and play, and we'd hop on our bikes and take off. Today, we don't let our children wander too far, their after-school activities are scheduled, and they have lots of electronic toys to keep them occupied.

According to the Mayo Clinic (www.mayoclinic.com/health/childhood-obesity/DS00698/DSECTION=3), in just two decades, the prevalence of overweight children in the U.S. between the ages of six and 11 doubled, and the number has tripled among American teenagers. The annual National Health and Nutrition Examination Survey by the Centers for Disease Control and Prevention found that about one-third of children in the U.S. are overweight or are at risk of becoming overweight. In total, about 25 million children and adolescents in this country are overweight or are nearly overweight.

This situation is leading to an even greater health debacle in the future because the population entering the workforce after college will be overwhelmed quickly by such risks for heart disease as diabetes, high blood pressure, and coronary artery disease. The time to start fighting this problem is now—before your kids are set in a couch-potato lifestyle and never discover the benefits of an active life. This is not a problem for your children, but a family problem that you can overcome together!

While food manufacturers are jumping on the "healthy food" bandwagon, they have only done so under the pressure of lawsuits. Slowly,

fast food is being kicked out of the school systems, and unless we continue to do more, our children may begin to die before we do. Perhaps
one number tells the story more succinctly. The annual worldwide rev-
enue of the children's food industry is over $600 billion.

You Can Overcome Obesity

Overcoming obesity is not simply about risk, or how and why we have
this problem. You have to learn about food, how it can be best used, and
how to avoid buying the foods that only cause you more distress.

There is good news and some evidence that a sea change is coming.
Like many of you, I shop at warehouse stores when I can. Until April 2007,
I never saw a product on the shelves that could remotely be considered
healthful. That has changed, albeit slowly. One-hundred-calorie snack
packs and organic produce now are being featured at these stores along
with environmentally conscious products like long-lasting light bulbs.

The other good news is that obesity is not a life sentence. In the next
section, you will find some steps you can use to begin to cope with your
weight problem. Obesity costs society billions of dollars each year in
health-care costs, lost productivity, and strain on our own psyches. Along
with family history and smoking, obesity is one side of a health risk tri-
angle. It does not have to be that way.

IN A SENTENCE:

> *While it's obvious that fat causes obesity, few of us recognize that
> exterior flab (cutaneous fat) is not as dangerous as the visceral fat
> that is wrapped around the liver, heart, and other vital organs
> deep in the body and that leads to increased plaque that clogs
> blood vessels.*

Losing Weight and Keeping It Off

IF YOU are obese or overweight, you probably have tried many weight-loss products; diet books; fitness programs; low-calorie, pre-packaged diet products or pills; and diet camps that guarantee the pounds will simply fall off. Having seen the happy, fit models on the packaging of many items, you might have concluded that the problem is you. At some point you may have just decided "Why bother?" and reached for the pint of Chunky Monkey ice cream, spoon in hand.

Well, it's not you. You are a victim of an insidious $30 billion industry with more than a 90 percent failure rate. Worse, all this diet noise you are exposed to has led you to believe that anything on the market is safe. Reports have shown that 64 percent of Americans think that if there are no side-effect warnings on diet products, the product possesses no side effects, and 54 percent of Americans think that those hundreds of diet products sold everywhere are approved by the U.S. Food and Drug Administration. They aren't. It's not uncommon for an individual to spend from $10,000 to $100,000 on a weight-loss program that results in a net loss of only a few pounds.

If this has happened to you, you should be furious. As an overweight person, you may have felt that you were discriminated against, and now you've discovered that cynical weight-loss scam artists keep you coming back for more. But as a formerly over-weight guy with heart disease, I can tell you that there *are* ways to re-duce your weight, keep it off, and improve your heart health. I have done it. While it is not easy, all that it required was *one single trait that every overweight person has: motivation*. The secret is to turn the switch to "on" and keep your motivation strong, even as you keep trying to lose weight. There is a way to harness your motivation and make it work for you.

Your Road forward Requires a Look Back

Every person who needs to lose weight arrived at this point through a different track, whether it's biology or behavior. For the first 45 years of my life, I was a short, relatively thin guy, 5'7", 145 pounds with a 33-inch waist. Fortunately (if that's the right word), my heart-health disas-ters and a 30-pound weight gain didn't happen at the same time. If they had, I might not have been alive to witness things that gave me great joy over the past decade.

Prior to my coronary artery bypass graft in 2000, my surgeon told me that I'd "do fine because I was young and in good shape." There is an in-teresting irony there, since being young and needing a quadruple bypass is not a good omen. But I did well and was told that, as a diabetic, I had to follow a specific diet that was carefully laid out for me. Still, after my surgery, I reverted to a poor diet: jars of candy on the coffee table, junk-food meals, consuming whole packages of Double Stuf Oreos in a single sitting, and ordering pretty much anything at a restaurant without con-sidering the effect of my conspicuous consumption on my already com-promised cardiovascular system.

Over the next several years, I was fortunate to have a very active lifestyle and a busy professional life that involved travel and long, hectic, calorie-burning hours. Since I was not gaining weight, as a natural-born "denier" I assumed that if my waist size remained stable, my interior car-diac pathways would keep functioning properly.

Here's the prime myth behind my rationale that you might also be buying into: I had a diet that wasn't adding weight, so I didn't need to go on a diet. This is the simple, key point to remember: Diet means more than one thing, especially if you are fighting heart disease and are over-weight or obese.

My lack of diet *compliance* (not awareness) caught up to me three years ago when I took an executive position, working in an office for the first time in a decade. This involved a long commute (snacks included), then lots of sedentary hours behind a desk. Before I knew it, two years later I was three sizes bigger. My so-called fitness was gone and, worse, my cardiologist, Dr. Rimmerman, became alarmed at my cholesterol levels and my overall condition. Two small vessels that had been used in the bypass had closed, and I was not a candidate for stenting. My diabetes worsened, and I had to give myself insulin shots for the first time. Three medications were added to stabilize my lipids and to help keep my sugars in control. The side effects, gastric and others, were unpleasant.

Slowly, it dawned on me that *I* was the problem, not the disease. I hated the way I looked. I was fat.

So How Do You Start to Lose Weight?

As a heart patient you can never forget that losing weight requires recognizing that a diet and dieting are really the same thing. In order to succeed, *you must have a clear idea of why you want to lose weight.*

1. To regain your health

You know now that you cannot recover from heart disease as long as you are obese. As you've read earlier, visceral fat is literally strangling your organs. If your blood is circulating through sludge or your blood vessels can throw off a clot that will kill you, it does not matter whether you can fit into pants of a certain size. This sounds harsh, but it was only the realization that my waist size was not going to get smaller until my cholesterol dropped, my blood pressure was normal, my glucose readings were acceptable, and I remembered to take medications each day, even if the side effects were unpleasant, that motivated me.

2. Pick a reinforcement that works for you

Everyone has secondary reasons for losing weight, which is very important because we all need reinforcement when we've accomplished something very difficult. Certainly, that is true for weight loss. I've met many people who have interesting approaches. My favorite was a cook-book author who had written several classic books. Every time she lost a certain amount of weight and kept it off for a length of time, she bought herself a nice ring. Gradually, she covered each finger several times.

Accumulating things as rewards is a common motivator, and if it works, there is no reason not to use it as a tool. While writing this book, I've spent considerable time with groups of people—mostly women—who are losing weight, and not one of them has cited vanity as the reason. All are concerned about their health, their family responsibilities, or trying to get their husbands, many of whom have had heart problems, on a better track.

"Changing Your Diet" vs. "Dieting"

When you have become clear in your own mind that you must lose weight to survive, you must recognize that you are not *going on* a diet. What you are going to be doing is *changing your diet*. This means that your diet is what you are going to eat for the rest of your life. It will be a major contribution to your heart health during the first year of your recovery.

Remember, *you cannot begin any sort of weight loss without talking to your doctor, a registered dietician, and other professionals, such as an exercise coach*.

Here's a secret that will boost your chances of success: *Enlist your spouse, partner, children, or a friend to support you in your effort*. Had I not had support in the past year, I would not have gotten healthier and lost weight. It doesn't take the proverbial village to lose weight, but it helps if you have a partner in the process.

Another problem that comes with changing your food lifestyle is having people around you who are eating foods loaded with saturated fat. Getting in control of the food served in your household and what your kids eat is important. Here are some tips from other people who have solved this problem:

- ○ One woman with grown children explained to me how she got so much support from her husband: "He eats what I cook or he doesn't eat."
- ○ With an active, growing family, dietary change is more difficult. A young mother in her mid-30s with three kids under age 12 used a somewhat devious approach. While learning to keep away from the

cookies and other things children normally want, she made healthy food that tasted good at mealtimes. She simply never told her family what was in it. Most important, she shared with them why she needed a healthy diet and why it was good for them, too. Gradually, they adjusted and, after learning about her need for good food, they became part of her support group.

○ An older mother with young teenagers worked a reward/treat system and good health behavior into one plan. The family lived about a mile and a half from the great local ice-cream parlor. The mother told them they could have ice cream if they walked there and back. The children walked along and Mom got a "no-sugar added" bowl for herself!

What Should Your Diet Be?

Your diet has to be targeted to your specific heart disease, and if you are overweight, that, too, will become part of the plan. For example, if you have congestive heart failure, you doctor will want to ensure that your sodium intake is reduced to lower the likelihood of retained fluid and to enlarge optimal heart function.

In some cases of severe obesity, gastrointestinal bypass (see below) may be an option for treatment. Your diet must maximize your recovery, but that is not as difficult as it sounds and it doesn't usually require some sort of diet of the month.

Get Up and Move!

Assuming your cardiac condition has been stabilized, the first thing you can do for your health and your weight is to get up and move around. You don't have to join a club or gym to start incorporating movement into your life. It has been proven that being active, more than dietary modification, is the most effective step you can take to lose weight and keep it off.

Simply using stairs instead of an elevator or taking a walk around the neighborhood will produce a change in your weight. (There is an added benefit if you can walk outside during the day, since sunshine can provide vitamin D and other benefits.) At first you may not be able to take long walks, but gradually build up your strength and then make walking a daily part of your life.

1. Learn to cook—the right way

Seriously, learning to cook is one of the best things you can do to help control your weight. Probably everyone reading this book knows how to cook on some level, especially if you have kids.

Cooking the *right* way is something else. It does not mean that you have wasted money on your expensive cooking lessons, or that you have to throw out Grandma's family recipes or make bland, low-cal dishes. It does not mean that you can't throw a dinner party or have a birthday party for your child. It may mean that certain "givens" in how you cook *will* have to be reconsidered.

It does mean that you have to learn to plan meals ahead. I plan a menu for the coming week so I know what I need to buy at the market. This prevents last-minute compromises, like a run to McDonald's or a quick microwave dinner.

You will have to try out some new things that you may have turned up your nose at in the past. For example, today's low-fat products taste just as good as the fatty, artery-clogging originals—if you know how to use them. My kitchen is filled with great pots and pans, and I love cooking. For years, I would fry chicken cutlets or deep-fry veggies. My salads would drown in my own creamy (i.e., lots of mayonnaise) dressings.

So I changed slowly. I determined what the worst saturated-fat product was that I used the most. The answer was easy: butter. I used it all of the time to sauté, on toast, and as a topping for mashed and baked potatoes.

I made changes. First I tried several spray butter substitutes, which, to my surprise, I liked. I went from using over one pound of butter a week to almost none. Then I found that there are dozens of sugar-free products, including chocolate! When it came to cooking, I started using non-stick cookware or cooking spray instead of butter. I turned to different techniques. I learned that you could brown chicken cutlets in a little olive oil, and then bake it for 15 to 20 minutes, and it would taste as good as fried chicken—if not better.

Is any of this news? Americans have been told for decades what makes a good, healthy meal and how to cook low-fat, nutritious, tasty food. Millions of people who have been using these techniques and others are not heart patients, and they are likely not obese.

One year ago, I began to eat differently, got off my butt, and lost 20 pounds. My blood values are close too or within normal range. My insulin level has been reduced by more than 66 percent. The difference: We learned a new way to cook that works and that has helped restore my health.

The news for you is that when you make these sorts of changes, you will see progress. You will lose some weight, your doctor will give you good news, and, pretty soon, these changes will become a natural part of your life. Today I walk through a supermarket and I never notice the cookies and cakes, but I certainly know my way around the vegetable section. I know how to pick lean meat, and how to cook tastier food. I feel good. You can do this, too. It's not hard, and the change will become evident very quickly.

2. Almost any recipe can be heart-healthy

In the early part of my period of recovery, I learned that any recipe could be converted into a heart-healthy one and that there are limitless sources for them. The Food Network has had a great influence on getting people to cook. It and dozens of online food and cooking sites have created an almost limitless database of recipes that you can search using virtually any set of parameters. If you want a chicken dish with a certain number of calories that can be made in a half hour, it is there. (See **Month Twelve** for a list of recommended websites.)

An easy step you can take to become a healthier cook is to read the Nutrition Facts labels mandated by the FDA. The label tells you what you are eating. It lists calories, total fat, saturated fats, trans fat, cholesterol, sodium, potassium, total carbohydrates, protein, vitamins, and other ingredients. It's important to make sure that what you eat is low in sodium (especially if you have high blood pressure) low in calories. If it says "low fat" or "fat free" on the package, make sure it says that on the label, too. You want any packaged food to be less than 5 percent fat, saturated fats, cholesterol, and sodium to give your heart a fighting chance.

It takes a little time to learn to convert what you read into a plan that meets your dietary needs. When you pick up a box of cereal, for example, you might see that it has 190 calories and only 15 calories from fat. Sounds great? However, beside the other ingredients, you have to look for the two *most* important numbers, sometimes in small print at the top or bottom: "serving size" and "number of servings" in the package. In my favorite cereal, the box has "ten 1-cup servings."

Think of what you are going to actually eat. A cup of anything is about the size of a tennis ball. When you sit down to eat breakfast, how many cups of food do you actually eat? Do you add milk or sugar or fruit that has substantial calories from sugar? Few people eat a good breakfast, and nutritionists generally believe that breakfast is a key part of a healthy diet. Perhaps going with a few cups of cereal and a nutritious topping is a good idea. The point is knowing what you are eating and incorporating it into your dietary life.

One of the most import aspects of learning to cook is recognizing the nutritional value of what you are going to eat and educating yourself about the healthy ingredients in a recipe. This will help you enormously in learning how to substitute ingredients. You do not have to turn to tofu only or to never eat a burger again. You can use very lean meat and a low-fat skim-milk cheese for occasional cheeseburgers. You can "bake" french fries and onion rings that taste just as good or better than the fat-drenched, artery-clogging version. Munch vegetables and low-fat popcorn instead of cookies and cake.

3. Be open to change!

Take an open approach as you develop your cooking skills and apply them to the foods you cook. I was not able to learn how to make changes from existing recipes at first, so I looked up dishes that already had those nutritional values listed in the recipes. Today, there are dozens of cookbooks—not necessarily low-fat-only books—that have picked up on the number of people who are in our position, who need to lose weight and recover from heart disease.

Also look for cookbooks in which the cooking techniques are basically healthy. You can find many excellent cookbooks on stir-frying, which is a very healthy, easy way to cook. Try books on slow cooking, pressure-cooking, and vegetarian cooking.

The value of a good cookbook is that it gives you an instant reference for a meal. You can assess what a dish contains and eventually learn to make substitutions. A good stir-fry menu can be developed into three meals just by switching between very lean sirloin, shrimp, and chicken, using the same types of vegetables for each. If shrimp is not on your list, stir-fried vegetables with tofu is great, too. (See **Month Twelve** for a list of great cookbooks.)

What Else Can You Do?

There are several basics for losing weight and eating for heart health. The FDA recommends that we eat a diet low in saturated fat, especially animal fats and palm and coconut oils; add foods high in monounsaturated fats, such as olive oil, canola oil, and seafood; and eat foods containing polyunsaturated fats found in plants and seafood (safflower oil and corn oil are high in polyunsaturated fats).

Avoid fatty foods like beef, whole milk, cheese, butter, palm oil, and coconut oils. Add fiber from fruits, vegetables, and grains that are reported to improve heart health. The more calories you take in, the more you have to burn off. Keep the scales tipped the right way. Sodium is something we need in limited amounts, but we usually add more on at the table, on popcorn, and in other dishes. Learn to live without it.

Are There Any Good Commercial Diet Programs?

Until 100 years ago, obesity was not a widespread problem in this country. We got plenty of exercise at work, doing manual labor or farming. At first, we got our vitamins in our food. Then the pre-packaged food industry began to flourish but required preservatives and used high levels of sodium, a problem that would eventually be part of our health problems. Health issues used to be more of a result of public health problems and basic hygiene, but those days, thankfully, are gone. We have life-saving medications and surgery. Unfortunately our diets have not changed for the better as life has become easier.

In some parts of the world, however, the people have consistently had healthy hearts, despite having the same rate of industrialization, leisure, and pace of living as the rest of the world. Their diet is the key.

The Food and Drug Administration
Also Recommends:

Instead of:	Do This:
whole or 2 percent milk, and cream	use 1 percent or skim milk
fried foods	eat baked, steamed, boiled, broiled, or microwaved foods
lard, butter, palm, and coconut oils	cook with unsaturated vegetable oils, such as corn, olive, canola, safflower, sesame, soybean, sunflower, or peanut
fatty cuts of meat, such as prime rib	eat lean cuts of meat or cut off the fatty parts
one whole egg in recipes	use two egg whites
sour cream and mayonnaise	use plain low-fat yogurt, low-fat cottage cheese, or low-fat or "light" sour cream
sauces, butter, and salt	season vegetables with herbs and spices
regular hard and processed cheeses	eat low-fat, low-sodium cheeses
salted potato chips and other snacks	choose low-fat, unsalted tortilla and potato chips and unsalted pretzels and popcorn

Mediterranean Diet

The most frequently cited of those is the **Mediterranean diet,** which has been studied and imitated over the past 50 years.

At the basis of this diet's success is that the countries that surround the Mediterranean Sea have very low rates of heart disease, along with low levels of elevated cholesterol, diabetes, and other problems common in the rest of the world. The diet is simple; it emphasizes fresh fruits and vegetables; foods high in fiber; limited meat; plenty of fresh fish, bread, and pasta made from complex carbohydrates; and the basic ingredient that seems to be used in everything, olive oil. The Mediterranean diet is basically a low-fat diet, and anyone who has ever traveled to France, Italy, or Spain can attest that the food was one of the most memorable parts of the trip.

DASH Diet

Another well-known diet is the **DASH (Dietary Approaches to Stop Hypertension) diet** created by the U.S. government more than two decades ago. It recently has been updated to match what we have learned about diet and high blood pressure. Because high blood pressure is a major risk factor in heart disease, this diet is very relevant to you. Researchers have found that "with DASH, blood pressures were reduced through an eating plan that is low in saturated fat, cholesterol, and total fat and that emphasizes fruits, vegetables, and fat-free or low-fat milk and milk products."

According to the National Heart, Lung, and Blood Institute, "this eating plan also includes whole grain products, fish, poultry, and nuts. It is reduced in lean red meat, sweets, added sugars, and sugar-containing beverages compared to the typical American diet. It is rich in potassium, magnesium, and calcium, as well as protein and fiber." To get more information, check out www.nhlbi.nih.gov/health/public/heart/hbp/dash/new_dash.pdf.

These two diets are not the only frameworks for good, healthful eating, which, when added to a doctor-approved exercise program, can help you. The American Heart Association offers dietary guidelines based on hundreds of studies that are similar to the Mediterranean diet. See www.americanheart.org/presenter.jhtml?identifier=1330.

Other Diet Plans

Numerous diet programs have remained popular for many years, and some, for decades. Do they work? If you had asked me that question in June 2006, I'd have laughed. I didn't believe in programs like that.

Well, I have changed my tune. Since June 2006, when I joined Weight Watchers, I have not attended any other program, but I have discovered, after interviewing people who have tried them, that there is no single best bet.

For Americans who want to lose weight, there's certainly no shortage of diets to choose from, with each claiming to offer the best weight-loss solution. The chart on pages 250–251 compares the basic elements of each diet profiled in the Public Broadcasting program "Diet Wars" (www.pbs.org/wgbh/pages/frontline/shows/diet/basics/compare.html).

Should You Join a Program?

When I realized that the reflection in the mirror was no longer what I remembered or wanted it to be, I panicked. I knew that I had to do something, and I was willing to do whatever I could. When you reach this point, one of the most important things to keep in mind is that you need someone to support your effort and help you to use what you've learned about diet.

At the time I was pondering this, I also did some research and found that many of the programs (including the ones in the chart following) were not necessarily a threat to my heart condition. A study printed in the *Journal of the American Medical Association* (January 2005) looked at a "Comparison of the Atkins, Ornish, Weight Watchers, and Zone Diets for Weight Loss and Heart Disease Risk Reduction" and concluded that "each popular diet modestly reduced body weight and several cardiac risk factors at 1 year." They noted that "increased adherence was associated with greater weight loss and cardiac risk factor reduction for each diet group." What this taught me was simple: Diet programs are associated with a lot of myths. Most of them work about as well as the others *if you follow the one you choose and stick with it.* In the case of the ones following, there seems to be little heart risk from the diet itself.

The study also reported that at any time there were over 1,000 diet books on the market, so the consumer has many choices. My decision was probably made the way most people make a choice—word of mouth and evidence that you can see in someone else.

This is exactly what happened when I was told that a man I worked with had lost more than 100 pounds. I was shocked because he was my size, and in much better shape than I was. I had not known him when he was heavy, and to look at him then you would never have guessed it.

Weight Watchers

DATE 1963

AUTHOR Jean Neiditch, housewife

PREMISE General goal of 10 percent weight loss with a "points" system to simplify calorie counting

LOGIC Every food is assigned a point value based on calories, total fat, and dietary fiber to meet a daily targeted point range. Weekly meetings create a supportive and educational community. There is an emphasis on exercise and making the diet part of a long-term lifestyle change.

CRITICISM Some members shy away from the weekly weigh-ins and meetings.

SAMPLE DINNER Chinese vegetables with chicken, tossed salad, brown rice (10 points)

Atkins

DATE *Dr. Atkins' Diet Revolution*, first published in 1972

AUTHOR Robert C. Atkins, M.D., cardiologist

PREMISE Achieve a "metabolic advantage" with a four-phase diet low in carbohydrates and high in protein

LOGIC By reducing the intake of carbohydrates, you will burn excess body fat for fuel and feel satiated from a diet that emphasizes fats and protein. Essential nutrients come from low-carbohydrate vegetables.

CRITICISM Critics, who range from vegetarians like Dr. Dean Ornish to proponents of cardiac health such as Nathan Pritikin, argue that the long-term effects of a diet high in protein and saturated fats are unknown.

SAMPLE DINNER From the preliminary "induction" phase: broiled steak, oven-fried turnips, arugula, and Boston lettuce salad

Pritikin

DATE First Longevity Center opened in 1976

AUTHOR Nathan Pritikin, engineer

PREMISE "Caloric Density Solution," a disciplined, low-fat approach designed to fighting heart disease and high blood pressure

LOGIC Strict adherence to low-fat, low-cholesterol diet, along with regular exercise, leads to better health and weight loss.

CRITICISM Early criticism was directed at what, at the time, seemed like an unscientific approach to fight heart disease. Today, proponents of good fats, like Walter Willett, M.D., criticize the diet's severe restriction of vegetable oils. Others question whether the diet is too severe and too hard to follow.

SAMPLE DINNER Salmon paella, baked plantain, onion basket stuffed with carrots and spinach, steamed asparagus

Ornish

DATE Studies of the theory started in the late 70s; *Eat More, Weigh Less* published in 1993

AUTHOR Dean Ornish, M.D., professor of medicine at the University of California

PREMISE "Eat more, weigh less" with a diet high in fiber, low in fat

LOGIC Fiber and soy reduce insulin and cholesterol levels, and eating less fat means less total calories consumed. Emphasis on antioxidants and avoidance of animal fats promotes overall health.

CRITICISM Like Pritikin, some critics feel that the diet is so low in fat, it's not practical for long-term maintenance. Others believe "good" fats, such as vegetable oils and omega-3 fatty acids, are unnecessarily avoided.

SAMPLE DINNER Rigatoni with tomato mushroom sauce, arugula fennel salad with cucumber and chick peas

South Beach

DATE Developed in 1996; *The South Beach Diet* published in 2003

AUTHOR Arthur Agatston, M.D., cardiologist

PREMISE Lose belly fat first with this three-phase plan

LOGIC Initial restriction of carbohydrates trains the body not to crave them. Mono- and polyunsaturated fats, whole-grain carbs, and fiber will improve blood chemistry, lower weight, and reduce bad cholesterol. Focus on realistic exercise plan.

CRITICISM Skeptics claim that all diets are tough to stick to, and despite its popularity, South Beach is not different. The Florida citrus industry is fighting against the diet's restriction of orange juice

SAMPLE DINNER From Phase One: Fish kabobs, oven-roasted vegetables, sliced cucumber with olive oil

Eat, Drink, and Be Healthy

DATE *Eat, Drink, and Be Healthy* published in 2001

AUTHOR Walter C. Willett, M.D., chairman of Department of Nutrition at Harvard School of Public Health

PREMISE Revise the food pyramid for healthy living

LOGIC Inverts USDA food pyramid by creating a foundation of "good fats" and whole-grain carbohydrates in combination with exercise. Emphasizes fruits, vegetables, and nuts, while putting refined starches at the top of the pyramid. Lose weight by reducing caloric intake on this regimen.

CRITICISM Critics argue Willett's "good" fats (e.g., olive oil) are laden with calories. Meanwhile, Atkins advocates do not agree with the good fat/bad fat distinction, saying that the risks from saturated fat are overblown.

SAMPLE DINNER Pork tenderloin with pistachio-gremolata crust, wild rice pilaf, steamed asparagus

I finally got up enough nerve and asked whether he minded telling me how he'd done it. Not only was he happy to tell me, but, it turned out, he had become a meeting leader at Weight Watchers. That was how he had taken the weight off and kept it off. I knew nothing about Weight Watchers except that it had evolved through many iterations, was very successful from a corporate viewpoint, and required members to weigh in every week in front of everyone.

At least, that's what I thought. I found a meeting at the local YMCA in my hometown. After an hour, I knew that Weight Watchers might help me in several ways. First, the program on which it is based does not require buying special foods or anything else that would make it easy for someone like me to find an excuse not to comply. The program is based on two different approaches to watching what you eat. One is a system of assigning points to any food, and controlling portion sizes. That's the "flex" plan. The key here is "tracking" your points, which you can do easily with the tools you are given when you register. The other is a "core" plan that enables you to choose from many foods as long as you keep within a caloric range.

While I chose to keep score, I didn't join the program for that reason. For me, the most surprising thing was the process. First, you weighed in, but it was not in front of dozens of people who would sneer at me. We were all in the same boat.

The meeting leader was a wonderful woman, Darleen, who had started, just as I had, as a member trying to lose weight. All of the meeting leaders are from the ranks and they, too, have to stick with the program to maintain their status. The meeting was great fun, and was not what I had expected. It was the epitome of support, a well-led exchange of ideas to help you change your food behavior, lots of cheers for those who lost weight that week, and stickers put in your membership card for trying. Our next leader, Becky, is just as wonderful, hilarious, warm, and motivating as Darleen had been. I look forward to the Thursday meetings.

In any weight-loss plan, the first few pounds come off rather easily, simply because of calorie reduction. Weight Watchers gives you goals, such as losing 10 percent of your body weight to begin with, and the leaders are knowledgeable and well trained.

They do sell food and they are hooked up with food manufacturers who assign point values to their supermarket products that make it easier to track your food points. I have not purchased anything beyond some of the snack food, and I have never needed nor felt pressure to do so. The cost per week of membership ($12) is minimal compared to what I've gotten in return: loss of 20 pounds and rebuilding much of my cardiac health. If I lose ten more pounds and become a life member, there is no weekly fee—as long as the weight loss is maintained.

It is very important to note that while I was following the Weight Watchers program, I was also involved in an exercise program that complemented the reduction in calories through my new eating patterns. Only the two aspects of my life, working together, could have produced those results. I knew how to exercise, but I didn't know how to eat well, and that is why this program worked for me.

One other thing that made a huge difference is that Weight Watchers has the best set of cookbooks I've seen for anyone trying to eat more healthfully. They are sold through the group, on its website, and at most bookstores. Several are listed in the "Top Cookbook Choices" in **Month Twelve.**

Lots of dietary tricks work in the long run, but they have to become part of your daily approach to eating. One is to eat smaller portions and don't go back for more—or, at least, don't go back for another "first" helping. Don't put yourself in a position to be around the types of foods that have gotten you into trouble: chocolate cake, ice cream, french fries, and other high-calorie foods.

You can do it! Once you see the health results, I promise that you will find you won't want those foods. You may crave them, and you may even have those fries once every few months, but you will find that the long-term feeling of good health is much better than the short-term sugar rush.

Gastric Bypass Surgery

Many people who are morbidly obese consider having gastric bypass surgery, which is a very serious procedure with potential complications. While preparing a book on this subject, I met with people who have had gastric bypass surgery. This procedure can provide a solution to people who have failed to reduce their weight through all other methods. While success rates for this surgery are improving, it still carries a complication and mortality rate. One reason is that not only are these patients hundreds of pounds overweight, but they frequently have heart disease, high blood pressure, and diabetes.

Any comprehensive gastric bypass program must include extensive pre-operative evaluation by a team that includes an endocrinologist, nutrition therapist, psychologist, nurse, and the surgeon. It also should include careful follow-up, regular meetings, and a support group to help with all the different aspects of recovery.

There are different types of bypass surgery. These include restrictive procedures that change the structure of your intestines, and malabsorptive procedures, which bypass the small intestine. About eight in ten procedures are gastric bypasses, which restrict the size of the stomach.

Almost every gastric bypass patient I talked with who had managed to keep the weight off (which is hard, since the amount of food eaten and the timing of meals is a difficult regimen) was very happy. Several of these patients had pursued a career in medicine on some level, and almost all were great promoters of the procedure. However, it can be very expensive—up to $40,000. Only recently has reimbursement become possible in certain private insurance and government programs.

In the long run, gastric bypass or bariatric surgery (or any other procedure) is not a great answer to obesity. Prevention and self-motivation to change eating habits are your best bets. However, if your physician recommends gastric surgery for you, the best way to choose a facility for this procedure is to check out the number of similar procedures they've done, the success rate, the pre-screening procedures, and post-surgical advice on plastic surgery and an exercise program.

IN A SENTENCE:

> *Weight loss requires an understanding that diet is what and how you eat, not a program to simply lose weight, and integral parts of a successful weight-loss program are exercise and learning what foods are good for you.*

Exercising the Right Way

BY THIS time in your first year of recovery, you should have a regular exercise plan that complements your weight-loss goals. However, you may feel overwhelmed by adding exercise to all the other things that you are being asked to do. If you are trying to stop smoking, your exercise tolerance may be low. If you are trying to lose weight by turning your eating habits around, you may be changing a lifetime of bad habits. Exercise: Something that may not have been at the top of your list before you were diagnosed. Certainly, it used to be low on mine.

The good news is that this is not your buff gym buddy's training program. You do not have to pump iron. Simple exercising for a healthy heart is something you can do that will make you feel good. That, in fact, has been the biggest surprise of my past year of recovery. Not only do I like exercising, but it has become an important part of my day.

Good news part two is that you also don't have to devote hours to exercise every day to help your heart in a significant way. If you exercise moderately for a half hour, at least five days a week, you'll see big benefits. Another great effect is that exercise keeps you young. Studies are beginning to appear that indicate that exercise may be able to affect your genetic structure, reversing aging. While these early studies were performed on a

65-plus age group, they are significant and open up the possibility that exercise may be a secret weapon for the life-extension/anti-aging movement.

Getting Started

According to Michael Crawford, M.S., supervisor of cardio-rehabilitation programs at Cleveland Clinic, you should not begin any long-term exercise program without an assessment of your current condition and physical capability. In general this occurs in, or prior to, your cardio-rehab class, and should include the following:

○ An exercise-rehab team member should take a complete history, going over your current medications and concomitant illness (e.g., diabetes).

○ A quality-of-life questionnaire is important and gives you an opportunity to express how you are feeling emotionally. Are you depressed or anxious? How is this affecting your health? After all, quality of life is one of the reasons you've gotten into exercise and cardio-rehab.

○ A stress test should be done about four to six weeks after surgery or two to three weeks after angioplasty to establish what level of exercise your heart can safely handle.

Some programs, Crawford says, have the patient begin light exercise, perhaps five to ten minutes a day, and start on a diet that enables them to establish new eating patterns.

During the cardio-rehab program, the main goal will be to teach you how to exercise properly and to establish some baselines. For example, you want to establish a target heart rate in a supervised exercise environment so that you will be able to work out on your own. You may be asked to wear a telemetry monitor, and your blood pressure will be taken at various intervals while you walk on a treadmill. Of course, if you are diabetic, your glucose levels should be monitored to avoid any sudden sugar-level drops.

Exercise Made Easy

The cardio-rehab program can run up to three months before your team has decided that you are safe to exercise in an unsupervised situation. Keep in mind that the reason you are doing this is to reduce your risk of death from cardiovascular disease, to get the cardiovascular system working, to reduce your blood pressure, to help keep your diabetes under control, to lower cholesterol levels, and, most importantly, to help you reduce body weight. All of this will come with even a moderate exercise program.

Your exercise program must have three basic components, says Crawford. "You have to have aerobic exercise, and it must be regular, and it must be, above all, safe." Another way to approach this is by creating a FITT program, which means that you construct a program that includes

F = Frequency

I = Intensity

T = Type of exercise

T = Time or duration

There are also specific exercise programs. For example, there is a program for women who suffer from leg problems such as cramping caused by peripheral artery disease. Your doctor can point you in the right direction for that.

Aerobic exercise increases the rate and depth of your breathing, raises your heart rate, and uses the large muscle groups. The most popular forms of aerobic exercise are walking, running, biking, and swimming. To be beneficial, a regular program of exercise begins in small increments and builds up to 30 to 40 minutes a day, five days per week. To ensure safety, any man over 40 with heart disease and any woman over 50 should have their exercise program reviewed by their cardiologist.

No matter what method or equipment you use, there are some guidelines to follow. Crawford suggests, "you should have a minimum of 30 minutes at each exercise session and aim for 200 minutes per week, which would be around six days. This will help a great deal in weight loss. Remember that exercise alone will not help you lose weight. If you can put together a longer exercise regimen with caloric reduction, that's the best thing you can do for yourself."

How Hard Should You Exercise?

Part of any exercise program is ensuring that it's intense enough to actually provide benefit. One way is a widely used device called the

RPE, or the Rated Perceived Exertion Scale. This scale is a simple way to measure the intensity of your activity or exercise. While the scale runs from 0 to 10 in benefit (10 being the most intense), it is somewhat subjective and uses phrases matched to numbers to help you measure your workout. Here's how it works:

The Rated Perceived Exertion Scale (RPE)

How intense is your activity?

```
   0  . . . .  Not at all
 0.5  . . . .  Just noticeable
   1  . . . .  Very light
   2  . . . .  Light
   3  . . . .  Moderate
   4  . . . .  Somewhat heavy
   5  . . . .  Heavy
   6  . . . .
   7  . . . .  Very heavy
   8  . . . .
   9  . . . .
  10  . . . .  Very, very heavy (maximum)
```

In general, keep your exercise level between 3 and 4, although you must first clear the type and intensity of exercise with your doctor. With this scale, you can keep track of how exercise is affecting you. If you find after a month or two that your exercise intensity is now a 2 instead of a 3, you can work out more often or with a little more intensity. One expert told me that an ideal level of workout would mean that "you are able to talk, but not sing, while doing it."

Your Exercise Plan

It's hard to avoid falling for gyms, workout programs, "as-seen-on-TV" machines, YMCA classes, yoga institutes, or multimedia products. Before you invest in anything, mold the elements of FITT and the other basics listed above into a program that is most likely to help you to succeed.

The following is an approach recommended by Mr. Crawford at Cleveland Clinic's Heart and Vascular Institute that you can modify to fit your exercise needs.

1. Make short-term goals

One of the things I liked about Weight Watchers is that it is goal-oriented and uses short-term changes like the weekly weigh-ins to mark progress. Start with short-term goals when you begin exercise to measure your improvement. One reason that walking on the street or a treadmill is a good start in an exercise program is that you can measure your progress.

A second, *very important short-term goal is to make exercise a habit*. Once you begin, continue to exercise regularly, and it will become a habit. It's important to remember to take your time, perhaps taking a few months, to develop your exercise habit. Don't expect results immediately. Ironically, some of the same physiologic, pleasure-seeking mechanisms that reinforce other bad habits kick in with exercise, but this is the best habit to have.

2. Choose the right time

Choose a good time to exercise, for you—not just when a club class begins—because you will, inevitably, miss classes, and then you will lose the benefit. Then you'll backslide. We've all been there.

Make your exercise into a daily appointment. Plan ahead so that if the weather is bad, you can walk in a place like the mall. Schedule exercise in your daily planner or PDA and keep to that schedule. If you miss it, do something else, like taking a walk around the block, so that you continue to make exercise a habit, enabling the benefit and positive feelings you gain from exercising to remain.

3. Keep a journal

Many diet programs suggest keeping track of what you eat. There is even more reason to keep an exercise log. This helps you to keep track of how your RPE has changed and to see what type of exercise works for you best.

4. Have fun

While exercise and fun may seem to be mutually exclusive, they do not have to be. To begin with, you don't have to pick one form of exercise. Ride a bike one day, hike around the block three times the next day, and drag someone from your family or a buddy to play tennis the third. Rekindling an old skill, such as dancing, tennis, or swimming, can break up the exercise pattern and can motivate you even more.

Exercise Safely

Any time you exercise, you want to make sure you do a few things to keep from hurting yourself or overdoing it.

- ○ Make sure you warm up before you begin: Stretch and move your arms around to loosen your range of motion, and begin slowly.
- ○ Wear loose clothing.
- ○ Keep the FITT formula in mind, noting the frequency, intensity, and duration each time you exercise so that you don't do too much.
- ○ Make sure that the type of exercise you choose actually helps you and that it relates to the weight problem you have, whether it's controlling your diabetes and hypertension or promoting your heart health.
- ○ Cool down as you finish your workout: Walk slower to get your heartbeat back to normal.

Take a Walk

There is no question that simple walking has enormous benefits, especially if you can't afford equipment or are not cleared for anything else. Studies carried out at Massachusetts General Hospital found that when women were given different aerobic exercise for several months, walking was, by far, their favorite. One good thing about walking is that it is a low-impact activity, and it is easy to get back into it when you've been a couch potato for a long time. Just stand up and take one step after another.

Be a Tortoise, Not a Hare

You've heard the old saying: Slow and steady wins the race. Well, it may also burn more calories, at least in the long run.

Researchers at Maastricht University in the Netherlands concluded that people who engage in moderate physical activity, such as walking and biking, had the highest overall physical activity levels.

Their study of 30 men and women over a two-week period also revealed that those who exercised vigorously for short periods of time compensated for that activity by spending a greater part of their day being sedentary.

Sure, vigorous exercise burns more calories, but the moderate exercisers tended to be more active overall.

Source: *Nature* 2001; 410:539

Walking has additional benefits. Low-impact exercise increases bone mass, and has a lasting effect, which is particularly important to women. A more high-impact exercise may stimulate more bone-mass growth; however, walking is beneficial and is less painful than the high-impact workout.

Involve your kids and your spouse or partner in working physical activity into your daily life. Exercise for heart health does not require anything more than an activity that gets your RPE up to 3–4, five or six times per week. Walk to the store and walk up stairs whenever you can. Clean the house, work in the yard—it doesn't matter. You've been much less active than you should be, and that's affected your heart. You will be surprised how much quicker you begin to recover.

IN A SENTENCE:

> *A good, effective exercise program to regain heart health begins with simple, moderate aerobic exercises, such as walking 30 to 40 minutes per day, five to six times per week, resulting in significant fitness improvement within a matter of weeks.*

Choosing the Right Equipment

YOU MAY have an expensive piece of exercise equipment sitting in the family room or basement where it's become more useful to you as a clothing rack or dust collector. It's also likely to be a stationary bike, since that has traditionally been the most popular piece of exercise equipment. However, exercise equipment has changed to meet the needs of its market, and much of that market is you, the heart patient. The secondary aspect of the new equipment industry is also aimed at you, but as a baby boomer looking for stress reduction, body toning, and overall fitness.

As you know, your main exercise goal is losing weight to relieve the strain on your heart. Joining a gym or buying a machine is not necessary as long as you have some sort of alternative activity that gives you the chance to burn more calories than you take in each day. However, there are good reasons to invest in a piece of exercise equipment, even if your old bike experience was not a good one. Today's exercise equipment is programmable to help you maximize its heart-health effect. In addition, it's reasonably priced for the ever-expanding, longer-living fitness-oriented population.

You may find that having the right mini-gym in your home becomes a magnet for you and a great opportunity to involve your family in your recovery program. Letting older children use the equipment is a chance to get them into a routine that they will use throughout their lives. In addition, if they want to stay in shape, exercise also will help prevent negative health behaviors like smoking.

Exercise has also been equated with athletic training, but it is important to remember that no one expects you to turn into a marathon runner, although many heart patients have recovered to the point where they do participate in competitive sports, including running, softball, golf, and tennis.

What Equipment Should You Consider?

You may be familiar with dozens of different exercise devices that you probably used in your cardio-rehab program. The first place to begin making a decision on an equipment purchase is to ask your rehab supervisor what he or she recommends. Another good source of information is a physical therapist, who may be familiar with the newest versions and best brands of equipment. Other sources include *Consumer Reports* (www.consumerreports.org) and trade organizations like the American Council on Fitness (www.acefitness.org). Also, search for sites that can give you feedback from customers.

My own experience with equipment has been very positive. Several years ago, we purchased a medium-priced, programmable treadmill that was on sale at Sears. I like swimming, but if you don't join a gym or a club, and you don't have a pool at home, you can't do it daily or on your own schedule. The treadmill was going to be an adjunct, but, instead, became our regular source of exercise. Recently, we added a recumbent exercise bike (see below) to break up our routines and because it also was easier on my aging knees. Our total investment has been less than $1,000. Amortized over five years, it cost no more per year than the cost of joining a gym.

Treadmills

Treadmills are an excellent way to burn calories, get your leg muscles in shape, and get a feel for how well you are doing. In fact, more than 11.6 million Americans use one regularly. Treadmills are, by far, the most popular pieces of exercise equipment, and they provide the type of aerobic exercise you need during your heart recovery.

Most treadmills give you a readout or graph of your distance, speed, calories burned, pulse, and other information. By increasing the incline of the treadmill surface, you burn more calories. A 60-minute workout, according to a study at the University of Wisconsin Medical School, will burn up to 865 calories.

When you use the treadmill, you can increase either distance or speed, which enables you to slowly build up your tolerance. As you get healthier, you'll want to increase the speed because that will burn more calories.

Over the years, I've done several different things. My favorite is the sprint. I begin at one speed and raise it for a specific distance. Next, I slow down the speed for a half minute, and then increase my speed again past where I had been for the same length of time. I repeat this process for at least 30 minutes. By the time I'm finished, I know I've burned some calories.

Another reason you may like the treadmill is that you can exercise regardless of the weather, so you have no excuses. Some people read or watch TV (I like the Food Network) while on the treadmill. Some treadmills have built-in music players.

Most important, the treadmill is a relatively safe device. It has a safety-stop key and side rails, and you don't have to worry about the hazards of running outside. Make sure you buy a machine that has a long enough surface for running if you are going to use it for jogging.

Because treadmills are relatively expensive ($600 to $3,500), you have to choose the right one. When you go to buy one, wear sneakers and try out more than one machine, each for more than a few minutes. If the store won't demo it, go elsewhere. Make certain that you can walk on it and that you can reach the controls easily. It should have at least a one-year warranty of durability.

Finally, consider where you are going to put the machine before you buy it. Treadmills are not light and small, although some fold up and can be maneuvered to the side of a room if necessary.

Recumbent Exercise Bike

The second-most-popular exercise device is the recumbent bike (or stationary bike), a bicycle-like device that has a seat on a level with the pedals and a backrest that provides support while you are pedaling. Like the treadmill, this machine provides the sort of aerobic exercise you need at this time in your recovery. To use it, you sit in the bike, adjust the pedals, and either program it or set the resistance to a level that gives you a good workout. Almost all of these bikes have programs and pulse- or speed-measurement functions.

There are multiple benefits to this machine. First among these is the cost. A good, top-of-the-line machine can be found for $250 to $350 and purchased online for less. However, many of these machines require as- sembly, and this is not a job for an amateur. I found that the best place to buy a recumbent exercise bike was not a sporting-goods store or big- box retailer, but the local bike store. If the bike shop near you doesn't regularly carry them, they can order and even assemble these bikes. They may also deliver one to your home, or you can pick it up, as they are not large.

Like treadmills, recumbent bikes are safe, but they put less of a strain on your knees, and they are also quieter. A recumbent bike can also serve as your primary exercise machine because it can be used indoors.

Ellipticals

Elliptical exercisers are designed to give you a multifaceted workout, simulating everything from climbing stairs to a sort of cross-country skiing workout. In 2003, sales of these machines jumped by 65 percent to 3.3 million home users. The basic activity comes from standing on two shoe- sized pedals that move in flattened circles (hence, the word "elliptical"). You climb up and down while pushing and pulling the handlebars. It takes a bit of time to get used to it, but it is not as hard as it sounds. According to Mr. Crawford at the Cleveland Clinic, the elliptical is "an excellent ma- chine because it is low-impact, good on your joints, and you use both your arms and legs at the same time. It is a good source of calorie burn."

The elliptical gives your upper and lower body a workout, and as a weight-bearing exercise, it helps protect you from osteoporosis. Unfortu- nately, ellipticals are not inexpensive. The models that work well at the gym usually cost about $5,000. Home machines, costing between $1,000 and $2,000, have not been rated as highly by users and are not as well made as gym-quality machines. Of course, there are all kinds of customized models with CD/MP3 players, cup holders, etc.

Choosing an elliptical pretty much follows the same process that you undertake for any other machine. In this case, you have to make sure it has adjustable and wide pedals, that the handlebars are designed so that you can reach them easily, and that it has the programmability that you need. This machine also occupies a lot of space.

Other Useful Devices

You can find other devices for general exercise, but you should begin your recovery with one of the "big three" machines we've discussed here, along with aerobic exercise. There are dozens of different abdominal and chinning/total-gym devices. These use angled boards with pulley devices that you use to raise yourself along the board. While this is good strengthening exercise, it is not aerobic, and, ultimately, while you will be able to lift your own weight, there is no way to increase the weight you are lifting since it's limited to your body weight.

Inversion tables, arm-curl machines, and other devices are designed to give you those taut arms or "six-pack" abdominals. Unless you are completely cleared by your doctor and you use these machines in a supervised manner to start, stay away.

Another popular tool is a rowing machine, which can give you a good workout on many levels. It is especially good for muscle toning. Fans claim that it is as close to swimming as non-impact exercises get. The downside of the rowing machine is that it can be hard on your back and can aggravate previous injuries. This is also a device that you have to adjust to fit you correctly.

Beyond these, there are resistance bands, giant exercise balls, and traditional bicycles. Biking is a great aerobic exercise, but people who are just recovering from heart surgery or a heart attack may be told to wait to start this form of exercise. There are dozens of good bikes for anyone of any age. I have met many people who ride bikes as part of their weight-loss program; however, bicycling is limited by the season and the weather. As good as a bike may be, it is not as effective as the other devices mentioned above. While they may be good for you after a certain period of recovery, a decent bike for comfort or fitness riding can cost between $300 and $600.

What about a Fitness Club?

Fitness clubs and community centers like the YMCA are popular, but are they right for you? There are 18,000-plus clubs in the U.S., and more than 32 million people shell out a considerable amount of money— $14.8 billion—each year to join. The fitness-club scene has increased by 39 percent in the past decade. Not surprisingly, more than 50 percent of the members are women, and the largest segment of the over-age-55 group has joined to lose weight.

The clubs have also gotten the health/diet/heart recovery message. Over half of the clubs offer some sort of dedicated diet and nutrition counseling, along with heart-safe exercise programs. One of the other strategies clubs use is to align themselves with diet programs, like Jenny Craig and Weight Watchers, that encourage exercise but that have no formal programs. These clubs work to get referrals and to encourage word-of-mouth endorsements in the diet programs. They set up special low-impact exercise programs that don't involve weights.

The downside of clubs is that you have to commit to go somewhere for exercise, which may interfere with last-minute meetings or family responsibilities. If the club is your only exercise source, then it can quickly slip away.

Other considerations are cost and hours of operation. On the positive side, clubs can be a good place to meet people, and you can get good, professional instruction. They are good places for step and Pilates classes, which you might not do on your own. The decision to join a club is very much an individual one. If you feel comfortable with the idea of club membership and you can justify the cost of a club against investing in home equipment, then the choice is yours.

Whether you invest in home equipment or join a gym, dedicating time to exercise is crucial to regaining your heart health.

IN A SENTENCE:

> *To meet your needs as a heart/weight-loss patient, new versions of treadmills, recumbent bicycles, and new devices, such as the elliptical machine, can provide a solid aerobic workout.*

living

Stressed Out!

ARE YOU a stress junkie? Is stress high on your list of unofficial risk factors that you read in **Day One**? Have you, like me, thrived on stress, using deadlines and unrealistic goals to amp your adrenaline? Or do you simply collapse, crawl into the corner, and curl up into a ball when you are stressed? You're not alone: Stress is a global problem with enormous economic impact. According to the Centers for Disease Control and Prevention and the National Institute for Occupational Safety and Health (NIOSH)

- ○ 25 to 40 percent of all U.S. workers are going to experience workplace burnout from stress.
- ○ Stress costs U.S. companies up to $300 billion a year on lost productivity, health-related problems, and absenteeism.
- ○ Medical expenses are twice as high for employees who are stressed out than for other, non-stressed workers.
- ○ Depression, frequently accompanied by stress, is predicted to be the leading occupational disease of this century, responsible for more lost work days than any other single factor.

Like many other factors that may have contributed to your heart disease, stress can add to the level of risk because we

---

Stress: It's a Worldwide Phenomenon

A recent Roper Starch Worldwide survey of 30,000 people between the ages of 13 and 65 in 30 countries showed that

○ Women who work full-time and who have children under the age of 13 report the greatest stress worldwide.

○ Nearly one in four mothers who work full-time and who have children under 13 feel stress almost every day.

○ Globally, 23 percent of women executives and professionals and 19 percent of their male peers say they feel "super-stressed."

Source: Stress Directions

---

are exposed to far more stressors than previous generations have been. We put in significantly more hours at high-stress jobs than did previous generations. This is particularly true for the highly competitive generation of baby boomers who perceive success in terms of how hard we work, how many awards we get, and who is the last man standing at a job.

Stress and its companion, anger, are part of the price we pay for today's lifestyle. According to the experts at the Cleveland Clinic Heart and Vascular Institute, stress and anger are a part of life; however, the body's reaction to uncontrolled stress and anger is a risk factor for heart disease. When the body senses danger, it releases epinephrine, a hormone that increases the heartbeat and makes the body ready for action. People who are stressed all the time also secrete a hormone called cortisol. This hormone raises blood pressure and causes the body to retain fluids. Together, these circulating hormones place more stress on the heart.

Anyone with stress on this level should seek help from a professional who can assist with behavior modification and anger management.

Stress has been linked to other negative health consequences beyond heart disease, such as lung cancer from smoking, obesity from compulsive eating, liver disease from alcoholism, immune deficiency, chronic headaches, ulcers, colitis, phobias, panic disorders, and depression.

What Is Stress?

You may think it's easy to tell when you're stressed, but it is not that simple. Stress expresses itself both mentally and physically. It is an insidious disease, like hypertension, that builds and then grabs you, before you're aware of it. Stress can be caused by a reaction to your environment or to a medical problem like an injury or accident. Stress doesn't show up as a specific change physically, so it's difficult to measure.

Stress manifests itself in different ways, such as anxiety or nervousness. According to the Stress Management Program at Cleveland Clinic, signs of stress include

○ Not feeling like yourself
○ Feeling overwhelmed
○ Being unable to cope with workloads that had been a snap
○ Uncalled-for anger, irritability, and tension
○ Headaches, tension in your muscles, jaw, or back
○ Inability to concentrate or to remember things
○ Stomach pain, nausea, unusual sweating
○ Heart palpitations, rapid heartbeat
○ Lack of energy and general disinterest
○ Insomnia
○ Drinking or using drugs to avoid your problems
○ Impulsiveness
○ Lack of intention
○ Obsessing
○ Bad judgment

If these symptoms become increasingly common in your life, you are heading for a crash and a possible burn. Worse, stress like this can cause you to turn off and pull back, rather than to seek help. Another thing to keep in mind when you encounter these symptoms is that what you're experiencing might not be stress. Many biological disorders, such as thyroid disease, provoke symptoms such as depression or stress. These are referred to as "mimickers."

Is There a Biological Basis for Stress?

You may have heard of a "fight-or-flight" response, a biological reaction that all animals share when we feel threatened. When we are

Is This You?

Take a look at the list of signs of stress on the previous page. How many symptoms can you identify as a part of your life today?

1._____
2._____
3._____
4._____
5._____

If you experience more than two or three of them regularly, it's time to start managing your stress.

confronted by something that scares us, the body sends a question to the brain: Do we take a stand or do we retreat?

Internally, our alarm is being read by the brain, which sends a signal to our adrenal glands, which are two organs situated next to our kidneys. The brain's signal to the adrenal glands, carried over the **sympathetic nervous system**, tells the body to give off adrenalin for energy, endorphins for pain killing, and cortisol for pain relief later on. Once your body is energized with adrenalin, your breathing rises, your pupils dilate, you begin to sweat—all the reactions you commonly notice when stressed. The internal pain from this will be alleviated by the cortisol.

This is what you go through when stressed. As a person with heart disease, all those high-test stress chemicals like adrenalin surging through your nervous system and your bloodstream add additional workforce to your compromised heart. If you have only partial heart function or if you are recovering from surgery or a heart attack, consider what potential harm more stress in the form of a strong, internal chemical reaction can cause.

If you and your body are constantly facing fight-or-flight moments, the process becomes overwhelming and habitual. Instead of controlling the situation, your body goes into overdrive whenever you face ordinary stress situations. This is when you enter the seriously dangerous land of chronic stress, a vicious circle that can compromise your health quickly.

What Sets off Stress?

Stress cuts across all genders, ethnic groups, ages, income levels, and geographic locations. It is an equal-opportunity risk factor. No one is immune. While many environmental, workplace, or personal experiences can create stress, and we understand the biological process it sets off, the cause of stress is a bit more complicated, every person reacts differently, and there is no diagnostic tool that can predict your specific stressors.

Stress is caused by triggers. Call them hot buttons, stressors, or pet peeves: you probably have a list of people, places, and things that set you off. Someone or something pushes the button and the chemicals start brewing in your brain. Just having heart disease can be a tremendous stressor, so, for you as a heart patient, it's important to remember the strong correlation between stress and cardiovascular risk. According to the American Heart Association, we don't know if stress acts as an independent risk factor for heart disease, but adding it to the risk factors you may already have (e.g., family history) is a must.

Stress can be addictive, and for heart patients like us, the pattern must be broken.

IN A SENTENCE:

> *Among the many risk factors that may have contributed to your heart disease is stress, which is caused by a number of external factors in your life and which sets off a biological reaction that can increase pressure on your heart and prevent full recovery.*

Getting a Grip on Your Stress

IF YOU believe you are stressed or your doctor has told you to "chill out," you may have spent as much time in the stress-management section of your library or bookstore as in the health-book section. Stress management advice is everywhere. A Google search will produce millions of links to advice pages, counseling services, yoga, and products that help in coping with marital problems or problems with your kids, work issues, and so on.

While all of this information is great, much of it is repetitive, and it often misses a salient point regarding your stress. Because you are a heart patient, you do not fit into a garden-variety stress-reduction program. Perhaps a close friend has told you how much stress she relieves with a jog after work. For many heart patients or people with some sort of orthopedic limitation, that's not an option.

The best thing that you can do when you are facing stress during your first year of recovery, especially now that you are getting healthier through diet and exercise, is to take a step back. Learn to take time for yourself. Find a way to change your lifestyle. This message has flowed through this book: *Recovery from heart disease requires changing the risk factors that caused it.* Whether stress is a major risk factor for you or not, the way to manage it—for you—is to eliminate it.

For other, healthier individuals, so-called stress-management programs might make sense; however, you should be approaching stress as an enemy to be removed completely from your life. Does this imply that you have to quit your job and move to a cave? As attractive as that may sound sometimes, it's not the solution.

The answer was provided by an author and psychiatrist I met many years ago. Drew M. Slaby, M.D., taught me that the secret to coping with stress is to make stress work for you, because we all have stress throughout our lives.

In Dr. Slaby's opinion, not all stress is bad. The question is: How can you make stress work for you?

How to Make Stress Your Ally

Dr. Slaby's main theory is that any specific stressor can be turned on its head and turned to advantage. In his book, *60 Ways to Make Stress Work for You*, Dr. Slaby suggests you take advantage of nine basic common issues. The brilliance of Slaby's concept is that it takes little work and anyone can change his or her behavior to reduce stress. Consider these ideas from Dr. Slaby:

- **Get organized**: Daily chaos, such as missed appointments and can't-find-it syndrome, is easy to change. Use an organizer, make lists, and don't let yourself get overextended.
- **Turn a crisis into an opportunity**: In every seeming disaster, there is a lesson. If you survive a heart attack, for example, you have the opportunity to change your diet and begin to recover.
- **Seek a more relaxing environment**: Feng Shui has been a hot decorating and environmental-design fad based on the belief that by combining the right elements in a space, you restore balance to your life. It's a great idea. By reducing the stress in your home through nice artwork or comfortable furniture, your personal stress will be eased.
- **Take control of your life**: Identify your goals, determine what actions you can take to achieve them, and avoid allowing yourself to create a crisis in your life, marriage, and work. Change is not easy

when you also have to perform the job that may have been causing your stress.

○ **Expect the unexpected:** If you have to do something or get somewhere, leave time for the unexpected. You will always be faced
with things that have to be done, so be prepared and don't be
caught short.

○ **Don't procrastinate:** Stress and procrastination go together.
Often, stress is caused by *anticipation* of something that causes
the stress. Step up, deal with the problem, and move on.

○ **Let it go:** If you dwell on the past, keep in mind that there is
nothing you can do about it. The old cliché that "today is the first
day of the rest of your life" is pretty accurate.

○ **You don't need any surprises:** This doesn't mean that you can't
have a good old-fashioned surprise party. This pertains to not
knowing all the information about something and suddenly finding yourself in a major mess. For example, getting to your destination and finding no parking can make you crazy. Plan ahead. You
are not infallible.

○ **Enlist friends to your side:** You need friends to help you recover,
and they can also be a great help in reducing your stress. They
support you, and they are there for you when you are depressed,
or in a quandary. You need great friends. Choose the ones who will
be there for you, not those who add to your stress.

Gain Control

The Cleveland Clinic's Stress Management Program also has many
excellent suggestions to help you regain control. For example:

○ Take note of your stressors.
○ Realize that you may not be able to change everything or everyone.
○ Learn to relax.
○ Exercise stress away.
○ Don't rush.
○ Dance.
○ Get enough sleep.

○ Avoid negativity.
○ Don't obsess about health issues. Call your doctor.
○ Keep a journal.
○ Maintain a good, healthy diet.

What about Stress-Management Programs?

Stress-management programs can be found anywhere at any price. You can find them at the YMCA, as part of cardio-rehab programs, and even on home-shopping TV shows. Most of them contain similar elements: relaxation techniques, muscle relaxation, visualization, and breathing exercises. The truth is that you can learn all of the above yourself through a book or a download from the Internet. The website www.intelihealth.com has complete descriptions of programs and instructions. For some people, group situations work well and are an incentive to attend.

Picking a stress-management program is related to how much you perceive your need for one. If you are very stressed or if you are more frequently stressed, you might benefit from a formal stress-relief setting. Once you have completed a stress-management program, you will take the techniques and information home to manage your stress.

The decision to join a program is personal, but, like all things you do during your recovery, make sure your doctor knows what you are doing. Your cardio-rehab program also can be a good referral source.

Getting Professional Help

Many people are uncomfortable with the idea of seeking counseling for a problem. Talking about intimate fears or issues is not easy, even for people who have previously met with a professional. I overcame those feelings, sought help for stress after my heart attack, and benefited from it. Although it wasn't easy, sometimes a tune-up is needed.

You have many options if you're looking for professional help for stress relief. After your diagnosis, your own doctor can be helpful, as he or she has years of experience in working with patients like you. A psychiatrist may prescribe medication and discuss deeper issues that you may have. Similarly, a psychologist can help you to change behavior and get family counseling, if necessary. A social worker can be a helpful counselor in helping you deal with practical problems and day-to-day family issues. You could also talk with a trusted priest, rabbi, or pastor, many of whom have experience in helping people through crises.

Regardless of the option you choose, your cardiologist can be helpful. If you have problems with stress, anger, depression, or any emotion that can increase your heart-health risk, you have to take measures to prevent them from worsening. This can run counter to your family attitude or your ethnic tradition, but you need to be pragmatic because your stress must be brought under control. If you can't do it yourself, get someone who can help.

A Final Word

In *60 Ways to Make Stress Work for You*, Dr. Slaby offers this final message: "Turning the natural stresses of life to your advantage involves combining awareness of physical health, nutrition, exercise, your home or workplace environment, and interpersonal relationships into a plan of your own for stress reduction. As you learn to make stress work for you, you'll see many new advantages to old situations you once thought were to be avoided at all costs."

This is especially true for us heart patients.

IN A SENTENCE:

> As a heart patient, getting control of your stress is vital, and the best way to do that is to choose the program and technique that best fits your lifestyle.

SIX MONTH MILESTONES

○ YOU HAVE LEARNED ABOUT WOMEN AND HEART DISEASE.

○ YOU HAVE LEARNED TO CREATE YOUR OWN RISK REDUCTION PROGRAM.

○ YOU HAVE STARTED SMOKING AND/OR DRINKING CESSATION PROGRAMS.

○ YOU HAVE LEARNED ABOUT CONTROLLING STRESS.

○ YOU HAVE SET SERIOUS WEIGHT LOSS GOALS AND HAVE BEGUN A PROGRAM.

○ YOU HAVE LEARNED HOW TO EXERCISE PROPERLY.

Alternative Medicine

WHETHER YOU call it alternative medicine, integrative medicine, holistic medicine or complementary medicine, until the last few decades, your doctor might have said, "Forget it!" if you had asked about an herbal tea all your friends were using. In 1997, if you asked about a popular new book like *Eight Weeks to Optimum Health* by Dr. Andrew Weil, which topped the best-seller lists, you might have received an even more vehement response.

Medicine's "old school" (also called "allopathic medicine") has changed slowly, but today, attitudes are different. The alternative-medicine message is no longer a controversial view, and the best-seller lists that once featured only mainstream advice now are loaded with books like Dr. Weil's. In fact, they now have their own category, "Health, Mind, and Body," and they explore every sort of cure.

It's important to understand the differences you may encounter when you look beyond conventional medicine and how they fit with your particular situation. Here are some quick definitions:

○ **Alternative medicine** is something that is used instead of something conventional. This can run the gamut from taking an herbal tea or cough drop to taking

Laetrile (which has not been proven to work) instead of chemo for cancer.

○ **Complementary medicine** is much more widely used today. For example, pain relief is often treated with medication and then physical therapy (PT). Frequently, medication is withdrawn and PT is used exclusively.

○ **Integrative medicine** is a combination of treatments from both the conventional and **complementary and alternative medicine (CAM)** world when each has been proven safe. A good example of this is using both medication and massage therapy to reduce stress or to unkink knotted muscles.

Why has this information become so widely accepted? Ten years ago, I was fortunate enough to have lunch with Dr. Weil. I'd followed his career, and wanted to know why his message had begun to catch on. He had recently been on the cover of *Time,* and *Eight Weeks to Optimum Health* was being carried into doctors' offices.

"What is integrative medicine?" I asked him. "What do you mean and why is it so appealing?"

"It's really quite simple," Weil explained. "If you are crossing the street and you get hit by a car, you need to go to the emergency room. However, there is no reason why you also can't live a healthy, balanced lifestyle, doing non-traditional things, leading the rest of your life differently. Integrative medicine simply brings both sides of the medical spectrum together."

Should You Consider a New Approach?

After you have reached a balance in your recovery where your body and mind are synchronized, functioning well at perhaps two to four months, you will need to focus on a lifestyle change. Exercise and diet will be key elements in this period, but it is likely you also will look for other ways to rebuild your heart.

There are hundreds of websites, books, magazines, DVDs, and classes that you can explore, but how reliable is the information? As a heart patient, you have to be especially careful, and you should always talk to your doctor before trying anything serious, such as an exercise program.

But can you be harmed by some mineral supplement? When should you try something on your own, perhaps on the recommendation of a fellow patient, especially since you may not feel comfortable about calling your doctor frequently?

This is a very understandable problem for a couple of reasons. We tend to give credence to something that appears in respected consumer media, such as the science section of the *New York Times,* The Discovery Channel, a widely publicized study published in a respected medical journal, or even an opinion in a blog or a website. You may also feel that your doctor will be angry that you doubt his word or you may fear that you won't even get an answer at all.

Another reason for considering a friend's opinion or experience with alternative medicine is that we are conditioned by advertising and marketing to believe "endorsements" as a source of valid information. One solution is to bring the report you've read with you and bring it up in your next doctor's visit. Physicians today are very aware of the impact of the media and the Internet, and they know that unless they can answer your questions, you may not comply with what they ask you to do.

Today, fortunately, treatment modalities that were ignored by the medical establishment are not only looked at with less skepticism, but are being seriously considered.

The National Center for Complementary and Alternative Medicine (NCCAM) is a part of the National Institutes of Health (NIH). The NCCAM defines and reviews "approaches to health care that are outside the realm of conventional medicine as practiced in the U.S."

The NCCAM's 2002 study of public attitudes toward CAM showed that 50 percent of people over 18 had used some sort of alternative medicine. Interestingly, one of the techniques cited by almost two-thirds of the population was prayer.

A decade ago, Dr. Weil's book rode the beginning of a wave that had been building for quite some time. Options such as chiropractic, herbal teas, and vitamins, although popular, were outside mainstream medicine at the time. Was this some sort of underground medical phenomenon?

In *Eight Weeks to Optimum Health,* Dr. Weil offered a simple philosophy of medicine that fits perfectly with NCCAM's goal of looking at other types of treatment in addition to traditional medicine.

"Health is a wholeness and balance, an inner resilience that allows you to meet the demands of living without being overwhelmed. If you have that kind of resilience, you can experience the inevitable interactions with germs, and not get infections; you can be in contact with allergens, and not suffer allergies; and you can sustain exposure to carcinogens, and not get cancer."

The Past Is the Best Predictor of the Future

Dr. Weil's vision of living a balanced life is being realized more frequently today; however, it is also not really a new development, even if traditional medical practitioners still reject some new approaches. Many tools that conventional medicine uses today are actually the products of medical advances that, in their time, were perceived in the same way today's alternative medical treatments have been perceived.

We now recognize that today's medical treatments are a result of the evolution of knowledge. This is especially true where the understanding of our cardiovascular system is concerned. Greek doctors identified the role of the heart's valves in 400 B.C. when they attempted the first open heart surgeries. Since the procedure did not catch on, it probably could have been labeled "alternative" at best.

By the 17th century, however, English physicians were able to describe how blood circulated through the veins and arteries, disproving previous theories that how much we ate influenced how our blood flowed.

Tragically, some of the most important medical breakthroughs sprang from treatments under the most horrifying conditions: on battlefields at Gettysburg, Omaha Beach, Dien Bien Phu, and Iraq. One of the first documented successful heart surgeries was performed in World War I by a German doctor who closed the heart wound in a German soldier. Similar techniques for shrapnel removal were developed 30 years later in World War II.

It's easy to come up with a quick list of medical breakthroughs that have changed your life that were, at one time, unproven, or that were developed for some other purpose, such as the following:

○ Anesthesia (Would you be able to have open heart surgery without it?) (1846)

○ Aspirin (A pain killer that helps keep blood from clotting) (1897)

○ X-ray (An important device that enables doctors to make a more accurate diagnosis) (1895)

○ Penicillin (Mold led to the discovery of antibiotic treatments and improved public health) (1928)

○ Blood transfusions (A procedure that makes successful surgery more likely) (1492)

○ Angiotensin-converting enzyme (ACE) inhibitors (Meds that treat heart failure and high blood pressure) (1950s–1970s)

○ Cardiopulmonary resuscitation (Improves survival when breathing or circulation stops) (1950)

Today, we take these discoveries for granted. A quick look at current medical practice reveals many more treatments that go back generations. Massage, meditation, acupuncture, and aromatherapy are therapeutic approaches that have been used in Asian countries for centuries. Today, they are as common here in the West as open heart surgery, clot-busting medications, and cholesterol-lowering drugs are.

Not surprisingly, NCCAM has helped to define and apply standards to new treatments that afford protection from unexpected side effects. The group has established a formal CAM program that explores the "complementary and alternative healing practices in the context of rigorous science; disseminating authoritative information to the public and professionals." This program acts as a national clearinghouse that provides research grants for a wide variety of programs and a source for the latest information.

Some Treatments Have Survived the Ages

Many of the studies funded by the NCCAM are large, multi-center efforts; some involve a single researcher. Some involve entire systems of alternative medical care.

For example, one major study is examining Ayurvedic medicine, a form of medicine practiced widely in India and contiguous countries for at least 5,000 years. "Ayurveda" derives from two Sanskrit terms: ayu (life) and veda (knowledge or science). The term was not widely known in the West until it was introduced by the Beatles' favorite guru, Maharishi

Ayurvedic Medicine

Dr. Deepak Chopra, a popular author and proponent of alternative medicine, has promoted Ayurvedic medicine: "Ayurveda is the science of life, and it has a very basic, simple kind of approach, which is that we are part of the universe and the universe is intelligent and the human body is part of the cosmic body, and the human mind is part of the cosmic mind, and the atom and the universe are exactly the same thing but with different form, and the more we are in touch with this deeper reality from where everything comes, the more we will be able to heal ourselves and at the same time heal our planet." (www.The Skeptic's Dictionary.com)

Mahesh Yogi. Because so much of India is rural and mainstream health care is not available, Ayurvedic medicine is the main method of health care for much of the country. Many larger cities have Ayurvedic colleges and hospitals.

Ayurevedic medicine is based on a specific diet, the use of herbs, and regulation of mind and body. Among its many tenets are promoting harmony (vata) to prevent anxiety, and pitta, composed of fire and water and governing all heat, metabolism, and transformation in the mind and body. It controls how you digest food, how you metabolize your sensory perceptions, and how you discriminate between right and wrong. By practicing Ayurveda you gain the power to bring back harmony and balance, which is the key to good health.

Many people totally discount Ayurveda as a treatment that embraces superstition; however, NCCAM, as an arm of the NIH, has seriously examined and validated the value and benefits of learning from the experience of whole regions of the world.

To learn more about NCCAM and CAM, visit http://nccam.nih.gov/.

How Do You Know What CAMs Are Legitimate?

One thing to keep in mind is that conventional physicians are usually focused on your body, its organs, and the body's system. Most physicians in this country practice **acute medicine**, which means they treat the cause of your symptoms. However, Dr. Weil and many others point out,

Anything Can Be "Alternative"

Did you ever wonder why everyone is smiling on those dance shows when they are waltzing? It's not just because they are having a good time. There is now scientific proof that waltzing is a beneficial treatment for heart disease—in a manner of speaking.

According to a study by Italian cardiologists presented at an American Heart Association scientific meeting in 2006, "Dancing improves the ability to function and quality of life among chronic heart failure patients and may be a good alternative to other aerobic exercises."

The research group said, "Dancing is the choice of exercise training for patients with heart failure. This is good news because if we want patients to take part in lifelong aerobic exercise at least three times a week, it should be something that's fun and makes them want to continue."

The results showed that "dancing improves the functional capacity and quality of life—particularly when it came to questions about emotions—among patients who underwent the dance protocol, while there was no improvement in these areas with patients who did not exercise." However, the study also showed that "quality of life was surprisingly more significantly improved in the dancing group vs. the exercise group."

While this study was small, it's hoped that it can be expanded, said the researchers. It is important to note that both slow and fast waltzes were judged to be safe for the patients. Like everything else—talk to your doctor. It's likely he'll be happy that you are looking for ways to stay active, even if it's an "alternative" form of exercise like this one!

and even the NIH has now agreed, conventional medicine is fine, but there is no reason not to consider taking it further.

Here are the basics of complementary and alternative medicine according to NCCAM:

○ **Whole medical systems** are built upon complete systems of theory and practice. Often, these systems have evolved apart from and earlier than the conventional medical approach used in the U.S. Examples of whole medical systems that have developed in Western cultures include homeopathic medicine and naturopathic medicine. Examples of systems that have developed in non-Western cultures include traditional Chinese medicine and Ayurveda.

What Others Think of Alternative Medicine

The NCCAM surveyed the American public on complementary and alternative medicine in 2002. According to the survey:

○ When *prayer* specifically for health reasons is included in the definition of CAM, the number of adults using some form of CAM in 2002 rose to 62 percent.

○ The majority of individuals (54.9 percent) used CAM in conjunction with conventional medicine.

○ Most people use CAM to treat or to prevent musculoskeletal conditions or other conditions associated with chronic or recurring pain.

○ That only 14.8 percent of adults sought care from a licensed or certified CAM practitioner suggests that most individuals who use CAM prefer to treat themselves.

○ Women were more likely than men to use CAM. The largest sex differential is seen in the use of mind-body therapies, including prayer specifically for health reasons.

○ Except for the groups of therapies that included prayer specifically for health reasons, use of CAM increased as education levels increased.

○ The most common CAM therapies used in the U.S. in 2002 were prayer (45.2 percent), herbalism (18.9 percent), breathing meditation (11.6 percent), meditation (7.6 percent), chiropractic medicine (7.5 percent), yoga (5.1 percent), body work (5.0 percent), diet-based therapy (3.5 percent), progressive relaxation (3.0 percent), mega-vitamin therapy (2.8 percent), and visualization (2.1 percent).

○ **Mind-body medicine** uses a variety of techniques to enhance the mind's capacity to affect bodily function and symptoms, such as patient support groups and cognitive-behavioral therapy. Other mind-body techniques include meditation, prayer, mental healing, and art, music, or dance therapies.

○ **Biologically based practices** use herbs, foods, and dietary supplements.

○ **Manipulative and body-based practices** are based on movement of one or more parts of the body, including chiropractic or osteopathic manipulation and massage.

○ **Energy medicine** involves the use of energy fields.

○ **Biofield therapies** are intended to affect energy fields that purportedly surround and penetrate the human body. The existence of such fields has not yet been scientifically proven. Some forms of energy therapy manipulate biofields by applying pressure or by placing the hands in or through these fields. Examples include qi gong, Reiki, and therapeutic touch.

○ **Bioelectromagnetic-based therapies** involve the use of pulsed fields, magnetic fields, and alternating direct-current fields.

IN A SENTENCE:

Alternative, holistic, integrative, and complementary medicine has now become so common that the National Institutes of Health and mainstream medicine now accept many of its claims and are studying these treatments to provide accurate data for patients to use in making choices.

What Alternative Treatments Can Help— or Hurt—My Heart?

IN THE last section, you had an opportunity to see the concept of alternative medicine through the lens of traditional medical organizations such as NIH. You have learned two important concepts: What is new and suspect can quickly become state-of-the-art, and you have more choices beyond what you may have been told.

At this point in your recovery, you are starting to feel very well, you understand many of the mind-body issues, and now you are intrigued by some alternatives. You may think some of the ideas that people have told you about are so obvious that you don't have to bother talking about them with your physician.

According to one American Heart Association study, 45 percent of heart patients were actually using herbal meds and vitamins, and only 39 percent of CAM users thought it was important to let their doctor know about the use of alternative therapies. Only half of the users in the study said they were aware of the risk of using these treatments, and most received their information from media or word of mouth. One of the most surprising aspects of this study was that three-quarters of the patients' families and half of their cardiologists weren't aware of what their patients were doing. *Be sure to consult your doctor before trying any alternative therapy.*

Alternative Medicine and Depression

Depression often accompanies heart disease and especially can appear in the aftermath of a heart attack or cardiac surgery. Proponents of alternative medication often suggest using "natural substances" (e.g., roots and herbs) to combat periods of sadness and the blues. Many of them are actually folk remedies that have been passed down for generations or that are part of a local culture.

Typical of these substances is St. John's Wort, which has actually been studied in several clinical studies. The data shows some possible effect on mild feelings of unhappiness, but not on major depression. While it doesn't appear dangerous, and is available over-the-counter, it can harm you in several ways. First, if you are really depressed, you need real medical treatment and you can't wait four to six weeks for St. John's Wort to take effect. Second, your depression-like symptoms may be caused by another problem that merits prompt evaluation.

Other alternative medications used to treat depression are omega-3 fatty acids, 5-HTP, folic acid, and SAM-e. As in everything you consider during your recovery from heart disease, ask your cardiologist before trying any herbal supplements, and always tell your physician what and how much of these supplements you are taking.

Are Vitamins a Good Alternative Treatment for Your Heart?

In the AHA study mentioned above, most of the patients were taking vitamins that they had heard had positive effects on heart disease. Everyone knows vitamins can be helpful, and dozens of products promise that you can get your minimum daily requirement of vitamins by drinking a few glasses of this juice or a bowl of that cereal.

Vitamins, which we do get from our food, are nutrients (i.e., something that nourishes) that affect daily metabolic processes. While our bodies do not have to have vitamin supplements to survive, some dietary vitamins, like vitamin K, act as catalysts in internal chemical reactions, such as blood clotting.

Vitamins have become a form of alternative medicine in an unconventional way. Until the early part of the 20th century, most of us ate fresh food from farms or gardens, a great many of us worked outside, and we got our vitamins the "natural" way. Today, the best way to get the vitamins you need is still through a good, balanced diet, yet there are stores full of vitamin pills, supplements, and other "natural" snacks.

As a heart patient, you have likely heard about several vitamins that are reputed to reduce heart disease. At the top of the list is probably vitamin E, which has been studied for more than five decades. At the basis of the studies are chemicals in our bodies called **antioxidants**, which attempt to prevent cancer. For some time, vitamin E intake, especially at high levels, has been thought to combat heart disease and cancer. Other vitamins (A and C) also have been grouped with vitamin E in this potential "magic bullet."

The consensus now is that vitamin E does not prevent heart disease, especially if it's being used to make up for a lack of proper nutrients in a balanced diet. Further, the AHA has now taken a strong stand on the matter: "Vitamins or mineral supplements aren't a substitute for a balanced, nutritious diet that limits excess calories, saturated fat, trans fats, and dietary cholesterol."

Still, the book isn't closed on the effect of certain vitamins on heart disease. The AHA points out that if you ask the question, "Will taking antioxidant vitamins replace the need to reduce your blood pressure, lower your lipids, stop smoking, or eat wisely?" the answer is a resounding "no."

What Alternatives Should You Consider?

Any alternative treatment might interact with medications you are taking. For example, St. John's Wort can interfere with digoxin (Digitalis), which affects heart rhythms, and warfarin (Coumadin; Jantoven), which affects blood clotting. Some herbal medication, like hawthorne

---

EDTA Chelation Therapy for
Blocked Arteries

One of the more controversial alternative therapies is **EDTA chelation therapy**. EDTA is a synthetic amino acid, an organic compound that is a building block of proteins, which has been proven effective in treatment of heavy metal poisoning. EDTA binds to dangerous metals and minerals in your body, and is eliminated with them intravenously.

For several years, there have been ongoing studies to determine if EDTA therapy could clear blocked arteries by removing calcium found in the plaque clogging your vessels. It's also thought that the process of chelation (binding one structure to another) would stimulate hormones to remove calcium. Most of the studies of the process have been small, anecdotal, or untested; however, advocates of EDT claim that several hundred thousand people currently use this procedure.

To bring things under control and to try to gain definitive information on EDTA, a large-scale, double-blind study was launched by NCCAM and the National Heart, Lung, and Blood Institute in 2003 at more than 100 sites in the U.S. The study results are not expected until 2010. For further information, go to www.nccam.nih.gov and www.clinicaltrials.gov.

---

berries, can interfere with blood pressure drugs. These herbals are often grouped in the natural supplements category that has become synonymous for something that is better than processed food. *The important point is that the interaction of herbal products with your medical treatment can be fatal.*

The NCCAM lists the following practices and concepts as the major areas that you may be considering. None of these should be attempted without first talking to your physician.

Acupuncture is a method of healing developed in China more than 2,000 years ago that involves stimulation of anatomical points on the body by a variety of techniques. American acupuncture incorporates medical traditions from China, Japan, Korea, and other countries. The acupuncture technique that has been most studied scientifically involves penetrating the skin with thin, solid, metallic needles that are manipulated by the hands or by electrical stimulation.

Aromatherapy involves the use of essential oils (extracts or essences) from flowers, herbs, and trees.

Chiropractic focuses on the relationship between bodily structure (primarily that of the spine) and function and how that relationship affects the preservation and restoration of health. Chiropractors use manipulative therapy as a treatment tool.

Dietary supplements are products other than tobacco taken by mouth that contain an ingredient intended to supplement the diet. Congress defined this term in the Dietary Supplement Health and Education Act (DSHEA) of 1994. Dietary supplements may include vitamins, minerals, herbs, or other botanicals; amino acids; enzymes; organ tissues; and metabolites. Dietary supplements are available in extracts, concentrates, tablets, capsules, gel caps, liquids, and powders. They have special requirements for labeling. Under DSHEA, dietary supplements are considered foods, not drugs.

Electromagnetic fields (EMFs) are invisible areas of force that surround all electrical devices. The earth produces EMFs when there is thunderstorm activity, and magnetic fields are believed to be produced by electric currents flowing at the earth's core.

Homeopathic medicine is based on the belief that "like cures like," meaning that small, highly diluted quantities of medicinal substances are given to cure symptoms, although the same substances, given at higher or more concentrated doses, would actually cause those symptoms.

Massage therapists manipulate muscle and connective tissues to enhance their function and to promote relaxation and a sense of well-being.

Naturopathic medicine or naturopathy proposes that there is a healing power in the body that establishes, maintains, and restores health. Practitioners work with the patient with a goal of supporting this power through nutrition and lifestyle counseling, dietary supplements, medicinal plants, exercise, homeopathy, and treatments from traditional Chinese medicine.

Osteopathic medicine is a form of allopathic medicine that, in part, emphasizes diseases arising in the musculoskeletal system. It is based on the belief that the body's systems work together and that disturbances in one system may affect function elsewhere in the body. Some osteopathic physicians practice osteopathic manipulation, a system of hands-on techniques to alleviate pain, restore function, and promote health and well-being.

Qi gong is a component of traditional Chinese medicine that combines movement, meditation, and regulation of breathing to enhance the flow of qi (an ancient term given to vital energy) in the body, improve blood circulation, and enhance immune function.

Reiki is a Japanese word representing universal life energy. Reiki is based on the belief that when spiritual energy is channeled through a Reiki practitioner, the patient's spirit is healed, which, in turn, heals the body.

Therapeutic touch is derived from the ancient technique of laying on of hands. It is based on the premise that the healing force of the therapist affects the patient's recovery, that healing is promoted when the body's energies are in balance, and that by passing their hands over the patient, healers can identify and correct energy imbalances.

Traditional Chinese medicine (TCM) is based on a concept of balanced qi or vital energy that is believed to flow throughout the body. Qi is thought to regulate the spiritual, emotional, mental, and physical balance in the body. It is influenced by the opposing forces of yin (negative energy) and yang (positive energy). According to TCM, disease results from the flow of qi being disrupted and the imbalance of yin and yang. Among the components of TCM are herbal and nutritional therapy, restorative physical exercises, meditation, acupuncture, and remedial massage.

IN A SENTENCE:

> *Many alternative treatments are available. They are frequently used by mainstream medical groups; however, never take non-prescription supplements without talking with your doctor first, no matter how innocent the product or therapy may seem.*

living

Taking Your Heart Medication

A MAJOR change in your life that comes with heart disease and that has probably caused you some concern is the number of pills you take. It's a strong possibility that you will be taking some of them within the foreseeable future and, possibly, forever. You might be on medications to help prevent or slow heart disease progression, regulate rhythms, or reduce your risk factors. Each year more and more medications come on the market, and, chances are, you may end up taking one of these drugs or substituting it for another.

Sometimes when I look at my daily pill case, I feel like I am running a pharmacy or a "Pills-R-Us" store. Right now, I take ten medications for heart disease, diabetes, and some unrelated orthopedic illness. I have been on at least four different cholesterol medications and different dosages of diabetes medication, including insulin, although my diabetes has improved through diet and exercise.

Some of these medications have unpleasant and unwanted side effects. To be honest, you may have bouts of nausea and other bowel and gastric side effects. When they say on TV that there is the "rare possibility" of sexual side effects, they're stretching the truth. Effects like this and others can and often do lead patients to skip doses or to discontinue taking the pills. *Do not do this! When you begin a new medication or develop side effects, call your doctor, talk to your pharmacist, or go to an emergency clinic if the side effects are severe or make you feel unusually ill. To add to that warning, remember not to simply stop taking a medication unless you are told by your doctor to do so: It can adversely affect your heart to suddenly stop taking your meds. Be able to describe your symptoms clearly.*

Prescription medications can be expensive and, too often, the cost makes people ask: Do I eat, take the pills, or buy gasoline to get to work? The pills may be the first to go. This is a horrible fact of life in our current medical system, especially for 40 to 45 million uninsured people in the U.S. Possible solutions to this problem are discussed in **Month Ten,** along with other strategies to help you keep health-care costs under control.

Using Medications

The rules for taking heart medications are pretty much the same as they are for any medications. Unfortunately, today we get our medications from many sources, and that has taken some of the interpersonal communication out of the prescribing process.

In addition, the doctor-patient interaction is frequently very short and anxiety provoking. Your focus is usually more on the medical aspects of your condition, and you may not have much opportunity to ask questions about medications prescribed for you.

Here are general rules about using medications:

○ Every medication today comes with a patient information sheet. *Read it carefully.* If you don't understand it, ask your pharmacist and your doctor.
○ Note the difference between **side effects,** which are expected, and **adverse reactions,** which are unexpected and very serious. For example, a side effect might be a stomachache or nausea, whereas an adverse effect might be severe swelling in your legs or severe shortness of breath.
○ Keep the patient information sheet in a file or somewhere handy for reference in an emergency.

O If you experience an adverse reaction, *immediately call your doctor or go to the emergency room.*

O Develop a system for taking your medication. Some people keep their morning pills in a vial of one color, their afternoon pills in another, and their evening pills in a third.

O Ask your pharmacist to help you set up a system for keeping track of your medications. Pharmacists often have special labels or ideas about when and how you should take each pill.

O There are commercial pill holders that allow you to deposit one to two weeks' doses in separate sections, one for each day. This system has worked for me. I have one for morning pills and one for evening pills. Every two to three weeks, I sit down with all of my pills and sort them for the next two-week period, and that helps me stay compliant.

O Many people have pill cases with timers to remind them when to take pills. I've never used one, but anything that makes this process easier is worth trying. Also, try to take your medication at specific times, such as before or after a meal.

O Ask your doctor when the medication should take some effect. If you don't notice the prescription becoming effective within the specified time, call your doctor ASAP.

What Are the Most Common Medications for Heart Disease?

Heart medications can be classified by their many uses and purposes. Depending on your type of heart disease, you have medications that are supposed to reverse your heart disease, treat or reduce symptoms, and prevent further cardiac deterioration. The following information from the National Heart, Lung, and Blood Institute summarizes the most frequently used medications for heart disease. More information can be found at www.nhlbi.nih.gov/actintime/hdm/hdm.htm.

Here's a short summary of the major heart medications. A complete chart can be found in the next section.

Aspirin helps to lower the risk of a heart attack for those who have already had one. It also helps to keep arteries open in people who have had a previous heart bypass or other artery-opening procedure, such as coronary angioplasty or stenting.

Because of its risks, aspirin is not approved by the Food and Drug Administration for preventing heart attacks in healthy individuals. It may be harmful for some persons, especially those who are not at risk of heart disease. Patients must be assessed carefully to make sure the benefits of taking aspirin outweigh the risks. Talk to your doctor about whether taking aspirin is right for you.

Anticoagulation medications prevent clotting. They include warfarin and heparin. These help prevent stroke in case of abnormal heart rhythm such as atrial fibrillation.

Digitalis is sometimes used when the heart's pumping function has been weakened. More importantly, it also slows some fast heart rhythms.

ACE (angiotensin-converting enzyme) inhibitors block the production of a chemical that makes blood vessels narrow and are used to help control high blood pressure. They are also used when the heart muscle is damaged. It may be prescribed after a heart attack to help the heart pump blood more effectively. It is also used in persons with congestive heart failure, a condition in which the heart is unable to pump enough blood to supply the body's needs.

Beta blockers slow the heart and make it beat with less contractile force, lowering the blood pressure and reducing the workload of the heart. It is used to control high blood pressure and chest pain, and to prevent another heart attack.

Nitrates (including nitroglycerine) relax blood vessels and relieve chest pain.

Calcium channel blockers relax blood vessels and are used to treat high blood pressure and chest pain.

Blood cholesterol–lowering agents decrease cholesterol levels in the blood.

Thrombolytic agents, also called "clot busters," are given during a heart attack to break up blood clots in a coronary artery and to restore blood flow.

High blood pressure medications keep your hypertension under control. There are a number of these drugs, including ACE inhibitors, alpha blockers, angiotension II receptor blockers, and beta blockers or calcium channel blockers.

Diuretics decrease fluid in the body and are used to control high blood pressure and congestive heart failure. Diuretics are sometimes referred to as water pills.

High blood cholesterol medications usually fall into the statin class, including lovastatin (Mevacor), simvastatin (Zocor), pravastatin (Pravachol), fluvastatin (Lescol), and atorvastatin (Lipitor). Statins are effective in lowering the LDL, and seem to do a better job than any other comparable class of medications. Importantly, these are not effective in all cases. Between 20 and 60 percent of patients find them effective.

How Much Do I Need to Know about My Medications?

As a recovering patient, you don't have to become an expert in medications. Also, you cannot obsess about daily reports about medications that are usually far less significant than they seem. Many news stories report on a new study, but when you look closely, it is usually a collection of studies, called a **meta-analysis,** that combine their raw data. From this, the researcher reaches conclusions that may or may not prove to be valid. The point is that some studies are meaningful and others may not be—for you. Talk to your doctor about what you read in the newspaper.

The five most important things you should keep in mind about your heart medications are

- ○ Learn about the one(s) you are taking, specifically the ones that are right for you.
- ○ Take them exactly as prescribed unless your doctor tells you differently.
- ○ Tell all of your doctors what you are taking, especially when visiting a new doctor.
- ○ Keep track of side effects and report them to your doctor to see whether a different dosage or drug will work for you.
- ○ Your medication is important, but it is a simple part of your recovery. Just take them as directed. Changing your lifestyle and reducing all the risk factors you may have is a more challenging, but equally important task.

Traveling with Medications: Current Rules

According to the Transportation Safety Administration you may bring all:

○ Prescription and over-the-counter medications (liquids, gels, and aerosols), including personal lubricants, eye drops, and saline solution used for medical purposes

○ Liquids, including water, juice, or liquid nutrition or gels for passengers with disabilities and other medical conditions

○ Life-support and life-sustaining products such as bone marrow, blood products, and transplant organs

○ Items used to augment the body for medical or cosmetic reasons, such as mastectomy products, prosthetic breasts, bras, or shells containing gels, saline solution, or other liquids

○ Gels or frozen liquids needed to cool medical or disability-related items used by persons with disabilities or other medical conditions
(Note: Check the TSA's web site, www.tsa.gov, before any trip as these guidelines may change.)

You are not limited in the amount of these items you may bring in your carry-on baggage, but if the medically necessary items exceed three ounces or are not contained in a one-quart, zip-top plastic bag, you must declare to the security officer at the checkpoint for further inspection.

If you refuse to allow examination of the medications, you will not be permitted to carry them out of the security area.

Non-liquid or gel medications of all kinds, such as solid pills or inhalers, are allowed through the security checkpoint once they have been screened. TSA recommends, but does not require, that medications be labeled to assist with the screening process.

TSA normally x-rays medication and related supplies, but you may ask that security officers visually inspect your medications and medical supplies.

You must ask for visual inspection before the screening process begins; otherwise, your medications and supplies will be x-rayed. If you want to take advantage of this option, separate your medication and associated supplies from other property in a separate pouch or bag before you approach the security officer at the walk-through metal detector. Ask the security officer to visually inspect your medication and hand it to him or her.

To protect your medication, medical supplies, or fragile medical materials from contamination or damage, display, handle, and repack your own medication and supplies during the visual inspection at the checkpoint.

Travel with Medication Can Be Complicated

Anyone who has flown anywhere within the past several years knows that you can only take certain things through security and in your carry-on luggage. In general, you can pack any medication in checked luggage, but the risk of losing it is not worth the convenience. You can carry any medication you need on board with you, but take time before your flight to find out the current regulations for doing so. You can easily find these on the Transportation Safety Administration's website: www.tsa.gov.

IN A SENTENCE:

> *As a heart patient, one of the biggest changes you may face is taking multiple medications daily, with varying side effects, for the rest of your life, and the most important task for you now is to learn about the meds you take and comply fully with that daily schedule.*

Quick-Reference Medication Chart

TODAY, YOU can find a great deal of information about medication. Your pharmacist will usually give you a patient package insert with each prescription and ask you if you understand how to use the product. The Internet, bookstores, and the media are other sources; however, common sense will tell you that if you have an adverse or bad side effect, you should contact your doctor. Don't depend simply on word of mouth, even if the source of information is a pharmacist or nurse. Always check with your doctor.

Keeping up to date on what and why various meds are used is helpful. The following is a quick-reference chart of the most frequently used heart medications.

ACE Inhibitors

The kidneys produce the enzyme renin, which releases the hormone angiotensin I. Angiotensin-converting enzyme (ACE) converts angiotensin I to angiotensin II, which constricts blood vessels and causes the kidneys to retain more fluid. The main function of angiotensin II is to increase the blood pressure. ACE inhibitors block the conversion of angiotensin I to angiotensin II, thereby reducing constriction and helping to reduce blood pressure.

Additionally, after a heart attack, the heart muscle tends to overcompensate for the damage caused by the infarction. This overcompensation can lead to an increase in heart-muscle thickness and size that can then make the heart function less efficiently, eventually leading to heart failure (inability of the heart to effectively pump blood). ACE inhibitors help to minimize this overcompensation and help prevent progression to heart failure.

What it is	What it is for
Benazepril (Lotensin)	BENAZEPRIL (Lotensin) is an antihypertensive (blood pressure–lowering agent) known as an ACE inhibitor. Benazepril controls high blood pressure (hypertension) by relaxing blood vessels; it is not a cure. High blood pressure levels can damage your kidneys, and may lead to a stroke or heart failure. Generic benazepril tablets are available.
Captopril (Capoten)	CAPTOPRIL (Capoten) is an antihypertensive (blood pressure–lowering agent) known as an ACE inhibitor. Captopril controls high blood pressure (hypertension) by relaxing blood vessels; it is not a cure. High blood pressure levels can damage your kidneys, and may lead to a stroke or heart failure. Captopril also can help to treat heart failure (heart does not pump strongly enough) and certain kidney disorders. Generic captopril tablets are available.
Enalapril (Vasotec)	ENALAPRIL (Vasotec) is an antihypertensive (blood pressure–lowering agent) known as an ACE inhibitor. Enalapril

controls high blood pressure (hypertension) by relaxing blood vessels; it is not a cure. High blood pressure levels can damage your kidneys, and may lead to a stroke or heart failure. Enalapril also helps to treat patients with congestive heart failure (heart does not pump strongly enough). Generic enalapril tablets are available.

Fosinopril (Monopril)

FOSINOPRIL (Monopril) is an antihypertensive (blood pressure–lowering agent) known as an ACE inhibitor. Fosinopril controls high blood pressure (hypertension) by relaxing blood vessels; it is not a cure. High blood pressure levels can damage your kidneys, and may lead to a stroke or heart failure. Generic fosinopril tablets are available.

Lisinopril (Prinivil, Zestril)

LISINOPRIL (Prinivil, Zestril) is an antihypertensive (blood pressure–lowering agent) known as an ACE inhibitor. Lisinopril controls high blood pressure (hypertension) by relaxing blood vessels; it is not a cure. High blood pressure levels can damage your kidneys, and may lead to a stroke or heart failure. Lisinopril also helps to treat patients with heart failure (heart does not pump strongly enough). Generic lisinopril tablets are available.

Moexipril (Univasc)

MOEXIPRIL (Univasc) is an antihypertensive (blood pressure–lowering agent) known as an ACE inhibitor. Moexipril controls high blood pressure (hypertension) by relaxing blood vessels; it is not a cure. High blood pressure levels can damage your kidneys, and may lead to a stroke or heart failure. Generic moexipril tablets are not available.

Perindopril (Aceon)

PERINDOPRIL (Aceon) is a medication that lowers blood pressure by relaxing blood vessels; it is not a cure. High blood pressure levels can damage your kidneys, and may lead to a stroke or heart failure. Generic perindopril tablets are not yet available.

Quinapril (Accupril)

QUINAPRIL (Accupril) is an antihypertensive (blood pressure–lowering agent) known as an ACE inhibitor. Quinapril controls high blood pressure (hypertension) by relaxing blood vessels; it is not a cure. High blood pressure levels can damage your kidneys, and may lead to a stroke or heart failure. Quinapril also helps to treat patients with heart failure (heart does not pump strongly enough). Generic quinapril tablets are available.

Ramipril (Altace)

RAMIPRIL (Altace) is an antihypertensive (blood pressure–lowering agent) known as an ACE inhibitor. Ramipril controls high blood pressure (hypertension) by relaxing blood vessels; it is not a cure. High blood pressure levels can damage your kidneys, and may lead to a stroke or heart failure. Generic ramipril capsules are not yet available.

Trandolapril (Mavik)

TRANDOLAPRIL (Mavik) is an antihypertensive (blood pressure–lowering agent) known as an ACE inhibitor. Trandolapril controls high blood pressure (hypertension) by relaxing blood vessels; it is not a cure. Generic trandolapril tablets are not yet available.

Angiotensin II Receptor Blockers

Angiotensin II constricts blood vessels and causes the kidneys to retain more fluid. The main function of angiotensin II is to increase the blood pressure. Angiotensin II receptor blockers (ARBs) inhibit the effects of angiotensin II by blocking the receptor, thereby reducing constriction and helping to reduce blood pressure.

Additionally, after a heart attack, the heart muscle tends to overcompensate for the damage that was caused by the infarction. This overcompensation can lead to an increase in heart-muscle thickness and size, which can then make the heart function less efficiently, eventually leading to heart failure (inability of the heart to effectively pump blood). ARBs help to minimize this overcompensation and help prevent progression to heart failure. ARBs are mainly used when ACE inhibitors are not tolerated by the individual.

What it is	What it is for
Candesartan (Atacand)	CANDESARTAN (Atacand) lowers elevated blood pressure. High blood pressure levels can cause you to have a stroke, get heart failure, or damage your kidneys. Candesartan helps prevent these things from happening. Generic candesartan tablets are not yet available.
Eprosartan (Teveten)	EPROSARTAN (Teveten) helps lower blood pressure to normal levels. It controls high blood pressure, but it is not a cure. High blood pressure can damage your kidneys, and may lead to a stroke or heart failure. Eprosartan helps prevent these things from happening. Generic eprosartan is not yet available.
Irbesartan (Avapro)	IRBESARTAN (Avapro) helps lower blood pressure to normal levels. It controls high blood pressure, but it is not a cure. High blood pressure can damage your kidneys and may lead to a stroke or heart failure. Irbesartan helps prevent these things from happening. Generic irbesartan tablets are not yet available.

Losartan (Cozaar)

LOSARTAN (Cozaar) helps lower blood pressure to normal levels. It controls high blood pressure, but it is not a cure. High blood pressure can damage your kidneys, and may lead to a stroke or heart failure. Losartan helps prevent these things from happening. Losartan is also used to improve symptoms in patients with heart failure. Generic losartan tablets are not yet available.

Olmesartan (Benicar)

OLMESARTAN (Benicar) helps lower blood pressure to normal levels. It controls high blood pressure, but it is not a cure. High blood pressure can damage your kidneys and may lead to a stroke or heart failure. Olmesartan helps prevent these things from happening. Generic olmesartan tablets are not yet available.

Telmisartan (Micardis)

TELMISARTAN (Micardis) helps lower blood pressure to normal levels. It controls high blood pressure, but it is not a cure. High blood pressure can damage your kidneys, and may lead to a stroke or heart failure. Telmisartan helps prevent these things from happening. Generic telmisartan tablets are not yet available.

Valsartan (Diovan)

VALSARTAN (Diovan) helps lower blood pressure to normal levels. It controls high blood pressure, but it is not a cure. High blood pressure can damage your kidneys, and may lead to a stroke or heart failure. Valsartan helps prevent these things from happening. Generic valsartan tablets are not yet available.

Antiplatelets

Blood clots that form in the blood vessels can block blood flow to the heart or brain, causing a heart attack or stroke. Antiplatelet medications work by preventing platelets from sticking together to form blood clots. Therefore, these medications can reduce the risk of heart attack or stroke, specifically in people who have already had a heart attack or stroke, or who have poor circulation to the legs that causes pain when they walk.

What it is	What it is for
Clopidogrel (Plavix)	CLOPIDOGREL (Plavix) helps to prevent blood clots. It reduces the chance of having a heart attack or a stroke in people who have already had a heart attack or a stroke. Clopidogrel can also decrease the chance of a heart attack or stroke in certain groups of people at high risk for these events. Generic clopidogrel tablets are not yet available.
Ticlopidine (Ticlid)	TICLOPIDINE (Ticlid) helps to prevent blood clots. Ticlopidine helps to prevent strokes in patients who have already had a stroke, or those who are at high risk of having a stroke. However, ticlopidine should not be used in patients who can take aspirin to prevent a stroke. Ticlopidine is sometimes used to prevent a heart attack in patients who have already had unstable chest pain or a heart attack. It is also sometimes given with aspirin after certain procedures used to open blocked blood vessels leading to the heart. Generic ticlopidine tablets are available.

Calcium-Channel Blockers

The expansion and contraction of the heart and smooth muscles of the blood vessels are dependent on the movement of calcium into muscle cells. Calcium-channel blockers interfere with the uptake of calcium, which then helps to relax and dilate blood vessels, and reduce resistance. Similarly, calcium-channel blockers interfere with the uptake of calcium in the heart muscle, slowing the contraction of the heart and making the contractions less intense. Because of how they work, calcium channel blockers are commonly used to treat hypertension and sometimes used to treat coronary heart disease.

Furthermore, because of slight variations in how various CCBs work in the body, the CCBs can be further categorized into one of two subclasses—the dihydropyridine (pronounced die-hi-dro-pie-rih-deen) CCBs and the non-dihydropyridine CCBs.

The dihydropyridine CCB subclass includes amlodipine, bepridil (no longer available in the U.S.), felodipine, isradipine, nicardipine, nifedipine, and nisoldipine.

The non-dihydropyridine CCB subclass includes verapamil and diltiazem.

What it is	What it is for
Amlodipine (Norvasc)	AMLODIPINE (Norvasc) is a calcium-channel blocker. It affects the amount of calcium found in your heart and muscle cells. This results in relaxation of blood vessels, which can reduce the amount of work the heart has to do. Amlodipine lowers high blood pressure (hypertension). It also relieves different types of chest pain (angina). It is not a cure. Generic amlodipine tablets are not yet available.
Bepridil (Vascor)	BEPRIDIL (Vascor) is a calcium-channel blocker. It affects the amount of calcium found in your heart and muscle cells. This results in relaxation of blood vessels, which can reduce the amount of work the heart has to do. Bepridil relieves chest pain (angina). It is not a cure.
Diltiazem ER (Cardizem CD, Cardizem LA, Cardizem SR, Cartia XT, Dilacor XR,	DILTIAZEM (Cardizem CD, Cardizem LA Cartia XT, Dilacor XR, Diltia XT, Tiazac, Taztia XT, and others) is a calcium-channel

Diltia XT, Taztia XT, Tiamate, Tiazac)

blocker. It affects the amount of calcium found in your heart and muscle cells. This results in relaxation of blood vessels, which can reduce the amount of work the heart has to do. Diltiazem reduces high blood pressure (hypertension). It is not a cure. Diltiazem may also be used to relieve angina (chest pain). Generic diltiazem extended-release capsules are available. Extended-release capsules from different companies do not always act the same way in the body. If you are used to one product, it is not a good idea to switch products without approval from your prescriber.

Felodipine (Plendil)

FELODIPINE (Plendil) is a calcium-channel blocker. It affects the amount of calcium found in your heart and muscle cells. This results in relaxation of blood vessels, which can reduce the amount of work the heart has to do. Felodipine reduces high blood pressure (hypertension). It is not a cure. Generic felodipine extended-release tablets are available.

Isradipine (DynaCirc)

ISRADIPINE (DynaCirc) is a calcium-channel blocker. It affects the amount of calcium found in your heart and muscle cells. This results in relaxation of blood vessels, which can reduce the amount of work the heart has to do. Isradipine reduces high blood pressure (hypertension). It is not a cure. Generic isradipine capsules are available.

Nicardipine (Cardene)

NICARDIPINE (Cardene) is a calcium-channel blocker. It affects the amount of calcium found in your heart and muscle cells. This results in relaxation of blood vessels, which can reduce the amount of work the heart has to do. Nicardipine (regular capsules only) reduces attacks of chest pain (angina) and helps reduce high blood pressure (hypertension). It is not a cure. Generic nicardipine regular capsules are available. Generic nicardipine sustained-release capsules are not yet available.

Nicardipine SR (Cardene SR)	NICARDIPINE (Cardene) is a calcium-channel blocker. It affects the amount of calcium found in your heart and muscle cells. This results in relaxation of blood vessels, which can reduce the amount of work the heart has to do. Nicardipine (regular capsules only) reduces attacks of chest pain (angina) and helps reduce high blood pressure (hypertension). It is not a cure. Generic nicardipine regular capsules are available. Generic nicardipine sustained-release capsules are not yet available.
Nifedipine ER (Adalat CC, Afeditab CR, Nifediac CC, Procardia XL)	NIFEDIPINE (Adalat CC, Procardia XL), is a calcium-channel blocker. It affects the amount of calcium found in your heart and muscle cells, and this results in relaxation of blood vessels, which can reduce the amount of work the heart has to do. Depending on the dosage form, nifedipine reduces attacks of chest pain (angina) and/or helps reduce high blood pressure (hypertension). It is not a cure. Generic nifedipine extended-release tablets are available.
Nisoldipine (Sular)	NISOLDIPINE (Sular) is a calcium-channel blocker. It relaxes blood vessels, which can lower blood pressure and reduce the amount of work the heart has to do. Nisoldipine reduces blood pressure and may reduce attacks of chest pain if you have angina. It is not a cure. Generic nisoldipine tablets are not available.

| Verapamil (Calan, Isoptin) | VERAPAMIL (Calan, Isoptin) is a calcium-channel blocker. By relaxing blood vessels, it can improve blood flow to the heart. Verapamil reduces attacks of chest pain (angina), lowers blood pressure (treats hypertension), and controls heart rate in certain conditions. Generic verapamil tablets are available. |
| Verapamil Extended-release (Calan SR, Covera-HS, Isoptin SR, Verelan, Verelan PM) | VERAPAMIL (Calan SR, Covera-HS, Isoptin SR, Verelan, Verelan PM) is a calcium-channel blocker. It affects the amount of calcium found in your heart and muscle cells. This results in relaxation of blood vessels, which can reduce the amount of work the heart has to do. Sustained-release verapamil helps reduce high blood pressure (hypertension) It is not a cure. Generic verapamil sustained-release tablets are available. It is not a good idea to change the brand of your sustained-release product. Your body may respond differently. If you do switch between products you will need careful supervision from your prescriber or health-care professional. |

Glycoprotein IIb/IIIa Inhibitors

Glycoprotein IIb/IIIa inhibitors are antiplatelet medications that work by preventing your blood from clotting during episodes of chest pain or a heart attack or while you are undergoing a procedure to treat a blocked coronary artery.

What it is	What it is for
Abciximab Injection (ReoPro)	ABCIXIMAB (ReoPro) prevents your blood from clotting during episodes of chest pain or a heart attack or while you are undergoing a procedure to treat a blocked coronary artery. Generic abciximab injection is not yet available.

Eptifibatide (Integrilin)	EPTIFIBATIDE (Integrilin) prevents your blood from clotting during episodes of chest pain or a heart attack or while you are undergoing a procedure to treat a blocked coronary artery. Generic eptifibatide injection is not yet available.
Tirofiban (Aggrastat)	TIROFIBAN (Aggrastat) prevents your blood from clotting during episodes of chest pain or a heart attack, or while you are undergoing a procedure to treat a blocked coronary artery. Generic tirofiban injection is not yet available.

Heparin

Blood clots that form in the blood vessels can block blood flow to the heart or brain, causing a heart attack or stroke. Anticoagulants such as heparin dissolve the blood clots. By dissolving the blood clots, anticoagulants can lower the risk for heart attack and stroke.

What it is	What it is for
Heparin Injection	Heparin is an anticoagulant, sometimes called a blood thinner. However, heparin does not thin the blood or dissolve clots that have already formed. Instead, heparin prevents clot formation and stops clots from getting bigger. Heparin helps to treat or prevent clots in the veins, arteries, lungs, or heart, and to prevent clotting during open heart surgery or dialysis, or in very sick patients who stay in bed. Generic heparin injections are available.

Low Molecular Weight Heparins

Low molecular weight heparins are a modified type of heparin used to prevent blood clots from forming. They work by stopping the formation of substances in the blood that cause clots. While low molecular weight heparins are given by injection, they do not require as much monitoring as heparin, and thus can often be given to patients at home.

What it is	What it is for
Enoxaparin Injection (Lovenox)	ENOXAPARIN (Lovenox) is commonly used after knee, hip, or abdominal surgeries to prevent blood clotting. Enoxaparin is also used to treat existing blood clots in the lungs or in the veins. Enoxaparin is similar to heparin. Enoxaparin is known as an anticoagulant, and is sometimes called a blood thinner; however, enoxaparin does not actually thin the blood, but decreases the ability of blood to form clots. Generic enoxaparin injections are not yet available.

Nitrates

Nitrates dilate the veins, bringing blood to the heart as well as the arteries in the heart itself. This process reduces the heart muscle's demand for oxygen and increases its supply.

What it is	What it is for
Isosorbide Dinitrate, Sublingual and Chewable (Isordil, Sorbitrate Chewable/SL)	ISOSORBIDE DINITRATE (Isordil, Sorbitrate Chewable/SL) is a type of vasodilator. It relaxes blood vessels, increasing the blood and oxygen supply to your heart. It relieves the pain you can get with angina. There are several different types of tablets and capsules. Each type has a special design to give the most effective action. Sublingual (under the tongue) or chewable tablets can also provide prompt relief as soon as chest pain indicates the start of an angina attack. Isosorbide dinitrate

can also help to prevent pain before activities that can cause an attack (such as climbing stairs, exercise, going outdoors in cold weather, or sexual intercourse). Isosorbide dinitrate is available as chewable or sublingual tablets. Generic sublingual tablets are available, but not generic chewable tablets.

Isosorbide Mononitrate (Imdur, Ismo, Isotrate ER, Monoket)

ISOSORBIDE MONONITRATE (Ismo, Imdur, Monoket) is a type of vasodilator. It relaxes blood vessels, increasing the blood and oxygen supply to your heart. It is effective in the long-term treatment of angina associated with coronary artery disease. Generic isosorbide mononitrate is available.

Nitroglycerin ER (Nitro-Bid Nitroglyn)

NITROGLYCERIN (Nitro-Bid, Nitroglyn) is a type of vasodilator. It relaxes blood vessels, increasing the blood and oxygen supply to your heart. Nitroglycerin sustained-release products are taken regularly to help prevent or relieve chest pain (angina). They are not suitable for immediate relief during an angina attack. Generic nitroglycerin sustained-release tablets and capsules are available.

Nitroglycerin Ointment (Nitro-Bid Ointment, Nitrol)

NITROGLYCERIN (Nitro-Bid, Nitrol) is a type of vasodilator. It relaxes blood vessels, increasing the blood and oxygen supply to your heart. Nitroglycerin skin ointment is used regularly to help reduce the number of angina attacks (chest pains). It is not suitable for immediate relief during an angina attack. Generic nitroglycerin skin ointment is available.

Nitroglycerin Skin Patches (Deponit, Minitran,

NITROGLYCERIN (Transderm-Nitro, Nitro-Dur, Nitrodisc, Minitran, Deponit) is

Nitrodisc, Nitro-Dur, Transderm-Nitro)	a type of vasodilator. It relaxes blood vessels, increasing the blood and oxygen supply to your heart. Nitroglycerin skin patches are used regularly to help reduce the number of angina attacks (chest pains). They are not suitable for immediate relief during an angina attack. Generic nitroglycerin skin patches are available.
Nitroglycerin Spray (Nitrolingual)	NITROGLYCERIN (Nitrolingual) is a type of vasodilator. It relaxes blood vessels, increasing the blood and oxygen supply to your heart. Nitroglycerin mouth spray is used for immediate relief of chest pain during an angina attack or to prevent pain before activities that can cause an attack, such as climbing stairs, going outdoors in cold weather, or having intercourse. Generic nitroglycerin mouth spray is not yet available.

Oral Anticoagulants

Blood clots that form in the blood vessels can block blood flow to the heart or brain, causing a heart attack or stroke. Anticoagulants dissolve the blood clots. By dissolving the blood clots, anticoagulants can lower the risk for heart attack and stroke.

What it is	What it is for
Warfarin (Coumadin, Jantoven)	WARFARIN (Coumadin) is an anticoagulant. Warfarin helps to treat or prevent clots in the veins, arteries, lungs, or heart. Warfarin stops clots from forming or getting bigger and lets the body naturally dissolve the clots. Sometimes warfarin is called a blood thinner because you may bleed more easily while taking it; however, warfarin does not actually thin the blood. Generic warfarin tablets are available.

Salicylates

Salicylates reduce pain and swelling by blocking the body's production of chemicals that cause inflammation.

Salicylates, especially aspirin, are also used to help prevent platelets from sticking together to form blood clots. Therefore, these medications can reduce the risk of heart attack or stroke, specifically in people who have already had a heart attack or stroke or who have poor circulation to the legs that causes pain when they walk.

What it is	What it is for
Aspirin (Acetylsalicylic acid, Acuprin, Alka-Seltzer, Ascriptin A/D, Bayer, Bufferin, Easprin, Ecotrin, Empirin, Zorprin)	ASPIRIN (Ascriptin, Bayer, Ecotrin, Empirin, Zorprin, and many others) treats fever, pain, and inflammation (swelling and redness) and reduces the ability of the blood to clot. Aspirin relieves the mild to moderate discomfort caused by a variety of conditions, including arthritis, headaches, infections, menstrual cramps or pain, and minor injuries. It can also be part of therapy to reduce the risk of a heart attack or stroke. Generic aspirin is available as tablets or caplets. Aspirin tablets can be enteric-coated, extended-release, or chewable.
Aspirin Gum (Aspergum)	ASPIRIN GUM (Aspergum) treats fever, pain, and inflammation (swelling and redness) and reduces the ability of the blood to clot. Aspirin relieves the mild to moderate discomfort caused by a variety of conditions, including arthritis, headaches, infections, menstrual cramps or pain, and minor injuries. It can also be part of therapy to reduce the risk of a heart attack or stroke.

Thrombolytic Agents

Blood clots that form in the blood vessels can block blood flow to the heart or brain, causing a heart attack or stroke. Thrombolytic agents work by preventing or breaking down blood clots that cause heart attacks. These agents work best when given soon after the onset of heart attack symptoms; thus, it is important to seek medical care quickly after the onset of heart attack symptoms.

What it is	What it is for
Alteplase (Activase)	ALTEPLASE (Activase) can dissolve blood clots that form in the heart, blood vessels, or lungs after a heart attack, or some other disease process. Alteplase is called a thrombolytic agent and works best when it is given soon after the onset of heart attack symptoms. Generic alteplase injections are not yet available.
Anistreplase (Eminase)	ANISTREPLASE (Eminase) can dissolve blood clots that form in the heart, blood vessels, or lungs after a heart attack. Anistreplase is called a thrombolytic agent and works best when it is given soon after the onset of heart attack symptoms. Generic anistreplase injections are not yet available.
Reteplase (Retavase)	RETEPLASE (Retavase) is a thrombolytic agent. Thrombolytic agents dissolve blood clots that form in certain blood vessels. Reteplase is used when a blood clot in a heart artery causes a heart attack. Generic reteplase injections are not yet available.
Streptokinase (Kabikinase, Streptase)	STREPTOKINASE (Kabikinase, Streptase) can dissolve blood clots that form in the heart, blood vessels, or lungs after a heart attack, or some other disease process. Streptokinase is called a thrombolytic agent and works best when it is given soon after the onset of heart attack symptoms. Streptokinase can also dissolve blood clots that form in intravenous catheters (tubing

that goes into a vein for the infusion of intravenous fluids or medicines). Generic streptokinase is not yet available.

Tenecteplase (TNKase)

TENECTEPLASE (TNKase) is a thrombolytic agent. Thrombolytic agents dissolve blood clots that form in certain blood vessels. Tenecteplase is used when a blood clot in a heart artery causes a heart attack. Generic tenecteplase injections are not yet available.

Urokinase (Abbokinase)

UROKINASE (Abbokinase) can dissolve blood clots that form in the heart, blood vessels, or lungs after a heart attack, or some other disease process. Urokinase is called a thrombolytic agent and works best when it is given soon after the onset of heart attack symptoms. Urokinase can also dissolve blood clots that form in intravenous catheters (tubing that goes into a vein for the infusion of intravenous fluids or medicines). Generic urokinase injections are not yet available.

NOTE: Beta blockers: These medications are primarily used in heart patients and others who have hypertension (high blood pressure). These drugs help reduce the risk of heart attacks. The major brands include Temormin (atenolol), Inderal (propranolol), and Lopressor (metorolol). Ask your doctor whether you should be using one of these, and make sure you tell him or her you have hypertension.

SOURCE: © Express Scripts Inc. Reprinted with permission.

Dining Out and Traveling

MOST OF my domestic and foreign travel over the past decades has been business-related, and I have lived in very exciting and vibrant urban and metropolitan areas. This has given me an opportunity to pursue one of my favorite hobbies: great food. Whatever the specialty of the area has been, I've sampled it with very little thought given to the health effects. My rationalization was simple: "Who knows when I'll ever have the chance to eat in this great restaurant again?"

Over the decades, this scenario repeated itself hundreds of times during my time working as the cookbook buyer at QVC and then as a cookbook publisher and editor. I met many of the top chefs in the country and sampled their wonderful, rich, fat-laden food.

It certainly was fun while it lasted! This lifestyle, with my other risk factors, caught up with me. Before I turned 50, my heart screamed, "Enough!" As you've seen in earlier sections of this book, it took another five years and a bypass for me to finally realize that you could have great food and still have a heart-healthy diet and lifestyle. Fortunately, just when it looked as if I couldn't find the strength to reform, I found help in the form of my family's support and further knowledge through Weight Watchers. I began to live a heart-healthy lifestyle.

One problem persisted. I still traveled to professional meetings in great cities, and still had a passion for good food. There was only one way to not fall off the wagon. I learned how to travel healthfully.

How to Travel Heart-Healthy

To eat well on the road, you have to learn to eat well at home and to sustain that effort long enough that it becomes second nature. For example, early on in my cardio-rehab period, I visited my daughter in New England, where I grew up. In my youth, I became a seafood addict: lobster drowned in butter, fried shrimp, fried clams, fried scallops, lobster rolls, and clam chowder—food of the gods! All those triggers were waiting for me as my daughter and I visited old hangouts, so I indulged myself for the weekend. Knowing that I should be eating differently, I realized for the first time that the seafood didn't taste quite as good as it used to.

What I didn't realize then was that no matter where you are, unless you can avoid or overcome the triggers that set off desire for food that can further harm your heart, you won't survive.

What do you do if you are in the same position as I was in a job that requires you to travel? What should you do when you visit family for holidays or celebrations that are an easy excuse to ignore healthy eating? It would be great if there were some sort of twelve-step program to help you stay on the wagon on the road, but there is not. There are several things you can do, however.

Step 1: Plan Ahead for Meals

Before you go to a new city, you usually do some research about the local sites, cultural attractions, and places to eat. This is where heart-healthy travel begins.

Contact the hotel where you will be staying, talk to the concierge, and explain what you are looking for. Not only will the concierge give you great suggestions, but you'll find out about restaurants that are not the usual tourist spots. This happened to me in San Diego and Washington, DC, and the restaurants were so good and they worked so well for our heart-healthy diet that I went back twice on the same trip.

The Internet also is a good place to start an overall survey. Many restaurants have photo tours and post their menus. With that information, you can decide where you want to eat and you can make reservations on-line or through the hotel concierge. If you can, select your dining spots before you begin your trip, so you'll know you can order healthful meals.

Step 2: Don't Go Hungry

Did you ever wonder why you spend so much money traveling? Certainly, you are aware of your hotel, dining, and shopping costs, but there are always some expenses you just can't track, and they're usually in cash, too. The answer is snacks.

Travel today, especially by air, involves long delays, and you may wind up missing meals or sitting on planes that have eliminated meals. You may find that your missing cash went for overpriced snacks purchased on your way to the flight gate.

Instead, pack low-calorie snacks, like 100-calorie snack packs that easily fit into your carry-on. Cut up some vegetables and put them in a plastic bag. Take along fruit. Look for sugar-free sweets and drinks and stash your snacks in small, soft thermal cases you can carry with you. The point, beyond saving the calories, is that if you have some healthy snacks while traveling, then you will not be famished by the time you have your first meal at your destination. Some airlines still serve food on long-distance flights. Call ahead to ask if they have a heart-healthy or low-fat meal.

I pack extra snack packs or low-cal treats in my suitcase so I don't buy junk in the hotel gift shop while I'm chilling out in the evening. This same approach works if you are traveling by car or train, except you can carry more snacks for the trip.

Finally, try to eat a full meal before you leave the house. Traveling hungry raises your risk for unhealthy snacking.

Step 3: Order Light Meals

Inevitably, sometimes where and what you eat on a business trip or even a family event is out of your hands. There are business luncheons in restaurants that someone else picks, banquets where you have limited choices, or a giant buffet that features food loaded with sauces and fried food. If there is a choice in the restaurant, order something that fits into your diet. If the menu is filled with fried food or pasta, ask if the chef can prepare something without a heavy sauce, and substitute a vegetable for the potatoes.

There also seems to be a restaurant trend that suggests that we are cavemen, craving woolly mammoths. Portions are enormous, so train yourself to not eat everything—perhaps half of what's on the plate—and have the rest packaged to take home. Remember that you may not feel full immediately because it takes about 20 minutes or so for you to feel satisfied. Eat slowly and you will find that you eat less. Today, with so many people following special diets, restaurants realize that they have to be flexible.

In the buffet situation, you actually may be better off. Almost every buffet I've been to recently has been huge, following the multi-course trends in many restaurants. This is one reason why you have to have established an ability to overcome your triggers so that your food choices will automatically be healthful. Because buffets offer so much food and because restaurants are aware of health trends, you probably will find some foods that work with your diet. However, you can do one more thing. Take a smaller plate from the dessert line and use that to hold your main courses, sampling what you like. You can satisfy your cravings while minimizing the negative effect.

Business trips also tend to include cocktail hours and after-dinner drinks. Booze is loaded with calories. I've heard people say that drinking "lowers your resistance to tempting foods," and I've rarely been in a bar that didn't have salty snacks to encourage you to order more drinks. One way or the other, it's not a positive diet step. Order soda water or diet soda.

Step 4: Burn Calories

I've been surprised by how many hotels have pools and exercise rooms that cater to business travelers. Along with Internet access, the workout room has become one of the bottom-line amenities hotels use to attract guests. Since fully equipped hotels are so plentiful, book one that has workout rooms with long hours that will accommodate your needs. If you jog, talk to someone at the hotel to make sure of where you can jog safely and not get lost.

You can't realistically expect to duplicate your home workout, but you can at least be active. Try to stay at hotels that are within walking distance of the convention center. The short five-to-seven-block walks allow you to window shop, help you get a good feel for the city, and give you exposure to fresh air and sunlight.

Step 5: Stop the Stress

Travel can be very stressful, physically and mentally. Just getting onto a plane these days or taking a road trip can leave you feeling wiped out. You may have passed through several time zones, are jet lagged, and feel like a pretzel sitting for hours on a crammed plane. Unfortunately, stress can increase your desire to eat more—at least that was my reaction for many years.

If you travel frequently, it would be a good idea to learn some stress-reduction exercises (**Month Six**) or try to hit the workout room soon after your arrival. Swimming is a great way to burn stress, as it uses many of your muscles, is aerobic in nature, and leaves you relaxed.

Step 6: Indulge in Occasional Celebrations

Not all travel is linked to business. Some may be for a celebration, such as a wedding or a party at someone's home. A wedding celebration presents many of the same problems as you will encounter on a business trip, so the same suggestions apply. The one difference may be the opportunity for total excess, along with the feeling that you want to have a good time.

Unless you are on an extremely limited heart/diabetic/high blood pressure diet, you probably can indulge yourself just a bit. The reality is that celebrations don't come around often, and you are working so hard that you can afford a short break from your program.

If you are going to a local party or a Thanksgiving celebration, bring a dish that you know is healthful and that you can eat. Mention to the host that you are on a heart-healthy diet and ask what the menu is going to be. Rarely will someone take offense at your asking ahead of time, compared to simply not eating the food offered.

Essential pointers for the road:

○ Bring healthy snacks for travel and to have in your room.
○ Pack for activity. Take your exercise outfit and sneakers.
○ Look for a hotel with exercise facilities and a pool, if possible.
○ Look for restaurants that have a varied menu.
○ Eat less at banquets and buffets if you must attend them.
○ Walk, walk, walk, walk whenever you can.
○ Avoid the open bar at celebrations.
○ Bring a healthy dish to a party or celebration when you can.
○ Loosen up once in a while—but not too much!

IN A SENTENCE:

Eating well when you travel is directly related to how well you have learned heart-healthy eating at home, so remember to avoid excess eating, carry your own food, make judicious restaurant choices, don't fall for stress-related eating, and keep in control at banquets and parties.

Living Alone

AS THIS book was being written, I met and talked to many heart patients who lived alone. Most were middle-aged, like me. Some were older. In that group, the majority were women. This is not surprising, as men have heart attacks earlier than women. The women often were widows, while most of the men were divorced. One thing that they did not have in common was the ability to cope well when living alone. (In this case, "living alone" means that you are not married or you do not have a partner. It means that with the exception of seeing friends or going to work, you come home to no one. This situation can, by itself, be a risk factor.)

Men, in my experience, don't like to be alone, and we also like being taken care of, although we may not be great patients. I was in the middle of a divorce at the time of my first heart attack, and living alone when I had my bypass. In fact, when I was released from the hospital after my surgery, a close friend drove me home and was speechless that I intended to spend my first day and night after open heart surgery by myself. At that time, probably still in some sort of mental shock, I thought I'd be fine. Previously, I'd lived alone for several years, and I was pretty domesticated. At that point, I think I just wanted some peace and distance from the hospital.

Living Alone Is Not Good for the Heart

There is not much data on the effect of heart disease on those who live alone; however, about 26 percent (73 million people of the U.S. population) are single people living with no roommate or partner. Studies show they tend to have poorer dietary habits, eating takeout food or eating in restaurants.

I can vouch for that. During my first years alone, food to go was my idea of a diet. Much of this was high in calories and sodium and low in vegetables.

A Danish study showed that people who live alone are twice as likely to have a heart attack or serious chest pain and sudden cardiac death as those who live with a partner or roommate. Researchers say the results suggest that doctors should take a patient's living situation, as well as age and other established risk factors, into account when assessing his or her risk of heart disease.

"(The researchers) say certain heart disease risk factors may be more common in the lifestyles of people who live alone, such as obesity, smoking, high cholesterol, and making fewer visits to the family doctor, and may help explain the findings. Using information on age, sex, education, and other demographic factors from population registers, researchers found age and living alone were the two strongest predictors of acute coronary syndrome."

Living Alone: The Reality

Data and stats are fine, but there is a reality to living alone after you have a heart attack and surgery that probably drives everything else. Certainly, beginning the cardio-rehab program is good and gives you something to do, but there is another underlying emotion that I experienced: fear. While I kept up a happy front, there were many emotions going through my mind that those of you who live alone might share.

For example, I was concerned about my "zipper," the badge-of-courage scar that all open heart patients get after the chest is closed. Your doctors will be very concerned that you don't sustain any chest injuries that might cause your incision to separate. You are warned to be extremely careful, and you're temporarily banned from bike riding, driving, or heavy lifting. That warning is enough to make you worry, and if you are alone, you are more concerned because there is no one there to help you should something happen.

That is at the crux of the problem with living alone: No one is there should anything happen. This is an especially acute concern when you are trying to sleep. I spent a great many sleepless nights worrying about "something" happening, whatever that meant.

I found myself forgetting things and was positive, despite what everyone told me, that I had expired during surgery and had had to be revived, causing brain damage. (Most of my friends said I was that way before surgery!) But nights were tough, and I finally got a mild sedative from my doctor, which saved me. Negative emotions lead to stress that leads to strain on your just-repaired heart or to any heart that is at risk.

If you live alone and you experience anxiety, sleeplessness, and heart palpitations, it is even more important that you talk with your doctor. People who have spouses or partners have a shoulder to lean on; you may not. You may also need more than just a prescription from a doctor. Strongly consider counseling of some sort, as described in the section on stress (see **Month Six**). After heart surgery or a heart attack, depression is common. It is dangerous, and you should not attempt to treat yourself for it.

Eventually, the fear begins to subside as you realize that you probably have been fixed pretty well by your doctor or surgeon and your strength is beginning to return. You may have overcome some of the immediate practical problems, such as getting a ride to the market, and you are sleeping well. Now, you have to adjust to life alone, as do many others, but with an extra burden, your cardiac health.

How Do You Stay with the Cardio Program?

There is no guidebook for living alone with heart disease. Everyone I've spoken to takes an approach based on their *life before their cardiac diagnosis or event*. If you are someone who has lived alone for a lengthy period, you probably have your own schedules, activities, and circle of friends.

Ultimately, that life can return very quickly. I was back at work and traveling within five weeks. What has changed is that you embrace the diet, exercise, and overall health program laid out for you by your doctor.

The only difference here between you and a married person is that you're the one who has to make sure you comply with everything. From my experience, and according to other patients, this is a greater challenge. To stay with the recovery program that's been laid out, you have to adapt your life to the new needs of your body and lifestyle.

Diet: Priority #1

Changing your diet is one area where you have to make changes. You have to learn to cook. Many people who live alone cook, but they may only prepare food that is not part of a heart-healthy diet. Here are a few tricks:

○ Learning to cook can make your mealtime easier because you can prepare large portions and store them in the refrigerator or the freezer. There are multiple ways to store food, and you will learn that the microwave is for more than popcorn. Pre-portioned cooked meals give you meals anytime.

○ Shop at farm-style markets where you can buy fresh vegetables, fresh meat, chicken, or fish. Talk to the people who work at the market, and you will be surprised at how much they know. As a single guy, I learned how to shop by just talking to people in the market.

○ Invite friends over to sample your cooking. Better yet, find a friend who is a great cook and who can teach you how to modify recipes and improve your culinary skills. I've learned knife skills, how to sauté, stir frying, and how to make nutritious soups.

○ If you can afford it, take some cooking classes, especially in healthy cooking. I can guarantee that you'll meet someone in your situation. The classes can turn into a social activity, which is a bonus.

Compliance with Medications and Exercise

When it comes to following your doctor's orders regarding medication and exercise, there is no difference between you and people who don't live alone, except that you don't have an immediate backup system or someone to remind you to take your meds or check to see that you have. Here are some tricks for you:

○ Taking your pills or medications is vital. When I lived alone, I put my pills in a place where I could not miss seeing them at any time of the day. I also bought some pill holders and laid out three weeks' worth of pills, which enabled me to keep track of them and ensured that I'd know when I'd taken them.

○ Every morning I make coffee and I put my pills next to the coffeemaker, actually under the bean jar. I can't miss them. At night, my pills are next to my razor and toothbrush. It may sound silly; however, if you stop taking your pills or if you miss doses, you can face some bad consequences.

○ Where exercise is concerned, many people would rather forget it, just as they did before they got sick. You cannot do that now. What has worked for me have been the things described in **Month Five** as a method; however, motivation is what you have to develop.

○ I quickly found an inexpensive gym membership, less than $150 per year. Search websites and the Yellow Pages. This is a competitive industry, and there are usually membership specials going on. In my case, I joined the YMCA and used all their facilities. Once I learned how to exercise properly from an expert, my motivation grew because I saw results, and that reduced my frustration with exercising.

○ Exercising with someone is the best way to exercise because it provides reinforcement, companionship, and fun.

Safety

If you are a heart patient and you live alone it is absolutely vital that you have some sort of around-the-clock lifeline. Your safety can be compromised in a moment.

Find one person or multiple people who will touch base with you every day, at least during the first six months of your recovery. Let them know the name of your doctor, what medications you take, and exactly what you have had in terms of surgery or other treatment. Make sure that your lifesaver knows where your medical records are if you have a copy at home.

Ask a string of friends whom you talk to frequently so they will know you are OK. Again, don't hesitate to call your doctor. Finally, if you have mobility problems, talk with your doctor about acquiring a heart-monitoring device in case something goes wrong.

IN A SENTENCE:

> *Living alone as a heart patient can be difficult because you may not have someone to give you help immediately or to keep you on your road to recovery; however, you can find inner strength and enjoy life more by participating in healthy activities that help your recovery.*

living

Keeping Your Costs in Check

WHEN YOU hear someone talking about keeping health-care costs in check, they are usually not talking about yours. The main concern about health-care costs actually seems to leave you—the patient—out of the equation, except when they talk about how much your health insurance costs your employer and why they have to raise the contribution from your paycheck.

About two-thirds of Americans get their health-care coverage through the workplace, and each year your contribution has gone up. While the costs to you have slowed somewhat in the last two years, the average share for a family of four is $2,700 per year. Remember, that amount is only for your share of the insurance plan; it does not necessarily cover costs of many other health-care needs. At the same time, health-care costs are rising faster than your paycheck is growing.

There do seem to be some disparities; however, a study published in 2005 in the *Journal of the American Medical Association (JAMA)* found that patients who needed ambulatory follow-up care with private insurance were more likely to get follow-up visits scheduled quickly than those who had Medicaid coverage were.

Can You Do Anything about Costs?

Keeping your personal health-care costs under control is not easy, but there are some places where you can make a difference.

Start with your insurance plan. If you have a workplace insurance plan, the human resources department, employee ombudsman, or the agents who work with the company are good sources of information. However, you have to be aggressive in talking with them. Make them read through the available policy or policies with you until you completely understand the benefits. Do they meet your needs as we discussed previously? Unless you really understand your insurance, something is likely to fall through the cracks.

Make sure you know what can happen to you if something catastrophic occurs and you are out of work for a period of time. Find out what treatments and services are covered.

Your doctor's office can be a great fountain of knowledge. There are people on staff who code procedures for the insurance companies and others who talk to insurance companies regularly. Ask them what your insurance will cover that might come up in your treatment.

The same goes for a hospital. It will have to pre-certify you before you are allowed to be admitted. Find out about their charges and confirm that there are no hidden charges—e.g., medication that you might be given that is not covered by your insurance.

If you have a chance to change policies annually at your workplace, you can make a decision about what type of plan you need at that time.

Keeping Medication Costs Down

Medication will be one of the most important parts of your healt care for the coming years. Drugs are expensive, and you may have to change your meds on occasion. Here are some cost-saving ideas:

○ Always ask if the medication can be given generically.
○ Our health-insurance company, Medical Mutual, has a program called Diabetes Advantage that provides all of my insulin, my blood glucose monitor, test strips, needles, and sterile wipes at no cost. Each month, I speak to a nurse who keeps records of my

progress and who provides information when I need it. I would not have known about the program if I had not asked.

○ Similarly, by asking, I found a discount drug program through the mail (www.medco.com) that provides my meds in bulk at a very good discount. There are many of these programs (see **Month Twelve**), such as www.drugstore.com, that can be found by searching online and by asking your doctor or the people you meet in cardio rehab.

○ It's not well known that many of the pharmaceutical companies actually have free medication programs for those with qualifying incomes. Your doctor or nurse will know about these. I was saved by this program during a rough financial period.

○ Ask your doctor for samples when you start a new drug, or ask the pharmacist to only partially fill the prescription to make sure that you can tolerate it without wasting money for a full prescription.

○ Finally, shop around for both prescription and over-the-counter drugs. Go to retail and warehouse stores and pharmacy chains that use medication discounts as a way to get people into the stores. Tell a pharmacist that you can get a better deal across the street and you might hear about a discount.

What Is a Health Savings Account?

In 2004, a new federal law created health savings accounts (HSAs) in the hope that this would give people an alternative method of insuring themselves and choosing (or changing) the doctor they wanted at any time. The HSA is similar to an IRA because it is a tax-free savings account, except that the money can be used only to purchase health care. In addition, health-care expenses are 100 percent tax-deductible. Current law allows you to deposit $2,850 as a single person and $5,650 as a family each year. If you don't use the money in a single year, you can continue to contribute to it, and your fund grows. When you reach age 65, it can go towards retirement or medical expenses.

The second part of this plan is that you can purchase a high-deductible point-of-service health-insurance plan that is usually an affordable plan with low co-pays once you have reached your deductible. The HSA approach enables you to build a tax-free nest egg for future medical expenses with coverage under an insurance policy in case you have a major medical problem.

Is There Any Guaranteed Way to Save Money on Health Care?

Health-care costs today are estimated to be 50 times higher than they were 50 years ago. You may feel that this is a runaway train that is one more thing to cope with, and that can harm your recovery. It's understandable, because we're all in the same boat.

While there are few ways to guarantee cost savings, one is obvious. Take care of yourself. I've saved money on pills by getting better and dropping them from my list. I take less insulin because I exercise and watch my diet, and my diabetes is under control.

Being well is the best way to navigate the health-care system and control the costs because it will give you the least contact with it!

IN A SENTENCE:

> *Controlling health-care costs requires a multi-front approach that includes making sure you have an insurance policy that covers your needs and the right access to medications, and exploring alternative methods of coverage, such as a health savings account.*

Navigating the Health-Care System

DURING YOUR recovery from heart disease, you will be called on to do many things that essentially lead to a total lifestyle change. Most of this is going to be a very positive experience in the long run because you will feel better. However, one thing is almost guaranteed to drive you slightly nuts, and that's the health-care system and your relationship to it.

There is no question that the health-care system in the U.S. is complicated, inconsistent, and probably the most unfair to those with lower incomes. However, even if you are in the middle class with a good job, you still may find yourself strapped financially due to uncovered medical costs.

If you are a heart patient requiring a variety of expensive procedures, continual office visits, cardio rehab, and multiple medications, you have an even more complicated challenge. Unfortunately, if you have certain kinds of insurance or if you are a Medicare or Medicaid patient, you may have limited options for paying for your care.

The U.S. is alone among almost all industrialized countries in lacking some form of guaranteed health coverage for its citizens. A 2007 report from the Centers for Disease Control and Prevention and the National Center for Health Statistics found that 43.6 million people (14.8 percent) had no health insurance in 2006. Worse, more than 54 million people (18 percent) were without insurance at some point during the year. Worse than all of this is that almost 9.3 million children under the age of 18 are uninsured. The numbers among minority groups are even higher: 32 percent of Hispanics lack health insurance, and 16 percent of African Americans were uninsured compared to 10 percent of Caucasians.

Within the groups most likely to suffer from lack of health insurance, the baby boomers, 13 percent of adults between the ages of 45 and 65 are uninsured. More men, who are likely to have cardiovascular problems early, report having no health insurance.

The *New York Times* reported in 2005 that "Life at the top isn't just better. It's longer." The reporter followed three different patients and learned that their social class determined "everything from the circumstances of their heart attacks, to the emergency care each received, the household they returned to, and the jobs they hoped to resume."

The goals of your insurance program should be to ensure the highest-quality care for your problem at a reasonable cost. Instead, the system serves us inconsistently. While there are strict standards of care, each doctor's practice and hospital operates differently. The amount of paperwork doctors and patients face makes health-care delivery more difficult each day.

What Are Your Insurance Options?

If you have been diagnosed with heart disease, you have already had multiple conversations with your health-care provider and your insurance company. You may think you are covered, and that all you have is a small co-pay, but then a bill shows up and you begin to wonder, "What the heck is this?"

This happened to me. I was asked by my doctor to have some tests and, after calling my insurance company, was confident that I was good to go. Wrong. About a month later, I got a large bill for "uncovered" tests. These were some things that I should have known about or thought about ahead of time, but I did not get approval in writing from the insurance company.

You can stop this from happening to you if you understand the system.

Do you know what type of insurance you have? Medical policies are not all the same. Most people who are insured today have one of four different types of health insurance, lumped under the general term "man-aged care." The purpose of managed care is to try to contain health-care costs. This is why many medical procedures have to be cleared and approved ahead of time by your insurer. Without this OK, you will not get care. This rule has become a point of contention for many years among health-care providers, insurance companies, legislators, politicians, and many other interest groups. Here are the four basic options you have:

1. Preferred Provider Organization (PPO)
2. Point-of-Service Plan (POS)
3. Health Maintenance Organization (HMO)
4. Fee For Service Plan

Each of these types of policies is available in many workplace insurance programs. In some cases, you are limited as to your choice of policy. Here are the basics of each one.

Health Maintenance Organization (HMO)

HMOs are the most restrictive type of insurance, but they also are the least expensive. The HMO contracts with groups of primary care doctors and specialists to form a "closed group." If you join an HMO, you can only see the providers in the group; however, you rarely have to pay more than a small co-pay for services.

You will be asked to choose a primary care physician who makes all your medical decisions. If the doctor does not to send you to a specialist, you can't go to one without paying more. If you are cleared to see a specialist, that physician will be someone who works for the HMO.

Some people like HMOs because they are fairly simple to deal with, and in some cases, you can get wellness care, checkups, and immunizations as part of your care.

Preferred Provider Organization (PPO)

PPOs are similar to HMOs in that they consist of a network of doctors approved by your insurance company. PPO doctors have agreed with your insurance company to accept that insurance and an amount they are paid for their services by the PPO, along with your co-pay. You also have to choose a primary care doctor from the network who will refer you to a cardiologist in the network.

If you stay within that network, your co-pay or deductible will be lower. If you go outside of the network, your costs can be very high, up to 50 percent of the bill.

While PPOs are less restrictive, you may have to pay more out of pocket at work as your employee contribution. Most PPOs offer preventative medical care, such as mammograms.

Point-of-Service Plan (POS)

POS plans are sort of an HMO linked to a PPO. This gives you the ability to choose which plan you want to use when you are in need of help. The doctors are part of a contract network and, depending on which doctor you pick, you may pay more. If you decide to go with a doctor in an HMO, you have to abide by those rules. You pay less, but you have fewer choices. If you choose a doctor who is in a PPO network, you have more flexibility, but a higher co-pay and deductible.

Fee for Service Plan

A Fee For Service plan is an "old-style" plan that still is somewhat popular. Basically, you pay premiums to an insurance company, you choose any doctor you want when you need one, and you are covered for most services.

The main problem is that you have to pay a high deductible before your insurance coverage kicks in. For example, if you have a $20,000 operation, the first $2,000 (if that is your deductible) must be paid, sometimes up front, before the surgery proceeds. Another problem is that the insurance company may have spending caps, and each year, the paid deductible reverts to $0 and begins over again.

If You Are Able to Choose Your Plan

One of the problems with the plans above is that most are only available through your workplace, unless you are over 65 and you are on

Medicare or you qualify for Medicaid because of low income. However, if you are covered in the workplace and you have the opportunity to change plans once a year, here are some things to consider about your current plan and alternate plans:

○ How high is the deductible?
○ What is the term of coverage?
○ Can you access the doctor you really want?
○ What does the policy cover and how comprehensive should it be?
○ What is the policy regarding specialists?
○ Are the doctors within easy access?
○ Are you organized to keep the records that may be required?
○ Are regular physical exams and screenings included?
○ What length of hospitalization is covered?
○ Is there a drug plan?
○ Can you get dental or vision coverage?
○ Are treatments for mental health or alcohol and drug abuse covered?
○ Are OB/GYN costs included?
○ Is chronic-care coverage available?
○ Does it cover alternative health care such as acupuncture and chiropractic procedures?
○ Is preventive care for children part of the plan?

Where to Seek Treatment

Trying to understand how the health-care system works can be overwhelming. For more details, there are countless books on this subject that you can check out from the library.

If you do not have insurance, you still have some options, although the reality is that it does make your life more difficult. One method is to start a Health Savings Account, which enables you to build a piggy bank to buy different kinds of insurance for a day when your health is at risk. Other options are free clinics run by community organizations. You can also contact the medical association that is most connected to your problem (e.g., the American Heart Association). All associations have local chapters, and they are there to help you.

Hospital emergency room doctors and staff must see you, but going to the emergency room for non-emergency care is not a good solution for people with chronic diseases. Sadly, the best option today is to go to the polls and vote for the candidate who actually has some credibility and who will, perhaps, institute national health care for everyone in the U.S., like people in most of the rest of the industrialized world have.

As a heart patient, the most important thing to keep in mind is *where you are going to seek treatment.* In **Day Four**, the process of choosing a doctor was discussed in some detail. However, choosing the facility for your care is just as important. So is making sure that your insurance coverage will take care of your expenses. Here are several things to think about when deciding on your treatment facility:

- ○ What are the heart-treatment facilities like?
- ○ Are they clean and up to date?
- ○ Does the facility publish its outcomes and procedural complication data?
- ○ Does it accept your insurance, and will the facility allow you to arrange a "pay-out" for extra expense?
- ○ Is the hospital accredited by the proper boards and government commissions?
- ○ Is this a comprehensive care facility? Will you have to go somewhere that doesn't take your insurance for outpatient care?
- ○ Does it offer education and rehab as part of the cost covered by your insurance?
- ○ If you need specialized care, is it covered?
- ○ Are all of your questions answered to your satisfaction?

Every year, the federal government promises new initiatives to reform the health-care system, and, consistently, these initiatives fail. In fact, virtually every U.S. president in the past 75 years has tried to introduce a universal health-care system.

People constantly point to Canada and England, where there are systems in place that make at least a certain level of health care available to everyone. These systems, while guaranteeing everyone basic levels of coverage, are not a panacea. In some cases, the only way you can see a doctor or other health specialist is in a hospital, and treatment for certain surgeries, like a cardiac bypass, may take many months to set up. The positive side of many of these programs is that they attempt to lower costs through wellness programs and childcare services. The absence of programs such as these is one of the reasons we lag behind many countries in the health of our children.

Now that you are a heavy consumer of health-care services and information, you will be affected by our health-care system, by the insurance plan you choose, and by the out-of-pocket costs you incur. If you have never been active in health-care issues, there is no better time to become involved than now. Contact your congressional representatives, learn what programs are being proposed, and decide for yourself, from your very unique perspective, what would benefit our country most.

Navigating any river requires a clear understanding of what is above and below the surface so that you have no surprises. The health-care system, as it applies to you now, is an uncharted river that you can navigate if you learn the system and make it work for you.

IN A SENTENCE:

> The health-care system is complex, but as a heart patient, you will have to learn how to choose the right insurance program, doctor, and treatment facility that meet your needs and are covered under the health-care plans available to you.

living

Will I Need a Heart Transplant?

AT SOME point, there is the possibility that the "T" word—transplantation—might have passed through your mind. Even if your doctor has never mentioned it or you were told that there was not even a remote chance that you needed anything as drastic as a heart transplant, the thought might still be lurking. It's likely that you do not need to worry because you would not be able to do too much on your own now. You would be quite sick.

In general, if you have had long-term heart damage or some sort of viral infection that has compromised your heart, you may need a transplant. It's also possible that a massive heart attack with significant cardiac muscle damage might put you at great risk of needing a transplant. Basically, if your heart no longer works well enough to keep you alive, then it is likely that you will be placed on the list of patients waiting for a donor.

Transplantation is no longer science fiction, but a fairly straightforward surgical procedure. In 2006, there were 2,125 heart transplants, up by about 100 from 2005. Almost three-fourths of the patients are males, and 70 percent of those are Caucasian. Almost half the patients are over age 50; however, 19 percent are under 50. Transplants work.

Over 85 percent survive 1 year, 75 percent survive 3 years, and 66 percent of women and 71 percent of men survive 5 years.

The Procedure

The transplant procedure is relatively straightforward. Most transplant patients have had long-term heart disease or sudden, catastrophic disease that damages the heart muscle almost totally. The heart simply can't carry the load. People who qualify for the surgery are carefully screened and tested at a medical center that specializes in transplantation and does many each year. The surgery itself will last between 4 and 12 hours. The donor heart is one that has been determined to be a good tissue match, which means the blood type and other genetic factors are the best possible match for the recipient.

The patient is put on a heart-lung bypass machine and the old heart is stopped. It's removed and the new one is transplanted in its place. Often, the new heart starts on its own as the bypass machine is withdrawn or an electrical shock is administered to get it restarted.

The recipient is usually up and around quickly after the surgery, although the main danger is rejection of the heart by the immune system. As a result, the patient must take an immunosuppressant "cocktail" of medications that have some side effects. For example, the face may become rounder, and the person may experience some weight gain, but altogether the patient is now able to live a very good lifestyle that had not been enjoyed in many years. The patient may be home within two weeks.

A heart transplant, like a kidney or corneal transplant, improves quality of life for many years to come and, in many cases, allows the patient to return to normal life.

Organ Donation

Needing a heart transplant and being able to get one are two different things. One of the greatest medical frustrations today is that, to a great extent, transplantation is a medical procedure that can take patients from "end-stage" heart failure and restore them to health, but organs are scarce. Unlike a kidney transplant, a viable heart can't be donated by a relative who might be a good tissue match. One of the great health failures in this country has been our inability to get enough people to agree to be organ donors when they die.

Right now, more than 96,000 people are waiting for an organ of some type, and over 4,000 need a heart. A national organ-sharing network called United Network for Organ Sharing (UNOS) (www.unos.org) has done a great job working with hospitals and potential donor families, to create a list of donors with those who are the sickest and who have been on the list longest.

There is no reason to not become an organ donor. Even if you have heart disease, you can be a donor. Organ transplantation has saved thousands and thousands of lives, some of them children who were born with defective hearts. As difficult an idea as this may be, organ donation is a priceless gift to society and the recipient.

IN A SENTENCE:

More than 96,000 people, including children, and 4,000 heart patients need transplants, and while it's true that they will live much better lives with transplants, it's important to recognize that donors are scarce, transplant patients require many medications, and transplant patients will have to work with their doctors closely to remain healthy.

What's on the Horizon?

IMAGINE ONE day receiving a call, opening the newspaper, or watching a report on TV telling you that heart disease has been cured. You would no longer have to take medication, and your diabetes or hypertension would be a thing of the past. We all wish that it would happen, but it won't any time soon.

Radical cures take generations to evolve, but in the meantime there is a solution. We now know how to prevent heart disease from becoming as devastating as it may be to you and your family. The idea of prevention is a great revolutionary treatment. The information in this book that you have absorbed over the last year has given you the tools you need. You can lower your risk factors, become active, and change your diet. You can reduce your stress and change the culture of your family, reducing the effect of risk factors you may have passed on through your DNA or your lifestyle to your children.

Teaching our Children

One of the things that can make the greatest difference in heart disease treatment would be to diminish the need for treatment. This will come from some sort of health-care policy reform—but not the one you might think, such as universal health coverage. *What must change is a focus on wellness for everyone, especially for our children.* This one change, which can be made quickly and simply, would change the economics of the health-care system and would create a better life for you.

We have to learn how to relax, how to use our vacation time, and how to make prevention of heart disease part of our daily lives. European workers take vacations, often an entire month, and they work a reasonable number of hours each day. Only recently, as our junk-food culture has spread throughout the world, has heart disease begun to increase worldwide.

As patients, some of the best things we can do for ourselves to increase heart health are to urge our country's leaders to focus on the health and well being of our children, put our knowledge to good use by working with the schools to eliminate junk food, and not patronize restaurants that do not offer healthy choices for our kids.

Wellness

One of the reasons wellness should be a part of our everyday lives is that our health-care system is rapidly getting maxed out. The aging baby boomer population and their growing medical needs will make matters more acute. In 25 years, twice as many people will be over age 65 as there are now, and the majority of them will be women. As a result, more care will be provided on an outpatient basis. Large hospitals will become medical centers that focus on high-tech procedures, and acute care will be distributed to outlying community-family medical centers. You will be able to see your primary physician, endocrinologist, gynecologist, cardiologist, and physical therapist in one building. Tests will be done on site. Electronic medical record systems already exist in virtually every health-care facility. Health care will be at a premium, so encouraging wellness will be the most cost-effective way to go.

More Accurate Diagnosis

Because your overall heart health depends on what affects your body's entire system, today cardiologists and other physicians are using more technology. The goal is not necessarily to simply create an overview of the body; in fact, the opposite is true. Today's medical technology focuses on having a better picture of specific sites where problems may appear, such as an artery in which blockages are beginning to build.

Scientists also are looking at new medications and genetic research for targeted treatment. A good way to track some of these new achievements is through some of the websites and electronic newsletters listed in **Month Twelve**. A few of the newest diagnostic tools are described below.

The CT Scan

You've probably heard of computed tomography (CT), which has been around for more than a decade. You may have had one of these scans to detect plaque buildup in your arteries and to determine whether you have atherosclerosis. New, super-fast CT machines enable your doctor to get a 3D view of your heart that is approaching the resolution of a coronary **angiogram**.

The CT machine can cost $1.5 million, much more than a coronary angiogram. It's also non-invasive, so the risk-to-benefit ratio of CT may be better. The benefit of this sort of technology is that if you begin showing symptoms of heart disease, your doctor may be able to make a quicker diagnosis without requiring you to go through the time-consuming angiography procedure. Unfortunately, the CT procedure can result in problems caused by the dye and radiation. It, too, can become a lengthy procedure at times.

Gene Therapy

Over the past decade, scientists have begun to detect genes that are implicated in different heart diseases, especially congenital heart disease. For example, researchers feel that there is a common gene at the root of DiGeorge syndrome, a disorder that causes birth defects. Detecting the genetic link to your potential heart problems suggests that in the future you could use genetic information or your genes themselves for treatment.

Genes are the functional units of heredity, which, when put in a certain sequence, create the basic protein we use to function each day. They influence not only how we live, but how we look, how we play a sport, and how we react to the environment around us. If our genes are altered or damaged, we cannot function normally. It stands to reason that since we have been able to study our genetic codes and determine why we are what we are in the mapping of the human genome we can turn that around and fix ourselves.

That dream is still only a dream, but scientists all over the world are working on making it a reality. Researchers at Johns Hopkins were able to transfer a gene for the G protein to cells of the AV node in pigs with atrial fibrillation with some success. Similar attempts to transfer genes to mice with heart-muscle problems have been tried with some success in Europe.

The goal of gene therapy at present is to repair, regulate (i.e., turn on and off), and maneuver your genetic structure to achieve improved heart function. Will this happen in your lifetime? The likelihood is not great, since research has, until recently, been mostly in the lab. There have been some isolated attempts in humans, where tissue from one part of the body was transplanted into another through a technique called **myoblast** transplantation. One trial in the late 1990s resulted in the death of a study subject, causing a setback to studies in humans.

There has been progress, however, in the continued ability to link specific genes to different diseases. By identifying these defective or mutated genes, medicines may be developed to correct the problem. Gene therapy offers one of the most exciting, and perhaps the most realistic, possibilities for new heart treatments. Some progress in this area has been made at Johns Hopkins, where scientists developed a gene therapy that seemed to work like a calcium channel blocker medication to stabilize arrhythmias, enlarged hearts, and high blood pressure.

What about Stem Cells?

Stem cell research cuts across many different issues. There is strong evidence that no one refutes that stem cell resources may produce cures for many chronic diseases. The basic arguments about stem cells are political and religious, and center more on where the stem cells would come from. Stem cells are actually part of your body's building blocks that function like an internal repair kit. In fact, there are multiple examples of someone's own (autologous) stem cells being transplanted with beneficial results.

Scientists are hopeful that there will be changes in the moral complexity surrounding stem cells, and that the public will understand that this is a complex issue that has become bogged down because of lack of knowledge and poor communication about the other potential sources of stem cells (such as muscle-derived and umbilical cells). The reality, except in some isolated cases, is that medicines or treatments for heart disease and other chronic conditions from stem cells are years, if not decades, away.

The good news is that there are private research labs and other organizations that do believe that stem cell research may be a true answer to many disorders, and they have not given up their research. One study on heart patients that has been going on in Europe involved three different sources of stem cells. Results are anticipated by the end of the decade.

The Future Is Now

Medical science changes frequently, as does medical opinion. This is one lesson about the future that you might want to keep in mind. As I've gone through the early stages of my recovery, as you are now, I was focused on my lifestyle changes, adjusting to medication, and regaining my spirits. After a decade, I've found that the changes in my treatment have remained fairly straightforward.

Certainly, medications have been replaced with new ones that seem to work better. However, my bypass was pretty straightforward, and was not much different seven years ago from how it's done today. Postoperative care and cardio-rehab are similar but are still dependent on how much you want to achieve.

The future for you as a heart patient is not going to change very much. It's unlikely that you will receive a bionic heart or some other miracle in the near future. However, *you* are the great breakthrough. With your doctor and your support group, your family and friends, you can decide that you are going to make the lifestyle changes you must make, and you will rise to the occasion.

IN A SENTENCE:

> *The future of heart treatment for you does not rest in the hands of scientists; rather, what you do now to improve your health will be the great breakthrough.*

living

Healthy Cooking, Healthy Living

AS YOU reach the end of your first year of recovery from heart disease, you will be able to take care of the basics. You'll see your doctor less frequently and your life will become more normal. You will have developed methods that help to rebuild your heart and to comply with your medication and exercise routines. A heart-healthy diet will be a normal part of your life. You are on the road back!

Building a Cookbook Library

One of the best parts of recovery for me was learning new skills in the kitchen and meeting experts through my profession who taught me a few cooking tricks, such as how to stir fry—a very healthy cooking method. I was fortunate to meet some of the best chefs in the country and watch them cook. If you can take some cooking classes, you'll meet people who have the same goals as you do and who can share your experiences.

Along the way, I have amassed an extensive library of cookbooks. Over the past year, I have added books that have taught me how to cook more healthfully and, to my amazement, to prepare better, more delicious food.

Another thing I discovered in my recovery—something that many home cooks already know—is that cookbooks are also great fun to read and to use. It's said that anyone who can read can cook. And anyone who can read can be a healthy cook.

I have more than 100 cookbooks in my collection, and I seem to get more each month. Only a few of the books I use frequently are books by famous chefs or culinary celebrities. Many of those books are really not created for the home chef who is trying to cook and eat healthfully. They're filled with recipes for foods drenched in butter and mayonnaise and many deep-fried foods.

When choosing a good cookbook, look for three elements:

○ The recipes are all on a single page or two opposite pages.
○ Ingredients are listed separately so you can make a shopping list easily.
○ In general, "prep"—cutting veggies, slicing chicken, etc., prior to putting something into the oven to bake or on the stove to sauté—should not take more than 30 minutes.

What about pictures? Today many cookbooks have lavish color pictures and you may find yourself attracted to them. Certainly, it is helpful to see what the dish is supposed to look like. The pictures in cookbooks usually do present the dish properly; however, they are styled, just like a photo of a cover girl on a fashion magazine. While this should not keep you from buying the book, be aware that the ingredients of the recipes—not only the way it looks—are what you are using to make your buy/no-buy decision. I have worked with cookbook publishers who have sold hundreds of thousands of books, and not one of them had a food picture in it.

Buying a Basic Cookbook

A basic cookbook is one that you will find useful in several ways. The recipes are easy to follow and, as the great cookbook author JoAnna Lund used to say, the ingredients are quickly found at your local supermarket. The ingredients are healthy and you only need basic kitchen utensils, pots, and pans to whip up a great meal. You will use these cookbooks over and over to plan your meals for the week, making shopping easier and keeping you focused on buying good things, not junk.

I have listed a good selection of basic cookbooks in this chapter. You can buy them online or at your local bookstore. There are many other books on the market that offer good recipes for heart health, but these are the ones I use most. They have become dog-eared and food-stained because I use them regularly to help us plan meals, cookouts, and dinner parties. You'll soon find that you can figure out how to swap a main ingredient or cooking technique to make recipes more heart-healthy— for example, substituting chicken for shrimp in a stir-fry recipe or browning veal cutlets and finishing them in the oven because baking is a much healthier way to cook than frying. Included in this (somewhat) alphabetical list are my recommendations and a suggestion or two of great dishes (with page numbers) we've enjoyed from these books.

Cooking for Two
Bruce Weinstein and Mark Scarbrough; Morrow Cookbooks, New York, 2004; ISBN: 0-06-052259-3

Weinstein and Scarbrough are very creative cookbook authors who say they have the answers for when you want to make a meal for just you and a friend, spouse, or partner. Usually, you have to cut down or halve a recipe for four, but the authors tell you what to buy and what you will need to prepare a meal for fewer people. They suggest substitutions and new methods to keep the meal and costs in check. This is a great book for every day: It gives you clear instructions and labels each recipe as quick, moderate, or leisurely to prepare.

Good Choices:
○ Steak Au Poivre (198)
○ No Fry Eggplant Parmesan (86)

Essentials of Healthful Cooking
Mary Abbott Hess, Dana Jacobi, and Marie Simmons; Williams-Sonoma, Oxmoor House, Tampa, FL, 2003; ISBN: 0-8487-2864-5

The Williams-Sonoma cookbooks are among my favorites. They are beautifully designed, and there are dozens that enable you to choose the foods you want to eat. This book teaches you and inspires you to cook healthfully. It suggests new ingredients that make each dish nutritious and flavorful. Many are classic dishes that have been designed to work in a heart-healthy diet.

Good Choices:
- ○ Oven Crisped Chicken (119)
- ○ Grilled Beef Fillets with Mushrooms and Red Wine Sauce (137)

Fifty Ways to Cook Most Anything

Andrew Schloss with Ken Bookman; Simon & Schuster, New York, 1992; ISBN: 0-671-734-51-2

This great book may not still be in print; however, you may find it in specialty or used bookstores. Contact the publisher for further information. If you can find this gem, hold on to it! I learned more about basic cooking from this book than from almost any other cookbook.

Good Choices:
- ○ Teriyaki Turkey Burger (204)
- ○ Stir Fried Sesame Asparagus (331)

Fish and Shellfish Grilled and Smoked

Karen Adler and Judith Fertig; Harvard Common Press, Cambridge, MA, 2002; ISBN: 1-55832-180-2

Many of us think that grilling fish is difficult and that the effort isn't worth it. The same goes for fish preparation in general. This book helps you prepare a healthier option to steaks and burgers on the grill. Fish and shellfish are healthier, lower in calories and fat, and actually easier to make on the grill. This book has more than 300 recipes, so almost anyone can find something to please the whole family. When the grill comes out in the spring, so does this book.

Good Choices:
- ○ Herb Grilled Grouper (51)
- ○ Stir Grilled Fish Tacos (60)

Food Network Kitchens Cookbook

Jennifer Dorland Darling, Ed.; Meredith Books, Des Moines, IA, 2005; ISBN-13: 978-0696227202

This book is from the people who make those Food Network chefs look good: the cooks, food stylists, tasters, researchers, and recipe creators. What you see on the shows comes from a talented crew of professionals who work behind the scenes and who have helped create this incredible TV phenomenon. This book gives you tremendous help in food preparation, with "Cook's Notes" on every page and exceptional illustrations. We have learned shortcuts that have improved our skills, and the recipes are simple and delicious. This is one cookbook that no kitchen should be without.

Good Choices:
- Chicken and Mushroom Quesadillas (43)
- Low and Slow Oven Barbecued Brisket (162)

Grazing

Julie Van Rosendaal; One Smart Cookie, Inc., Calgary, Alberta, Canada, 2005; ISBN: 0-9687563-1-X

Good Choices:
- Hummus (66)
- Curried Peanut Shrimp (91)

One Smart Cookie

Julie Van Rosendaal; Rodale Books, Emmaus, PA, 2004; ISBN-13: 978–1579549442

Good Choices:
- Classic Lemon Bars (101)
- Turtle Brownies (133)

Julie Van Rosendaal has an inspiring personal story of weight loss. After a family illness, she adopted a healthy lifestyle that led to an amazing 165-pound weight loss through diet and exercise. Since that time, she has become a widely known teacher and food writer. These books contain simple, low-fat, easy-to-make and easy-to-eat snacks and wonderful cookie recipes that you will swear are bad for you. These are the best healthy alternatives to the traditional junk or party-food snacks that you can pull out of the freezer.

Looney Spoons

Janet and Greta Podleski; Granet Publishing, Waterloo, Ontario, Canada, 1997; ISBN: 0-9680631-1-X

Good Choices:
- Mac Attack (macaroni and cheese) (96)
- Veal of Fortune (veal scaloppini) (119)

Crazy Plates
Janet and Greta Podleski; Granet Publishing, Waterloo, Ontario, Canada, 1999; ISBN: 0-9680631-2-8
Good Choices:
- Lawrence of Arrabbiata (penne) (86)
- Takin' Care of Biscuits (53)

Eat, Shrink and Be Merry
Janet and Greta Podleski; Granet Publishing, Waterloo, Ontario, Canada, 2005; ISBN: 0-9680631-3-6
Good Choices:
- Born To Be Wild Mushroom Pizza (76)
- Wowie Maui Meatballs (130)

These three books are part of a series created by two amazing Canadian sisters, Janet and Greta Podleski. They're icons in Canada and are known throughout the U.S. for their hilarious TV appearances. Almost a decade ago, Janet and Greta decided to quit their jobs, sell everything, and write a book that made low-fat cooking fun. After being turned down by dozens of publishers, they partnered with Dave Chilton, author of *The Wealthy Barber*, and they took their message on the road. Within months, they had reached the top of the best-seller lists in Canada and the U.S. Today, their family-friendly cookbooks are snapped up, and the Podleski sisters have launched their own low-fat frozen-food line. The recipes are funny, cleverly written, and, above all, healthy: proof that cooking well can be a riot *and* good for you!

Learning to Cook with Marion Cunningham
Marion Cunningham, Alfred A. Knopf, New York, 1999; ISBN-13: 978-0375401183

The author is one of the best-known cookbook authors in the country, and in this book has taken 150 recipes that are so simple that anyone can make them. As a teacher, Cunningham knows how to get the message across and teach you what you need to know. There are great illustrations that show you techniques and how to read a recipe. This book helped me develop my cooking skills and demystified cooking jargon and techniques. The tone is reassuring and the food is practical enough for any rookie.

Good Choices:

○ Tiny Red Roasted Potatoes with Rosemary (15)

○ Ginger Chicken Breasts (106)

The New Basics Cook

Julee Rosso and Sheila Lukins; Workman Press, New York, 1989; ISBN-13: 978-0894803413

The title may be a bit misleading because it isn't a beginner's cookbook *per se*, but it is a classic with great recipes. At more than 850 pages, it is fascinating to read. You will find recipes that interest you and that you can make for special occasions or a regular dinner. The authors created a food phenomenon with their first book, *The Silver Palate Cookbook*, spun off from their famous New York gourmet take-out store. The recipes, according to one reviewer, seem trendy but are really classics. This is another must-have for any kitchen collection.

Good Choices:

○ Arugula Pesto Pasta (64)

○ Not So Sloppy Joe (523)

Prevention's Quick and Healthy Low-Fat Cooking

Gene Rogers, Editor; Rodale Press, Emmaus, PA, 1993; ISBN-13: 978-0875961743

This cookbook focuses on the well-known Mediterranean diet, which is considered to be among the healthiest cuisines in the world. While this might seem like a difficult cookbook, most of the recipes can be prepared in 30 minutes. The heart of the Mediterranean diet is fish, fruit, seafood, vegetables, pasta, grains, and olive oil. This book is valuable to anyone on a heart-healthy diet because it gives you new ideas and choices to explore. This book might be a little hard to find; however, try contacting the publisher or *Prevention* magazine.

Good Choices:
○ Greek Orzo (204)
○ Couscous Salad (100)

The last three books on this list were acquired over the past year during my ongoing, very rewarding Weight Watchers membership. I use these books virtually every day and cannot recommend them more highly. Beyond the value of the healthy nature of the recipes, the books are high quality, beautifully produced, and easy to use. They are also inexpensive. For those on Weight Watchers, the meals correlate with the system, but you certainly don't have to be on the program to benefit. Although a few are only available through Weight Watchers, most are available in stores. If you are going to buy one book to start your new life as a heart-healthy cook, the *Weight Watchers New Complete Cookbook* would be our choice.

Here are the ones I like best:

Pure Comfort
Weight Watchers International Inc., New York, 2007 (only available through Weight Watchers)
Good Choices:
○ French Potato-Leek Soup (93)
○ Tuna Noodle Casserole (151)

Stir It Up
Weight Watchers International Inc., New York, 2006 (only available through Weight Watchers)
Good Choices:
○ Veal Piccata (46)
○ Shiitake-Chicken Stir Fry (66)

Weight Watchers New Complete Cookbook
Wiley Publishing, Hoboken, NJ, 2006; ISBN-13: 978-0-7645-7350-7
Good Choices:
○ Cold Sesame Noodles (286)
○ Tacos with Salsa (198)

The Low GI Diet Cookbook
Dr. Jennie Brand-Miller, Kaye Foster-Powell, and Joanna McMillan-Price; Marlowe & Company, New York, 2005; ISBN: 978-1-56924-359-6

This cookbook is by the authors of the *New Glucose Revolution,* which made the "glycemic index" a household term. The book focuses on "Smart-Carb" recipes as a weight-loss and healthy-diet method.

Good Choices:
- Barley and Vegetable Soup (75)
- Chicken and Bok Choy Stir Fry (111)

Heart Books

Put simply, no heart patient's home should be without these books. There are dozens of good reference books on heart disease, although none are focused in the same way that this one is. However, you may be looking for something different, or comparing information. In the next section, there are Internet resources you can use.

These books on heart disease are on my bookshelf. Several reflect the work of the top heart treatment centers in the U.S.

Cardiovascular Diseases and Disorders Sourcebook
Sandra J. Judd, Ed.; Omnigraphics Inc., Detroit, MI, 2005; ISBN: 0-7808-0739-1

Heart Attack: A Cleveland Clinic Guide
Curtis Mark Rimmerman, M.D.; Cleveland Clinic Press, Cleveland, OH, 2006; ISBN: 159-6240148-014-8

Mayo Clinic Heart Book
Bernard J. Gersh, M.D.; Morrow, New York, NY, 2000; ISBN: 0-688-17642-9

Your Heart: An Owner's Manual
American Heart Association; Pocket Books, Simon & Schuster, New York, NY, 1995; ISBN: 0-671-53081-X

General Health Books

Along with the books listed previously, I always like to have some general reference books at hand. These are a few that you can rely on for accurate and interesting information about general health.

8 Weeks to Optimum Health
Andrew Weil, M.D.; Alfred A. Knopf, New York, NY, 1997; ISBN: 0-679-44715-6

The 30-Minute Fitness Solution
JoAnn Manson, M.D., and Patricia Amend, MA; Harvard Press, Cambridge, MA, 2001; ISBN: 0-674-00479-5

You: The Owner's Manual
Michael F. Roizen, M.D., and Mehmet C. Oz, M.D.; Harper Resource, New York, NY, 2005; ISBN: 0-06-076531-3

IN A SENTENCE:

> *One of the best parts of recovery for me has been educating myself in the area of good nutrition while learning to cook great food; thus it's important to build a good library of health and wellness books and cookbooks.*

Organizations and Websites

AS YOU move forward past your first year of recovery, you'll want to keep up with what's new in heart disease and other health issues you may have. Remembering that you always want to talk to your doctor before changing anything, you also want to remain as educated as possible. Fortunately, there are many ways to do this, beyond simply learning how to cook well, exercising regularly, and maintaining other lifestyle changes.

Many people simply search for a word or subject on any number of search engines like Google, Yahoo, and Ask.com, and open everything, hoping for some good information. What you find, more often than not, are hundreds of articles, ads, and strange things.

The best rule, at least as a starting point, is to look at websites with the suffix "org" or "gov." That indicates that the site is probably backed by a legitimate not-for-profit institution. Be very careful when using sites that are "edited and corrected," like Wikipedia, that have no serious authority behind them. Remember that health information can change quickly, and that today's breakthrough may be reversed tomorrow. Your life can be affected if you put too much faith in something found at random on the Internet.

Where Do You Look for Reliable Information?

Look for associations and organizations that regularly update their websites with new information. These include

The American Heart Association (www.americanheart.org) generally is one of the best places to go for reliable information about heart disease and stroke. The site is content-rich, with a "heart encyclopedia" and buttons for "I am looking for (Spanish translation, news updates, information for professionals and patients, what's new in the field, etc.)." The AHA also reports its scientific positions on virtually every subject, such as cholesterol or exercise. The site has a simple, reliable search engine, and it offers suggestions if you are not quite sure of what you are looking for.

The AHA as an organization is also well organized, and can be very helpful. The key to getting help is to search for the local chapter (there is a place on the home page where you can enter your ZIP code). You'll find the AHA helpful and responsive. A secret to getting help and attention from a local chapter is, if you don't get a response immediately, write or call and ask for the public relations/media person. Even though you may not be a reporter, PR people are very sensitive to the reputation of their organizations, and they're very responsive.

The AHA also has several newsletters that you can get either via e-mail or in print. You can find them on the website by simply searching under "newsletters." You can also request helpful brochures. If you do any online searches for heart-related subjects, notice how often the AHA comes up. This is the best place to start.

The America Diabetes Association (www.diabetes.org) and **The American Stroke Foundation** (www.americanstroke.org) have good information on diabetes and stroke, but they're not the only ones who do. In this case, ask your doctor or cardio-rehab specialist for guidance.

Academic medical centers are great places to look for information. The Cleveland Clinic, the Mayo Clinic (Rochester, MN), Brigham and Women's Hospital (Boston), Johns Hopkins Medical Institutions (Baltimore), Massachusetts General Hospital (Boston), New York–Presbyterian Hospital, Texas Heart Institute (Houston), Duke University Medical Center (Durham, NC), Stanford Hospital and Clinics (Stanford, CA), and Barnes-Jewish Hospital (St. Louis) are the top ten heart centers in the U.S. All have excellent websites. A simple word search will get you there, and all have phone numbers or e-mail addresses so you can easily find answers to your questions. As with any other place, if you're not being helped, ask for the PR department, and you will get results.

Online newsletters are everywhere, and many people feel that by subscribing, they'll end up on every spam list in the world, if not on every advertising-agency and drug-company mailing list. In these days of identity theft, it's wise to consider that risk. Further, the continual flood of irrelevant e-mail is annoying enough.

WebMD (www.webmd.com) is a good source for overall views of subjects, and it has a good search engine. Their news is usually up to date, and their content comes from legitimate institutions. The content is usually reviewed by medical experts, and you may find this e-newsletter worth searching. You do not really need to be on an e-mail subscription list if you are concerned about security.

There are a few other e-letters, like Aetna Intelihealth (www.inteli heath.com), that I read and receive by e-mail. Although it has commercial sponsorship, almost all of this newsletter's content is from the Harvard Medical School. It has a very wide variety of information on virtually every medical problem, from dental health to medication to interactive tools. It has an "ask the doctor" button and other user-friendly features like "today's news." I get this one daily and I recommend it.

One little-known site is the U.S. Government Accountability Office, or GAO (www.gao.gov). Commonly thought of as the investigative arm of Congress or the congressional watchdog, GAO is independent and nonpartisan. It studies how the federal government spends taxpayers' dollars. GAO advises Congress and the heads of executive agencies such as the Environmental Protection Agency, the Department of Defense, and the Department of Health and Human Services about ways to make government more effective and responsive. GAO evaluates federal programs, audits federal expenditures, and issues legal opinions. When GAO reports its findings to Congress, it recommends actions. Its work leads to laws that improve government operations and save billions of dollars.

I enjoy receiving the GAO updates posted on the organization's website. You can sign up and have newsletters about medical matters sent to you whenever they are posted. I find them fascinating, and you may, too, as they give you an interesting view of how our system works where medicine is concerned.

Is There Too Much Information?

We live in a world in which information is abundant on virtually everything. It's at your fingertips and on your cell phone and computer whenever you want it. It's impossible to say that this is a bad thing.

As someone who grew up assuming that the world of science fiction would come true by the time I reached middle age, the computer age is a wonderful time in which to live. But, like anything else, information is a product that is good only when used well and correctly. Luckily, we have sounding boards in our cardiologists and other medical specialists.

Fifty years ago, I probably would not have survived my medical ordeal. Now I survive and thrive. I know what I have to do and I know that, regardless of what someone says on the Internet or in a book, it is up to me to make those changes—and it is up to you to take charge of yourself and your cardiovascular risks to live well.

IN A SENTENCE:

> *With so many sources of information on the Internet and in the daily news, it's best to have reliable sources at your fingertips when you need help, and some of the best places to begin are professional associations and medical-research websites.*

Glossary

Adverse Effects: Unexpected effects of a medication that indicate that you should contact a doctor immediately or go to an emergency room.

ACE Inhibitors: Originally developed for high blood pressure, this medication affects the angiotensin levels and a hormone called renin. High levels of renin can cause vasoconstriction and narrow the arteries. Ace inhibitors block the renin angiotensin system and relax the pressure on blood vessels, lowering blood pressure.

Adrenal Glands: Located near the kidneys, these glands secrete hormones such as estrogen and cortisol and help keep the body's liquid and salt levels in balance. In addition, they excrete norepinephrine, which helps modulate blood pressure.

Angiogram: An x-ray that creates an image of the veins, arteries, and heart chambers that physicians use to judge the condition of your cardiovascular system. A radiographic substance known as an iodine dye is injected into an artery through a catheter to help create the contrast when the x-ray image is read.

Angina Pectoris: Marked by sharp pains felt in the center of the chest, with a choking feeling and possible pains in the left arm, angina may cause a "doomed" feeling. Usually a signal of worsening clogged heart arteries, it can be tripped off by cold and exercise. It normally subsides in a few minutes with medication or rest.

Arteries: Arteries carry oxygenated blood away from the heart to various parts of the body, except for the pulmonary artery, which carries oxygen-depleted blood to the lungs.

Beta-Blockers: These medications are primarily used in heart (and other) patients who have hypertension or high blood pressure. These drugs help reduce the risk of heart attacks. Ask your doctor whether you should be using one of these, and make sure you tell him you have hypertension.

Body Mass Index: This is a number that is either found on a chart or determined by a calculation of height and weight. This is generally accepted as a measure of how close to a proper weight a person may be.

Brachycardia: When the heartbeat is slowed and the pulse is under 60 beats per minute.

Calcium Channel Blockers: Generally effective medications for angina. While how they work is not exactly known, it appears they prevent the passage of calcium ions across the cellular membranes, relieving the symptoms of angina. They are often given together with beta-blockers or used in the treatment of arrhythmias.

Capillaries: Tiny blood vessels that connect the veins and arteries when blood is exchanged and routed to and from the heart.

CAT Scan: Known correctly as Computed Axial Tomography, a CAT scan device creates a computerized x-ray picture of "slices" of the body that enables the doctor to read the body structures, fluids, tumors, and other aspects of your body in a full 3-dimensional manner.

Cardiac Arrest: If the heart suddenly stops and all function ceases, the victim may die within four to six minutes of cardiac arrest onset. Often, it is unexpected, due to undiagnosed heart disease or an accident. The cause may also be disruption of the electrical impulses of the heart or an abrupt slowing of the beat of the heart muscle. Some victims can be revived through an electric shock; however, the chances of successfully doing so diminish with each minute that goes by.

Cardiac Arrhythmias: A disorder of the heart's rhythm that often occurs in people with heart disease or post-heart attack, usually caused by inadequate blood supply to the heart. There are atrial arrhythmias (upper chamber) and ventricular arrhythmias (lower chamber).

Cardiac Catheterization: A common procedure used by cardiologists to determine the blood flow in the coronary arteries and the condition and efficiency of the heart chambers and valves. A thin, flexible tube—a catheter—is guided into your blood vessels to the heart. If they are blocked by plaque a **balloon** on the end of the catheter can open them, a procedure called **percutaneous translu-minal coronary angioplasty (PTCA)** or **angioplasty.** Two other procedures may be performed during catherization: **stenting,** in which a small wire mesh tube is inserted to keep the artery open, or **atherectomy,** in which a small, spinning blade or laser cuts away the plaque.

Cardiovascular Disease: Often referred to as CVD, this occurs when both the blood vessels and the heart are compromised by blockages and lack of blood flow to the heart.

Cardiologist: A physician who is trained in internal medicine who also special-izes in treating cardiovascular disease. Cardiologists receive specialized training and must pass an extensive examination to achieve board certification.

Cardiomyopathy: In general, this is a disease that primarily affects the heart muscle and occurs when a heart chamber becomes dilated or enlarged, causing the heart muscle to become thickened and inflexible. There are multiple types of cardiomyopathy, depending upon the cause.

Cardio-rehab Classes: Organized exercise, nutrition and behavior/lifestyle modification classes, lasting from one to three months, and recommended for most heart disease patients or post-heart-surgery patients.

Cholesterol: A complex chemical present in all animal fats and in various organs in the body. If the levels are too high, it can clog arteries, leading to heart attack and stroke.

Collateral Arteries: Tiny arteries that connect to larger cardiac arteries; however, they do not carry significant blood flow unless the main arteries begin to narrow. At this point, the collaterals come into use and serve as a backup system for the main arteries to carry blood to the heart.

Congenital Heart Disease: Less than 1 percent of all children are born with some sort of heart problem, usually an imperfection of some kind that can be repaired or cured through surgery or medication. Most congenital heart disease is linked to environmental or genetic factors that can't be predicted. However, lifestyle factors, such as maternal smoking, drinking, and drug use, may cause prenatal damage.

Congestive Heart Failure (CHF): Usually occurring after a heart attack, CHF is signified by a buildup of fluid and congestion that is found in the blood vessels, lungs, and elsewhere due to the heart's inability to pump sufficiently.

Coronary Artery Bypass Graft: Also known as a "CABG," this is an open-heart surgical procedure in which the surgeon takes one or more arteries, such as an internal mammary artery or long vessel from your leg, and uses it to route blood past clogged coronary arteries, leading to improved or restored blood flow to the heart. These are called grafts, and usually more than one graft is performed during a single operation.

Coronary Artery Disease: Referred to as CAD, this is generally a term for hardening of the heart arteries or atherosclerosis. The occurs when plaque builds up on and narrows the inner walls of the arteries, resulting in reduced oxygenated blood flow to the heart, often leading to a heart attack.

Cutaneous Fat: Fat that accumulates under the skin and is visible.

Dipyridamole: A medication used to reduce blood clot risk after heart valve surgery.

Diuretics: Medication used to decrease excess body fluid by increasing urine output in patients with edema or high blood pressure.

Electrocardiogram: An electrocardiogram (or ECG) is a record of the electrical activity generated by the heart and recorded on a machine called an electrocardiograph. The information on the heart is expressed as "waves" such a P Wave, or Q Wave. This provides information on the rhythms or possible damage to the heart and is repeated regularly to chart changes.

Epicardium: The inner layer of the three layers of membranes that surround the heart.

Erectile Dysfunction: Inability to attain and/or sustain an erection, caused by lack of blood flow to the penis, often a result of hypertension, medication side effects, high cholesterol levels, diabetes, or emotional problems, such as depression, that may occur after cardiac surgery or heart attack.

Ejection Fraction: The percentage of blood that is expelled by the left ventricle of the heart after it contracts. It is indicative of the severity of heart muscle damage or weakening.

Endothelial Dysfunction: The endothelium is the layer of cells that coat the inner surface of all the veins and arteries and assist in normal functions such as coagulation and platelet adhesion. Disease or lifestyle behaviors, such as smoking, can cause the endothelium to become dysfunctional, resulting in heightened risk of atherosclerosis and heart attack development.

Fibrillation: Very quick and rapid contractions of the heart muscle that can occur in the atria or ventricles, leading to heart damage from decreased blood supply. This can be reversed by "defibrillation," applying prompt shock to the heart.

Fibrin: A protein that binds together red and white blood cells and platelets that can form blood clots.

Gastric Bypass Surgery: A serious surgical procedure also referred to as bariatric surgery. A surgical specialist creates a small stomach pouch that enables food and liquids to literally bypass the small intestine, reducing the number of calories that the body will absorb. This changes eating patterns and leads to weight loss. This procedure usually is only performed on carefully selected patients.

Gastrointestinal Distress: Generally any sort of severe stomachache, vomiting, diarrhea, or constipation causing severe pain.

Glucose: A simple sugar that is found in virtually all fruits and also is a byproduct of carbohydrate metabolism. Glucose is absorbed into the bloodstream and is used by the body; however, if too much is absorbed, the glucose level will be too high and may contribute to type 2 diabetes.

Heart Murmur: An irregular sound produced by the heart and heard on examination of the heart sounds by stethoscope. The heart murmur may be caused by an abnormal (or leaky) heart valve. This may also simply be a normal function of the heart pumping blood, a so-called functional murmur.

High Blood Pressure: Also called hypertension, high blood pressure is a chronic condition. Physicians measure blood pressure using a scale that measures this pressure. If your systolic (top) number is above 140 mm Hg and your diastolic (bottom number) pressure is above 90 mm Hg, you are at risk for a stroke, eye problems, heart attack, or kidney disease. The source of hypertension is often multifactoral and can include dietary (too much salt intake), genetic, or hereditary causes.

Hypercholesterolemia: Excess amount of cholesterol in the bloodstream.

Inferior Vena Cava: The large vein that returns blood back to the heart from below the diaphragm.

Intravenous Clot Busters: These medications, also known as thrombolytics, are used widely in emergency rooms when a heart attack is suspected. They are most effective when administered within sixty to ninety minutes after the first symptoms of a heart attack. They are very effective in disrupting a clot causing a heart attack; however, they have to be given under very strict hospital-setting guidelines.

Lipid Profile: A measurement of levels of total cholesterol, HDL, LDL, triglycerides, and other lipid parameters in the blood that provides the doctor with an impression of the patient's vascular risk and what treatments may be needed to reduce any levels that are elevated.

Magnetic Resonance Imaging: Known as an MRI, this procedure produces pictures of living tissue inside the body in a non-invasive manner.

Mitral Valve Prolapse: A form of heart valve disease that causes the leaflets or flaps of the mitral valve to flop back into the left atrium as the heart contracts, sometimes allowing leakage of blood through the valve opening. Although the majority of cases need no treatment at all, severe cases can be repaired surgically.

Myocardium: The thick middle layer of the heart muscle.

Myocardial Infarction: Also known as a heart attack, this condition is caused by a blockage in one or more of the coronary arteries, leading to reduction of oxygenated blood flow to the heart. This, in turn, leads to reduced ability of the heart to circulate blood.

Negative Health Behavior: Negative health behavior includes poor diet, lack of exercise, smoking, and excessive use of alcohol that leads to or exacerbates heart disease.

Nitroglycerin: Relieves the symptoms of angina when placed under the tongue. This is called a vasodilator medication because it expands the veins and reduces the pressure from blockages.

Nuclear Stress Test: Heart disease can often be diagnosed more accurately if the heart is put under stress by exercising, usually on a treadmill or bicycle. The patient walks while attached to an electrocardiograph machine that shows changes in breathing, heart rate, or pain as the speed is increased. In a nuclear stress test, an image is created by injection of a radioactive dye (thallium) into your blood that enables your doctor to obtain a "live" picture of your cardiovascular system's efficiency.

Palpitation: Rapid heartbeat that occurs, especially, for example, when a person is either frightened or startled. It may also indicate a heart condition.

Pericardium: A double-layered, sac-like structure that surrounds the heart and blood vessels going to and from the heart. The pericardium is strong and protects the heart, and contains a small amount of lubricating blood.

Plaque: A substance that builds up on the inner wall of your blood vessels causing atherosclerosis. Generally, this is caused by a buildup of lipids: fats that come from food that do not dissolve normally, but form clogs.

Pulmonary Embolism: A blood clot (thrombosis) lodged in the pulmonary artery; the artery that carries deoxygenated blood from the right ventricle of the heart to the lungs for refreshing. This is a serious situation that can cause severe chest pain and can lead to death.

Pulmonary Valve: Controls the flow of deoxygenated blood from the right ventricle to the pulmonary artery, sending blood to the lungs for oxygen.

Radiologist: A physician whose specialty is working with x-rays, including administering, reading, and interpreting tests.

Right and Left Atria: The upper chambers of the heart where blood flows from and through the tricuspid and mitral valves into the ventricles.

Right and Left Ventricles: The lower chambers of the heart where blood is pumped out into the bloodstream or lungs.

Side Effects: Expected, common, or annoying consequences of a medication, such as stomach distress.

Silent Heart Attack: Some people (three to four million) may have restricted blood flow to the heart (ischemia) without knowing it or without having obvious symptoms. This may cause a heart attack abruptly without symptoms such as angina. Diabetics and those who have a history of heart attack may have silent ischemia.

Sinoatrial Node: Specialized nerve fibers located near the atrium that generates electrical impulses and functions as an internal, natural cardiac pacemaker.

Superior Vena Cava: The vein that brings blood from the upper half of the body to the right atrium of the heart.

Sympathetic Nervous System: A large part of the body's nervous system that supplies the involuntary muscles, such as the heart, blood vessels, and sweat glands.

Tachycardia: When the heartbeat rises above 100 beats per minute. This can reflect either a normal physical response such as fear or emotional excitement, or it can signal any number of serious disorders of the heart, such as a disruption in the heart's electrical system.

Thrombus: A non-mobile blood clot that is attached to the interior wall of an artery or vein.

Toxemia: Blood poisoning caused by bacteria in the blood.

Tricuspid Valve: Located between the right atrium and right ventricle of the heart. After blood flows through the valve, it shuts as the ventricle contracts to prevent blood from flowing back into the atrium with the contraction.

Trans Fats: A commercially created product, widely used in food preparation, that is inexpensive and gives the food a longer shelf life and enhances flavor. Trans fats have been found to increase cholesterol, lower HDL, and increase risk of type 2 diabetes and heart disease. Trans fats are now being widely removed by most food manufacturers and restaurants.

Tunica Media: The middle muscular coating of an artery.

Type 2 Diabetes (Diabetes Mellitus): Also called adult onset diabetes, this is a chronic disease that usually appears in people over age fifty, but is now being seen in many younger people including adolescents in greater numbers. Type 2 diabetes occurs when the pancreas fails to secrete enough insulin and the body develops tissue or cellular resistance to the effects of insulin. In addition, there is less than optimal processing of peripheral glucose, which is required by the body to help regulate certain metabolic functions that help generate energy. Type 2 diabetes may have a strong hereditary factor, and is a major risk factor for heart disease.

Type 1 Diabetes: Formerly known as juvenile diabetes, this usually appears in childhood and often is discovered when the patient begins to show symptoms of constant thirst, frequent urination, or weight loss. The type 1 diabetic's pancreas does not produce insulin, which can lead to serious adverse effects on the heart, vision, mouth, and nervous system. It is usually diagnosed by a simple blood test.

Vasculitis: Inflamed blood vessels due to a systemic disease or a possible allergic reaction.

Visceral Fat: Located near or attached to internal organs, visceral fat creates a strong risk for increased cardiovascular disease.

Bibliography

Adams, Jesse, MD, and Apple, Fred, PhD, DABCC. "New Blood Tests for Detecting Heart Disease." *Circulation*, 109 (2004):12–14.

Aetna InteliHealth. "Drug-Coated Stents Falling from Favor." Aetna InteliHealth website. *http://www.intelilhealth.com/IH/ihtIH/ EMIHC267/333/8011/508365.html.*

Aetna InteliHealth. "Health A to Z: High Cholesterol (Hypercholesterolemia)." Aetna InteliHealth website. *http://www.intelil-health.com/IH/ihtIH/EMIHC267/9339/10157/201972.html.*

Aetna InteliHealth. "FDA Probes Safety of Popular Heart Stent." Aetna InteliHealth, Inc. website. *http://www.intelihealth.com/ IH/ihtPrint/EMIHC267/333/8011/510789.html.*

American Heart Association. "African Americans and Cardiovascular Diseases–2007 Statistical Fact Sheet." American Heart Association website. *http://www.americanheart.org/presenter.jhtml? identifier=3000927.*

American Heart Association. "American Heart Association Challenges One Million Women to Know Their Heart Disease Risk at GoRedForWomen.org!" American Heart Association website. *http://www.goredforwomen.org/newsroom/02_02_2007.html.*

American Heart Association. "American Indians/Alaska Natives and Cardiovascular Diseases–2007 Statistical Fact Sheet." American Heart Association website. *http://www.americanheart.org/presenter.jhtml?identifier=3000929.*

American Heart Association. "Angioplasty and Cardiac Revascularization Statistics." American Heart Association website. *http://www.americanheart.org/presenter.jhtml?identifier=4439.*

American Heart Association. "Asian/Pacific Islanders and Cardiovascular Diseases–2007 Statistical Fact Sheet." American Heart Association website. *http://www.americanheart.org/presenter.jhtml?identifier=3000931.*

American Heart Association. "Common Heart Defects." American Heart Association website. *http://www.americanheart.org/presenter.jhtml?identifier=158.*

American Heart Association. "Congenital Heart Defects in Children Fact Sheet." American Heart Association website. *http://www.americanheart.org/presenter.jhtml?identifier=12012.*

American Heart Association. "Heart Failure in Children and Adolescents." American Heart Association website. *http://www.americanheart.org/presenter.jhtml?identifier=3016405.*

American Heart Association, "Heart Valves." American Heart Association website. *http://www.americanheart.org/presenter.jhtml?identifier=4598.*

American Heart Association. "Hispanics/Latinos and Cardiovascular Diseases–2007 Statistical Fact Sheet." American Heart Association website. *http://www.americanheart.org/presenter.jhtml?identifier=3000934.*

American Heart Association. "International Cardiovascular Disease Statistics–2007 Statistical Fact Sheet." American Heart Association website. *http://www.americanheart.org/presenter.jhtml?identifier=3001008.*

American Heart Association. "Menopause and the Risk of Heart Disease and Stroke." American Heart Association website. *http://www.americanheart.org/presenter.jhtml?identifier=4658.*

American Heart Association. "Response to Heart and Estrogen-Progestin Replacement Study Follow-up (HERS II) published in July 3, 2002 *Journal of the American Medical Association (JAMA)*." American Heart Association website. *http://www.americanheart.org/presenter.jhtml?identifer=3003570.*

American Heart Association. "Risk Factors and Coronary Heart Disease." American Heart Association website. http://www.americanheart.org/presenter.jhtml?identifier=4726.

American Heart Association. "Sexual Activity and Heart Disease or Stroke." American Heart Association website. *http://www.americanheart.org/presenter.jhtml?identifier=4714.*

American Heart Association. "Whites and Cardiovascular Diseases–2007 Statistical Fact Sheet." American Heart Association website. *http://www.americanheart.org/presenter.jhtml?identifier=3000939.*

American Heart Association. *Your Heart: An Owner's Manual: American Heart Association's Complete Guide to Heart Health*, Pocket Books, a division of Simon & Schuster, Inc. 1995.

American Public Health Association. "Fact Sheets: Disparities in Heart Disease." Medscape.com website. *http://www.medscape.com/viewarticle/472720.*

Brookfield, Ernest G., MD. "Bacterial Endocarditis." *CHASER News. http://www.csun.edu/hcmth011/chaser/article2.html.*

Chilnick, Lawrence, Ed. *The Pill Book of Heart Disease: Drugs and Treatment*, Bantam Books Inc., 1985.

China Daily "Heart Disease, Cancer Top Killers in China." *China Daily* website. *http://www.chinadaily.com.cn/english/doc/2005–09/15/content_478073.htm.*

Cleveland Clinic Heart & Vascular Institute. "Cholesterol Guidelines." Cleveland Clinic website. http://www.clevelandclinic.org/heartcenter/pub/guide/prevention/cholesterol/cholesterolguidelines9_0.1htm.

Cleveland Clinic Heart & Vascular Institute. "Coronary Artery Disease Diagnosis and Treatment: Cardiac Catheterization and Coronary Interventional Procedures." Cleveland Clinic website. http://www.clevelandclinic.org/heartcenter/pub/guide/disease/cad/treatment_interventional.htm

Cleveland Clinic Heart & Vascular Institute. "Estrogen and Heart Disease." Cleveland Clinic website. http://www.clevelandclinic.org/heartcenter/pub/women/estrogen.htm.

Cleveland Clinic Heart & Vascular Institute. "Heart Surgery Recovery." Cleveland Clinic website. *http://www.clevelandclinic.org/heartcenter/pub/guide/disease/recovery_ohs.htm.*

Cleveland Clinic Heart & Vascular Institute. "Thoracic Aortic Aneurysm." Cleveland Clinic website. *http://www.clevelandclinic.org/heartcenter/pub/guide/disease/aorta_marfan/aorticaneurysm.htm.*

Cleveland Clinic Heart & Vascular Institute. "Cleveland Clinic Finds Raising Levels of 'Good'Cholesterol With Statins May Be as Beneficial as Lowering 'Bad.'" Cleveland Clinic: Heart & Vascular Institute website. *http//www.clevelandclinic.org/heartcenter/pub/news/archive/2007/hdl2_09.asp.*

Coulis, Louie, MD. "Silent Heart Attacks Are a Concern." St. Nicholas Hospital website. *http://www.stincholashospital.org/newsweekly_silentheartattacks.htm.*

Every Day Health. "Aspirin and Cardiovascular Health." Every Day Health website. *http://www.everydayhealth.com/publicsite/printview.aspx?puid=8F234643-2e73-4fdb-86b4-55316486fa48&p=1.*

Harvard Health Publications. "Two New Erectile Dysfunction Drugs: How They Measure up Against Viagra." Harvard Medical School: Harvard Health Publications website. *http://www.health.harvard.edu/press_releases/new_erectile_dysfunction_drugs.htm.*

Heart Failure Society of America. "Common Symptoms of Heart Failure." Heart Failure Society of America website. *http://www.abouthf.org/questions_symptoms .htm.*

Heart Health iVillage. "Pregnancy & the Heart." Heart.Health.iVillage.com website. *http://heart.health.ivillage.com/common/articleprintfriendly.cfm?artid=34.*

HeartPoint. "Cardiac Catheterization." HeartPoint website. *http://www.heart-point.com/cath.html.*

Imperatore, Giuseppina; Cadwell, Betsy L.; Geiss, Linda, et al. "Thirty-year Trends in Cardiovascular Risk Factor Levels among US Adults with Diabetes." *American Journal of Epidemiology*, vol. 160, no. 6 (2004):531–539.

Judd, Sandra J. Health Reference Series (Third Edition). *Cardiovascular Diseases and Disorders Sourcebook*, Omnigraphics, Inc. 2005.

Loren, Karl. "How Doctors Diagnose Heart Disease." The Atlantic Cardiology Group, P.C. website. *http://www.karlloren.com/ultrasound/p33.htm.*

"Study Says Hispanics Have Higher Rate of Heart Disease." Lubbock *Avalanche-Journal* website. *http://lubbockonline.com/news/031897/study.htm.*

March of Dimes."March of Dimes Quick References and Fact Sheets for Professionals & Researchers." March of Dimes website. *http://www.marchofdimes.com/printableArticles/14332_1212.asp.*

March of Dimes. "Genetic Cause of Heart Defects Identified by March of Dimes Grantee." March of Dimes website. *http://www.marchofdimes.com/printableArticles/791_9212.asp?printable=true.*

Mayo Clinic. "Cardiac rehabilitation: Building a Better Life after Heart Disease." MayoClinic.com website. *http://www.mayoclinic.com/print/cardiac-rehabilitation/HB00017.*

Mayo Clinic. "Heart Attack: First Aid." Mayo Clinic.com website. *http://www.mayoclinic.com/print/first-aid-heart-attack/FA00050.*

Mayo Clinic. *Mayo Clinic: Heart Book (Second Edition)*. William Morrow and Company, Inc., 2000.

Mitcham, Mary Lynn. "Staying Slim on Business Trips." Weight Watchers website. *http://www.weightwatchers.com/util/prt/article.aspx?articleID=25811.*

National Heart, Lung, and Blood Institute. "Heart and Vascular Diseases." National Heart, Lung, and Blood Institute website. *http://www.nhlbi.nih.gov/health/public.heart/*

National Institute of Mental Health. "Depression and Heart Disease." Mental-Health-Matters.com website. *http://www.mental-health-matters.com/articles/print.php?artID=319.*

"Neighborhood Heart Watch: Depression Linked to Heart Disease." Neighborhood Heart Watch website. *http://www.neighborhood-heart-watch.org/newsletter/printer_45.shtml.*

"Hospitals Join to Speed Care in Treating Heart Attacks." The *New York Times* (November 13, 2006).

Pick, Marcelle, OB/GYN NP and Mills, Dixie, MD, FACS. "Risk Factors for Heart Disease." Women to Women website. *http://www.womentowomen.com/heartdiseaseand stroke/riskfactors.as?id&campaigno.*

Pilote, Louise, MD. "Heart Differences Appear in Men and Women." Heart-CenterOnline by Healthology website. *http://heart.health.ivillage.com/newsStories/newsprintfriendly.cfm?newsid=85121.*

Rimmerman, Curtis Mark, MD. *Heart Attack: A Cleveland Clinic Guide*, Cleveland Clinic Press, June 2006.

Rodriguez, Liliana. "Preventing Coronary Heart Disease Through Diet Modification Among Hispanic Adults Living in the Barrio of Magnolia in Houston, Texas." University of Texas School of Public Health. http://www.sph.uth .tmc.edu/courses/CHP/ph1110/LRodriguezdraft2.htm.

Sharma, Vijai P., PhD. "Some Behaviors and Emotions Can Worsen Heart Problems." Mind Publications website. *http://www.mindpub.com/art082.htm.*

Slaby, Andrew E., MD, PhD, MPH. *Sixty Ways To Make Stress Work For You*, The PIA Press, 1988.

Stein, Rob. "Estrogen Doesn't Raise Heart Risk for Women in Their 50s, Study Finds." *Washington Post* website. *http://www.washingtonpost.com/wp-dyn/content/article/2006/02/13/AR2006021301263_print.*

Sternberg, Steve. "Stents Under New Scrutiny: Safety Concerns for Drug-coated Devices 'far from resolved.'" *USA Today* (February 13, 2007).

Taubert, Kathryn A., PhD and Dajani, Adnan S., MD. "Preventing Bacterial Endocarditis: American Heart Association Guidelines." *American Family Physician*, vol. 57,no. 3 (February 1, 1998).

Texas Heart Institute. Cooley, Denton A., M.D. (ed.). *Heart Owner's Handbook*, John Wiley & Sons, 1996.

Texas Heart Institute at St. Luke's Episcopal Hospital. "Heart Conditions: Recovering from a Heart Attack." Texas Heart Institute website. *http://texas-heart.org/HIC/Topics/Cond/recovery.cfm?&RenderForPrint=.*

Texas Heart Institute at St. Luke's Episcopal Hospital. "Surgical & Medical Procedures: Coronary Artery Bypass." Texas Heart Institute website. *http://texas-heart.org/HIC/Topics/Proced/cab.cfm?&RenderForPrint=1.*

The Society of Thoracic Surgeons. "STS Patient Information: What to Expect after Your Heart Surgery." The Society of Thoracic Surgeons website. *http://www.sts.org/doc/3563.*

U.S. Department of Health and Human Services. "High Blood Cholesterol: What You Need to Know." National Heart, Lung, and Blood Institute Health

Information Center website. *http://www.nhlbi.nih.gov/health/public/heart/chol/wyntk.htm.*

U.S. Department of Health & Human Services. "The Surgeon General's Call to Action to Prevent and Decrease Overweight and Obesity." United States Department of Health & Human Services website. *http://www.surgeongeneral.gov/topics/obesity/calltoaction/fact_adolescents.htm.*

U.S. Department of Health and Human Services. "What is Coronary Angioplasty?" National Heart, Lung, and Blood Institute Diseases and Conditions Index website. *http://www.nhlbi.nih.gov/health/dci/Diseases/Angioplasty/Angioplasty_All.html.*

U.S. Department of Health & Human Services. "Heart Disease Deaths in American Women Decline: 17,000 Fewer Women Died of Heart Disease; Awareness Continues to Climb." National Institutes of Health: NIH News website. *http://www.nhlbi.nih.gov/new/press/07-02-01.htm.*

U.S. Department of Health & Human Services "WISE Study of Women and Heart Disease Yields Important Findings on Frequently Undiagnosed Coronary Syndrome." National Institutes of Health: NIH News website. *http://www.nhlbi.nih.gov/new/press/06-01-31.htm.*

U.S. National Library of Medicine and the National Institutes of Health. "Medical Encyclopedia: Arrhythmias." Medline Plus website. *http://www.nlm.nih.gov/medlineplus/print/ency/article/001101.htm.*

University of Iowa Hospitals & Clinics. "Children and Heart Disease." University of Iowa Hospitals & Clinics website. *http://www.uihealthcare.com/topics/cardiovascularhealth/card3024.html.*

Valentine, Diane, BSN, RN, CCRN; Byers, Jacqueline F., PhD, RN, CNAA; and Peterson, Janice Z. PhD, RN. "Depression as a Risk Factor for Coronary Heart Disease: Implications for Advanced Practice Nurses." Medscape website. *http://www.medscape.com/viewarticle/408416_print.*

Walsh, Bryan. "Asia's War with Heart Disease." *Time* website. *http://www.time.com/time/magazine/article/0,9171,501040510-632135-2,00.html.*

Walsh, S. Kirk. "Tips for the Traveling Set." Weight Watchers website. *http://www.weightwatchers.com/util/prt/article.aspx?article ID=26251.*

Weil, Andrew, MD. 8 *Weeks To Optimum Health: A Proven Program for Taking Full Advantage of Your Body's Natural Healing Power,* Alfred A. Knopf, Inc. 1997.

Index

Abbokinase. *See* Urokinase
Abciximab injection (ReoPro), 313
Academic medical centers, 363–364
Accupril. *See* Quinapril
ACE inhibitors, 42, 94, 285, 299, 307
 benazepril, 304
 captopril, 304
 enalapril, 304–305
 fosinopril, 305
 lisinopril, 305
 moexipril, 305
 perindopril, 306
 quinapril, 306
 ramipril, 306
 trandolapril, 306
Aceon. *See* Perindopril
Acetylsalicylic acid. *See* Aspirin
"Act in Time" campaign, 34, 91
Activase. *See* Alteplase
Acuprin. *See* Aspirin
Acupuncture, 285, 293–294, 341
Acute medicine, 286
Adalat CC. *See* Nifedipine ER
Addiction
 kicking, 217–220
 psychological, 216–217
 smoking, 216–220
 tolerance and, 216
Adler, Karen, 355
Adrenal glands, 215, 271

Adult onset diabetes. *See* Type 2
 diabetes
Aerobic exercise, 14, 114, 126, 257,
 260–261, 263, 265–267, 287,
 325
Afeditab CR. *See* Nifedipine ER
African Americans, 12
 diabetes in, 18
 HBP in, 15
 heart-disease statistics and,
 190–191
 obesity and, 234
 smoking and, 213
 women and death rates, 125, 160
Against Medical Advice (AMA), 4
Agatston, Arthur, 251
Age, 196, 199–200, 227
Aggrastat. *See* Tirofiban
AHA. *See* The American Heart
 Association
Alcohol, 2, 45, 73, 172, 179, 213,
 220, 269, 341
Alka-Seltzer. *See* Aspirin
Altace. *See* Ramipril
Alteplase (Activase), 319
Alternative medicines, xxiv, 281
 acupuncture, 285, 293–294, 341
 ancient treatments and, 285–286
 aromatherapy, 285, 294
 Ayurvedic, 285–286, 287

Alternative medicines (*continued*)
 Bioelectromagnetic-based therapies, 289
 biofield therapies, 289
 biologically based practices and, 288
 body-based practices and, 288
 chiropractic, 294
 choices, 292–295
 considering new approaches and, 282–284
 depression and, 291
 dietary supplements, 294
 digoxin, 43, 292
 EDTA chelation therapy and, 293
 EMFs, 294
 energy and, 288
 heart treatments and, 290–295
 homeopathic, 294
 integrative and, xxv, 282
 legitimate CAMs and, 286–289
 manipulative-based practices and, 288, 294
 massage, 282, 285, 288, 294, 295
 mind-body and, 288
 naturopathic, 287, 294
 osteopathic, 294–295
 qi gong, 289, 295
 reiki, 289, 295
 St. John's Wort, 291, 292
 statistics, 283, 288
 TCM, 287, 295
 therapeutic touch, 295
 using past to predict future and, 284–285
 vitamins and, 291–292
 warfarin, 293, 317
 what others think of, 288
 whole medical systems and, 287
AMA. *See* Against Medical Advice
AMBS. *See* The American Board of Medical
 Specialties
Amend, Patricia, 361
American Board of Internal Medicine, 68, 80
American Board of Surgery, 68
American College of Cardiology, 20
American Council on Fitness, 263
The American Board of Medical Specialties
 (AMBS), 68, 69
The American Diabetes Association, 16, 17,
 20, 145, 363
The American Heart Association (AHA), 2–3,
 11, 12, 34, 45, 46, 69, 83, 90, 112, 132,
 139, 160, 226, 361, 363
 guidelines for resuming sex, 153–154
 recommendations, 172

The American Stroke Foundation, 363
Amlodipine (Norvasc), 94, 310
Amniotic fluid embolism, 176
Anesthesia, 284–285
Aneurysm, 50, 99
Anger, 10, 277, 269–271
Angina pectoris, xix, 26, 27, 33, 36, 48, 90, 225
 causes, 30
 diabetes, shortness of breath and, 16
 medicines, 31
 pain, 3
 statistics, 25
 symptoms, 29
 treatment, 30–31
Angiogram, 4, 65, 349
Angiography. *See* Cardiac catheterization
Angioplasty, 5, 6, 43, 91, 92
Angiotensin II receptor blockers
 candesartan, 307
 eprosartan, 307
 irbesartan, 307
 losartan, 308
 olmesartan, 308
 telmisartan, 308
 valsartan, 308
Anistreplase (Eminase), 319
Antibiotic prophylaxis, 38
Anticoagulation medications, 299
Antiplatelets
 clopidogrel, 309
 ticlopidine, 309
Anxiety, 135–136
Aorta, 62, 97
 coarctation of, 180
Aromatherapy, 285, 294
Arrhythmias, 36–37, 94, 167, 174. *See also*
 Cardiac arrhythmias
Arteries
 aorta, 62
 arterioles, 62–63
 arteriosclerosis, 27
 blockage reasons, 27–28
 capillaries, 63
 circulatory system and, 62–63
 coronary, 63
 pulmonary, 63
Arterioles, 62–63
Arteriosclerosis, 27
Ascriptin A/D. *See* Aspirin
Asian Americans, 12
 diabetes in, 18

heart disease statistics and, 190–191
smoking and, 213
Aspergum. *See* Aspirin gum
Aspirin (Acetylsalicylic acid, Acuprin, Alka-
    Seltzer, Ascriptin A/D, Bayer, Bufferin,
    Easprin, Ecotrin, Empirin, Zorprin), 34,
    91, 93, 94, 169, 170, 171–172, 191, 285,
    298, 299, 309, 318
Aspirin gum (Aspergum), 318
Atacand. *See* Candesartan
Atenolol, 94
Atherosclerosis, 13
Athletes, 46
Atkins diet, 250, 249
Atkins, Robert C., 250
Atorvastatin, 229, 300
Avapro. *See* Irbesartan
Ayurvedic medicine, 285–286, 287

Bacterial endocarditis (BE), 37–38
Bacterial pericarditis, 43
Balloons, heart attack, stents and, 95–100
Bayer. *See* Aspirin
BE. *See* Bacterial endocarditis
*Be Smart About Your Heart: Control the ABCs
    of Diabetes,* 20
Behaviors. *See* Health habits
Benazepril (Lotensin), 304
Benicar. *See* Olmesartan
Bepridil (Vascor), 310
Beta blockers, 31, 43, 94, 299
Bhatt, Deepak, 98
Biofield therapies, 289
Biolelectromagnetic-based therapies, 289
Biologically based practices, 288
Birth control pills, 166, 214
Blood
    circulatory system and, 61–62
Blood cells
    bone marrow and, 62
    circulatory system and, 61–62
    plasma and, 62
    platelets and, 62
    red and white, 61
Blood cholesterol, contributing risk factors
    and high, 20–21
Blood clots, 39, 61, 176. *See also* Thrombus
    busters, 93–94
Blood lipids
    panel, 226
    target levels, 20

Blood pressure (BP), 3, 14, 15, 38, 235
    high, 14, 15–16, 20–21, 38, 235, 299
    measuring, 16, 58–59
    medicines, 299
Blood tests, 83
Blood transfusions, 285
Blood vessels, 32
Blurred vision, 22
BMI. *See* Body Mass Index
Board certification, 68
Body Mass Index (BMI), xv, 14
    calculating, 232–233
    statistics, 234
    table, 233
Body shape, 235
Body-based practices, 288
Bogues, Muggsy, 11
Bone marrow, 62
Bookman, Ken, 355
BP. *See* Blood pressure
Bradycardia, 37
Brand-Miller, Jennie, 360
Breast cancer, 25, 150, 161–162
Breath
    diabetes, angina and shortness of, 16
    shortness of, 5, 16, 26, 29, 41, 90
Brown, John M. III, 76, 77
Bufferin. *See* Aspirin
Bundles of Kent, 53
Bupropion, 219
Bypass surgery. *See* Coronary artery bypass

CA. *See* Cardiac arrhythmias
CABG. *See* Coronary artery bypass graft
CAD. *See* Coronary artery disease
Calan. *See* Verapamil
Calan SR. *See* Verapamil, extended-release
Calcium channel blockers, 299
    amlodipine, 310
    bepridil, 310
    diltiazem ER, 310–311
    felodipine, 311
    isradipine, 311
    nicardipine, 311–312
    nicardipine SR, 312
    nifedipine ER, 312
    nisoldipine, 312–313
    verapamil, 313
    verapamil extended-release, 313
Caldwell, Ron, 15
Calories, burning, 324–325

CAMs. *See* Complementary and Alternative Medicines
Cancer, 43, 44, 61, 113, 141, 160, 178, 212, 214, 236, 282, 284, 292
  breast, 25, 150, 161–162
  lung, 13, 199, 269
Candesartan (Atacand), 307
Capillaries, 52, 62, 63
Capoten. *See* Captopril
Captopril (Capoten), 304
Cardene. *See* Nicardipine
Cardene SR. *See* Nicardipine SR
Cardiac arrest, 33. *See also* Heart attack
Cardiac arrhythmias (CA), 36–37, 94, 167, 174
Cardiac catheterization, 4, 87–88. *See also* Angiogram
Cardio rehab. *See also* Exercise
  heart attack and, 111–114
  living alone and, 329–330
Cardiologists, 22, 28, 31, 51, 59, 82, 96, 122, 225
  board certification and, 68
  cardiology and, 66
  choosing, 65–75
  finding specialists and, 67–69
  first visit with, 72–73
  making choices with, 69–72
  offices of, 71
  online research about, 79–80
  preparing to meet with, 73–75
  relationship with, 70, 290
  second opinions and, 76–80
  treatment plans and, 71–72
Cardiology, what's, 66
Cardiomyopathy, 38–40
Cardiopulmonary resuscitation (CPR), 89, 91, 285
Cardio-rehab classes, xxi
Cardiovascular disease (CVD), xx, xxiii, xxiv. *See also* Heart disease
  statistics, 3
Cardiovascular Diseases and Disorders Sourcebook (Judd), 360
Cardiovascular system, 52
Cardizem CD. *See* Diltiazem
Cardizem LA. *See* Diltiazem
Cardizem SR. *See* Diltiazem
Carmona, Richard H., xx, 12, 212
Cartia XT. *See* Diltiazem
CAT scan. *See* Computed tomography

Caucasians, 167–170
  heart disease statistics and, 190–191
  smoking and, 213
  women and death rates, 25, 160
CBC. *See* Complete blood count
Celebrations, dining out and, 325–326
Cells
  blood, 61–62, 83
  stem, 350–351
Center for Sexual Health, 158
Chantix, 219
Chest pains, xix, 3, 26, 27, 29, 31, 33, 36, 48, 90, 225. *See also* Angina
Chest x-ray, 41, 84
CHF. *See* Congestive heart failure
Children
  acquired heart disease in, 181–182
  cigarettes and, 221–222
  congenital heart defects in, 178–184
  heart disease and educating, 347–348
  obesity and at-risk, 236–237
  other heart problems in, 183
  smoking statistics and, 221–222
Chilton, Dave, 357
Chinese medicine, 287, 295
Chiropractors, 294
Cholesterol, xv, 3, 196, 198
  contributing risk factors and high blood, 20–21
  good and bad, 224
  HDL, 7, 20–22, 197, 201, 224–225, 226, 227, 228, 229, 235
  heart disease and, 224–225
  hypercholesterolemia and, 240
  LDL, 7, 20–22, 27, 83, 164, 169, 172, 201, 224–226, 227–229, 235, 300
  lipids and, 225
  lowering, 223–230
  managing, 227–228
  medicine, 229–230, 299, 300
  right levels, 225–227
  total, 226
  trans fats and, 228
  triglycerides and, 20, 21, 225, 226, 227
  what's, 224
Cholestyramine, 229
Chopra, Deepak, 286
Cigarettes, 221–222. *See also* Smoking
Circulation. *See* Circulatory system
Circulatory system
  arteries and, 62–63

blood and, 61–62
blood cells and, 61–62, 83
circulation and, 62–64
heart and, 53–58
understanding, 60–64
veins and, 63–64
Clofibrate, 229
Clopidogrel (Plavix), 94, 309
CME. *See* Continuing medical education
Coagulants, anti, 317
Coarctation of aorta, 180
Cocaine, 35
Colesevelam, 229
Colestipol, 229
Complementary and Alternative Medicines
    (CAMs), 282
  legitimate, 286–289
Complete blood count (CBC), 83
Computed tomography scan (CAT scan), 88,
    349
Congenital heart defects, 40–41. *See also*
    Congenital heart disease
  causes, 179
  children and, 178–184
  coarctation of aorta, 180
  heart valve abnormalities, 180
  hypoplastic left heart syndrome, 181
  most common, 180–181
  patent ductus arteriosus, 180
  pregnancy and, 176–177
  septal, 180
  tetralogy of Fallot, 181
  transposition of great arteries, 181
Congenital heart disease
  acquired and, 178–184
  causes, 179
  defects, 40–41
Congestive heart failure (CHF), 41–43
Constipation, xx, 22, 124
Constrictive pericarditis, 43
Consumer Reports, 263
Continuing medical education (CME),
    69
Contributing risk factors
  diabetes, 16–20
  HBP, 15–16
  heart disease, 12–21
  high blood cholesterol, 20–21
  obesity and lack of exercise, 13–15
  smoking, 13
Control. *See* Getting control

Cookbooks
  buying basic, 353–354
  library of, 352–353
Cooking
  buying basic cookbooks and, 353–354
  cookbook library and, 352–353
  diets and meals, 243–246, 352–361
  good food choices and, 354–360
  healthy lifestyles and healthy, 243–246,
    352–361
  heart and general health books and, 360–361
Cooking for Two (Weinstein and Scarbrough),
    354
Coronary arteries, 63
Coronary artery bypass
  heart attack and, 100–105
  reducing, 104
  statistics, 100
  surgery and recovery, 106–127
Coronary artery bypass graft (CABG), 6
  having, 120–123
  heart-head link and, 120
  recovery from, 106–127
Coronary artery disease (CAD), 26, 81, 101
  blocked arteries and, 27–28
  pain, 28
  statistics, 25
  treatment, xxiii, xxiv, 28
Cortisol, 269, 271
Coumadin. *See* Warfarin
Covera-HS. *See* Verapamil, extended-release
Cozaar. *See* Losartan
CPR. *See* Cardiopulmonary resuscitation
Crawford, Michael, 256, 257, 259, 265
Crazy Plates (Podleski, J., and Podleski, G.),
    357
Crestor, 94
CT scan. *See* Computed tomography
Cunningham, Marion, 358
Cutaneous fats, 234, 235
CVD. *See* Cardiovascular disease

Dancing, 287
Darling, Jennifer Dorland, 355
DASH diet (Dietary Approaches to Stop
    Hypertension), 248
Death
  heart disease and sudden cardiac, 46–47
  statistics, 25, 46–47, 92, 160, 162, 185,
    188–189, 231
Denial, 137, 167–168, 196, 203, 239

Deponit. *See* Nitroglycerin skin patches

Depression, 22, 110, 124, 129–130, 144, 150, 169, 277, 269–270, 329
  alternative medicines and, 291
  emotions and, 131–134
  statistics, 132–133
  stress and, 268
  symptoms, 132

DES. *See* Drug-eluting stents

Diabetes, 12, 196, 199
  blood lipid target levels and, 20
  contributing risk factors and, 16–20
  diabetic dyslipidemia and, 19
  HDL, LDL and, 20
  heart-disease link and controlling, 19–20
  heart-disease statistics and, 16–17, 18
  insulin resistance and, 19
  obesity and, 18
  shortness of breath, angina and, 16
  triglycerides and, 20
  type 1, 18–19
  type 2, 5, 17, 18, 19, 175
  what's, 18–19

Diabetes Advantage, 334

Diabetic dyslipidemia, 19

Diagnosis, heart transplants and more accurate, 348–349

Diarrhea, xx, 22

Dietary supplements, 294

Diets, xxiv, 22. *See also* Weight loss
  Atkins, 250
  cooking meals and, 243–246, 352–361
  DASH, 248
  dieting and changing, 241–242
  Eat, Drink and Be Healthy, 251
  family impact and, 140–141
  FDA recommended, 247
  HBP and high-sodium, 15
  journals, 259
  living alone and, 330
  Mediterranean, 246–247
  Ornish, 251
  other, 248–251
  Pritikin, 250
  programs, 246–251, 249–253
  South Beach, 251
  statistics, 238
  TLC, 228
  Weight Watchers, 248, 250, 249
  work and, 116–117, 130

Digitalis, 299

Digoxin, 43, 292

Dilacor XR. *See* Diltiazem

Diltia XT. *See* Diltiazem

Diltiazem (Cardizem CD, Cardizem LA, Cardizem SR, Cartia XT, Dilacor XR, Diltia XT, Taztia XT, Tiamate, Tiazac), 94

Diltiazem ER, 310–311

Dining out
  burning calories, 324–325
  celebrations and, 325–326
  not going hungry, 323
  ordering light meals, 323–324
  planning ahead for meals, 322–323
  traveling and, 321–326

Diovan. *See* Valsartan

Diuretics, 94, 300
  African American, Hispanics, smokers and, 15
  contributing risk factors and, 15–16
  heart disease's link to, 38
  high-sodium diets and, 15
  measuring, 16
  Mexican Americans and, 15
  obesity and, 14, 235
  pregnancy and, 175
  statistics, 15, 235

Dizziness, 22

Doctors, 65, 66. *See also* Cardiologists
  ancient Greek, 284
  finding specialists and, 67–69
  first visit with, 72–73
  getting control/recovery and point of view from, 200–202
  jargon, 121
  making choices with, 69–72
  mnemonics and, 121
  offices of, 71
  online research about, 79–80
  preparing to meet with, 73–75
  relationship with, 70, 290
  second opinions and, 76–80
  treatment plans and, 71–72

Down's syndrome, 179

Drinking, 2

Drowsiness, 22

Drug-eluting stents (DES), 98

DynaCirc. *See* Isradipine

Easprin. *See* Aspirin

Eat, Drink and Be Healthy diet, 251

Eat, Shrink and Be Merry (Podleski, J., and Podleski, G.), 357

ECG. *See* Electrocardiogram

Echocardiogram, 5, 37, 40, 41, 85

Ecotrin. *See* Aspirin

ED. *See* Erectile dysfunction

EDTA chelation therapy, 293

Education, knowing about personal health and, 22

Eight Weeks to Optimum Health (Weil), 281, 283, 361

Ejection fraction, 59

Electrocardiogram (ECG), 28, 30, 41, 73, 84, 85, 87, 92

Electromagnetic fields (EMFs), 294

Electronic medical records (EMR), 73, 82

Elliptical machines, 265–266

Embarrassment, 80, 129, 135, 137, 151

Embolus, 39

EMFs. *See* Electromagnetic fields

Eminase. *See* Anistreplase

Emotions, 108

  anger, 10, 277, 269–271

  anxiety and, 135–136

  denial, 137, 167–168, 196, 203, 239

  depression and, 22, 110, 124, 129–134, 144, 150, 169, 277–270, 291, 329

  embarrassment, 80, 129, 135, 137, 151

  heart disease and, 128–146

  intimacy and, 125, 134, 149–159

  low self-esteem and, 129, 134–137, 211

  recovery and, 124–125

  resentment, 129, 136–137

Empirin. *See* Aspirin

EMR. *See* Electronic medical records

Enalapril (Vasotec), 304–305

Endocardium, 52–53

Endothelial dysfunction, 13

Energy medicine, 288

Enoxaparin injection (Lovenox), 315

Epicardium, 52–53

Epinephrine, 269

Eprosartan (Teveten), 307

Eptifibatide (Integrilin), 314

Erectile dysfunction (ED), xx

  meds, 155–159

  statistics, 155

Erectile dysfunction meds

  functions, 156–159

  sex and, 155–159

Essentials of Healthful Cooking (Hess, Jacobi and Simmons), 354

Estrogen, women, heart disease and, 163–165

Exercise, 196, 200

  aerobic, 14, 114, 126, 257, 260–261, 263, 265–267, 287, 325

  contributing risk factors and lack of, 13–15

  equipment, 262–267

  FITT program and, 257, 258, 260

  getting started, 256

  having fun with, 260

  journal, 259

  living alone and compliance with medicines and, 330–331

  made easy, 256–257

  measuring intensity of, 257–258

  plan, 258–260

  right time to, 259

  right way to, 255–267

  RPE and, 258

  safety and, 260

  short-term goals, 259

  statistics, 261, 264

  walking, 260–261

  weight loss and, 242

Exercise equipment

  choosing right, 262–267

  ellipticals, 265–266

  fitness clubs and, 267

  other kinds of, 266

  recumbent bike, 264–265

  treadmills, 263–264

  types of, 263–267

Exhaustion, 108–109

F.A.C.C. *See* Fellows of the American Academy of Cardiology

Family history, 2, 3, 169, 196, 198, 223, 227

Family impact, 203

  diet and, 140–141

  getting with program and, 139

  independence and, 143

  medical problems and, 144–145

  medicines and, 143–144

  mobility and, 142–143

  recovery and, 138–146

  recovery time and, 145–146

  smoking and, 141–142

  support team and, 139–140

Fatigue, 48

Fats, 227

  cutaneous, 234, 235

  healthy cooking and, 243–246

  obesity and, 232, 234–236

Fats (*continued*)
  trans, saturated, monounsaturated and
    polyunsaturated, 228
  visceral, 234, 235, 236
FDA. *See* Food and Drug Administration
Fear, xxiv, 6
Fee For Service plans, 340
Fellows of the American Academy of
    Cardiology (F.A.C.C.), 68
Felodipine (Plendil), 311
Feng Shui, 274
Fertig, Judith, 355
Fibrates, 229
Fibrillation, 37
Fifty Ways to Cook Most Anything (Schloss
    and Bookman), 355
Fight-or-flight response, 270, 271
Fish and Shellfish Grilled and Smoked (Adler
    and Fertig), 355
Fitness clubs, 267
FITT program, 257, 258, 260
Fixx, Jim, 46
Fluvastatin, 229, 300
Food and Drug Administration (FDA),
    recommended diet, 247
Food Network, 244, 264, 355, 356
Food Network Kitchens Cookbook (Darling),
    355
Foods
  cooking and choosing good, 354–360
  FDA recommended diet and, 247
  junk, 196, 200
Fosinopril (Monopril), 305
Foster-Powell, Kaye, 360
Framingham Heart Study, 145
Fungal pericarditis, 44

Gastric bypass surgery, 242, 253–254
Gastrointestinal distress, xx
Gemfibrozil, 229
Gene therapy, 349–350
Genetic disorders, 183–184
Gersh, Bernard J., 361
Getting control
  assessing inventory and, 197–198
  back in business with, 207–208
  doctor's point of view and, 200–202
  game planning and, 203–210
  goals (long-range) and, 208–210
  goals (medium-range) and, 207
  goals (short-range) and, 206–207

health inventory and, 196–197
  inventory-taking and, 195–202
  recovery and, 195–210
  risk-factor replacement and, 198–200
  setting goals and, 205–206
  strategy development for, 204–205
Global perspective
  gaining, 185–192
  heart disease and, 186
  heart disease worldwide and, 187–190
  risk factors of U.S. ethnic population and,
    190–192
Glycoprotein IIb/IIIa inhibitors
  abciximab injection, 313
  eptifibatide, 314
  tirofiban, 314
"Go Red For Women," 161, 170, 171
Goals
  exercise, 259
  getting control with, 206–210
  long-range, 208–210
  medium-range, 207
  short-range, 206–207
Grazing (Van Rosendaal), 356
Guilt, 10

Hawaiians. *See* Native Hawaiians
HBP. *See* High blood pressure
HDL cholesterol (High-Density
    Lipoproteins), 7, 20–22, 197, 201,
    224–225, 226, 227, 228, 229, 235
Health
  general books on heart and, 360–361
  getting control and inventory of, 196–197
  weight loss and regaining, 240
Health care
  choosing insurance plans and, 340–341
  Fee For Service plans and, 340
  HMOs and, 339
  HSAs and, 335–336, 341
  insurance options and, 338–339
  keeping costs in check, 333–336
  keeping medicine costs down and,
    334–335
  navigating, 337–343
  POS plans and, 340
  PPOs and, 339–340
  saving money on, 336
  statistics, 338
  what to do about cost of, 334
  where to seek treatment, 341–343

Health habits, 1
  negative, 106
  not learning about medical condition and, 22
  overcoming bad, xxiii–xxiv
Health illiteracy, xx
Health Maintenance Organizations (HMOs), 339
Health Savings Account (HSA), 335–336, 341
Heart, 51
  alternative medicines for treatment of, 290–295
  basic structure, 47–48
  bundles of Kent in, 53
  bypass surgery, 119–127
  CABG and link between head and, 120
  capillaries, 52
  cardiovascular system's, 52
  chambers, 56
  circulatory system and, 53–58
  diagrams, 49, 56, 57, 97, 103
  ejection fraction, 59
  epicardium, myocardium, endocardium in, 52–53
  general books on health and, 360–361
  His-Purkinje system and, 53
  insides, 54–57
  living alone not good for, 328
  mechanics, 52
  as perfect machine, 52–54
  size, shape, location, 52
Heart and Estrogen-progestin Replacement Study (HERS), 164–165
Heart attack, 22, 28, 29, 196, 198
  acute response to, 92–100
  balloons, stents and, 95–100
  cardio rehab and, 111–114
  causes, 27, 34–35, 114
  coming home from hospital after, 108–109
  coronary artery bypass and, 100–105
  establishing home schedule after, 110
  feelings/emotions with, 108
  first days at home after, 109–114
  how to survive, 89–105
  life after, 107–108
  medicines, 93–94
  MI and, 89–105
  recovery, 106–127
  sex and, 151–152
  "silent," 33
  statistics, 25, 33
  symptoms, 31–33, 89–92

what to do in case of, 34, 91
  working after, 114–118
Heart Attack: A Cleveland Clinic Guide (Rimmerman), 361
Heart beats
  arrhythmias, 36–37, 94, 167, 174
  bradycardia, 37
  fibrillation, 37
  mechanics, 53–54, 58–59
  tachycardia, 37, 42
  Woff-Parkinson-White syndrome and, 53
Heart catheterization, 41
Heart defects
  congenital, 40–41, 178–184
  infants and, 40
  statistics, 41
Heart disease
  acquired, 178–184
  angina pectoris and, xix, 3, 16, 25–27, 29–31, 33, 36, 225
  arrhythmias and, 36–37
  bacterial endocarditis, 37–38
  blocked arteries and, 27–28
  blood tests for, 83
  CAD, 26–28
  cardiac catheterization and, 87–88
  cardiomyopathy, 38–40
  chest X-rays and, 84
  cholesterol and, 224–225
  congenital, 40–41, 178–184
  congenital heart defects, 40–41
  contributing risk factors of, 12–21
  diabetes control and link to, 19–20
  diagnosis, 82–88
  echocardiogram and, 85
  electrocardiograms and, 84
  emotions and, 128–146
  estrogen and, 163–165
  HBP's link to, 38
  heart attack and, 31–35
  heart failure, 41–43
  holter monitors and, 84–85
  major risk factors of, 11–12
  men and, 11
  organizations and websites, 362–365
  other kinds of, 36–50
  patent foramen ovale (hole in heart), 44
  pericarditis, 43–44
  pregnancy and, 174–177
  recognizing, 81–88

Heart disease (*continued*)
red flags, 1–8
reliable information about, 363–365
rheumatic heart disease, 44–45
risk factors, 9–23
silent ischemia, 45
statistics, xix, 3, 9, 11, 16–17, 18, 25,
185–186, 190, 191
stress and, 3–4
stress tests and, 85–87
sudden cardiac death, 46–47
symptoms, 26, 29, 31–33
teaching children about, 347–348
tests, 41
valvular disease, 47–50
waltzing, dancing and, 287
what's, 24–35
women and, xxiv, 11, 160–177
Heart failure
symptoms, 41–42
treatment, 42–43
Heart medicines
most common, 298–300
taking, 296–320
things to know about, 300
traveling with, 301–302
using, 297–298
Heart murmurs, 167, 175
Heart transplants, 38
CT scan and, 349
future, 347–351
gene therapy and, 349–350
more accurate diagnosis and, 348–349
organ donation and, 345–346
procedure, 345
statistics, 344–345
stem cells and, 350–351
teaching children and, 347–348
wellness and, 348
who needs, 344–346
Heart valves, 56
abnormalities in, 180
Hemoglobin, 83
Heparin, 94
enoxaparin injection, 315
injection, 314
low molecular weight, 315
Heroin, 217
HERS. *See* Heart and Estrogen-progestin
Replacement Study
Hess, Mary Abbott, 354

High blood pressure (HBP)
cholesterol and, 20–21
contributing risk factors and, 15–16
heart disease and, 38
high-sodium diets and, 15
medicines and, 299
obesity and, 14, 235
red flags and, 15–16
statistics, 15, 235
Hispanics
diabetes in, 18
HBP in, 15
heart disease statistics and, 190–191
smoking and, 213
His-Purkinje system, 53
hMaxi-K, 158
HMOs. *See* Health Maintenance
Organizations
Holter monitor, 84–85, 174
Homeopathy, 294
Hormone replacement therapy (HRT),
164–165
Hospitals. *See* Academic medical centers
HRT. *See* Hormone replacement therapy
HSA. *See* Health Savings Account
Hypercholesterolemia, 223
Hyperlipidemia, 224
Hypertension, 15–16, 58. *See also* High blood
pressure
pre, 16
Hypertrophy, 42
Hypoplastic left heart syndrome, 181

Imdur. *See* Isosorbide mononitrate
Incentive spirometer, 77
Infants, 40
Inferior vena cava, 64
Insulin, resistance, 19
Insurance, health care, 338–339
choosing plans, 340–341
Fee For Service plans, 340
HMOs and, 339
Medicare, Medicaid and, 337, 341
options, 338–339
POS plans and, 340
PPOs and, 339–340
statistics, 338
Integrative medicine, xxv, 282
Integrilin. *See* Eptifibatide
Intimacy, 125, 134
ED meds and, 155–159

resuming, 152–154
returning to sex and, 149–159
Intravenous clot buster, 4
Irbesartan (Avapro), 307
Iron, 83
Ismo. *See* Isosorbide mononitrate
Isoptin. *See* Verapamil
Isoptin SR. *See* Verapamil, extended-release
Isordil. *See* Isosorbide dinitrate
Isosorbide dinitrate (Isordil, Sorbitrate),
    sublingual and chewable, 315–316
Isosorbide mononitrate (Imdur, Ismo, Isotrate
    ER, Monoket), 316
Isotrate ER. *See* Isosorbide mononitrate
Isradipine (DynaCirc), 311

Jacobi, Dana, 354
Jantoven. *See* Warfarin
JFJ. *See* Junk food junkie
Job stress, 116, 268
Journal of the American College of Cardiology,
    33, 100
Journal of the American Medical Association,
    98, 164, 333
Judd, Sandra J., 360
Junk food junkie (JFJ), 196, 200
Juvenile diabetes. *See* Type 1 diabetes

Kanovsky, Marty, 200–203
Karo, Gus P., xvii
Kawasaki disease, 182
Kidney failure, 42
Koh, Howard, 215

Laetrile, 282
Latino Americans
    diabetes in, 18
    smoking and, 213
LDL cholesterol (Low-Density Lipoproteins),
    7, 20–22, 27, 83, 164, 172, 201,
    224–226, 227–229
    very, 21
Learning to Cook with Marion Cunningham
    (Cunningham), 358
Lescol, 94
Leukemia, 61
Leukocytes. *See* White blood cells
Lifestyles
    creating less intense, 23
    diet and changing, 241–242
    healthy cooking and, 352–361

living alone, 327–332
recovery and changing, 106–127,
    202–210
weight loss, past history and, 239–240
Lipids, 225
    profile, 226
Lipitor, 94
Lisinopril (Prinivil, Zestril), 305
Living alone
    compliance with medicines and exercise,
        330–331
    diet and, 330
    lifestyles, 327–332
    not good for heart, 328
    reality of, 328–329
    safety and, 331–332
    statistics, 328
    staying with cardio program and,
        329–330
Looney Spoons (Podleski, J., and Podleski, G.),
    357
Losartan (Cozaar), 308
Losing weight. *See* Weight loss
Lotensin. *See* Benazepril
Lovastatin, 229, 300
Lovenox. *See* Enoxaparin injection
Low molecular weight heparin, 315
Low self-esteem, 129, 134–137, 211
The Low GI Diet Cookbook (Brand-Miller,
    Foster-Powell, McMillan-Price), 360
Lukins, Sheila, 358
Lund, JoAnna, 353
Lung cancer, 13, 199, 269

Magnetic resonance imaging (MRI), 41, 88
Maharishi Mahesh Yogi, 285–286
Major risk factors
    age and sex, 11
    family history and ethnic background,
        11–12
    heart disease, 11–12
Make the Link! program, 20
Manipulative-based practices, 288, 294
Manson, JoAnn, 361
Maravich, Pete, 46
The March of Dimes, 40, 179
Marijuana, 217
Massage, 282, 285, 288, 294, 295
Mavik. *See* Trandolapril
Mayo Clinic Heart Book (Gersh), 361
McMillan-Price, Joanna, 360

Meals. *See also* Diets; Dining out
  healthier recipes and, 244–246
  ordering light, 323–324
  traveling and planning ahead for, 322–323
  weight loss and cooking, 243–246, 352–361
Medic Alert bracelets, 91
Medicaid, 337, 341
Medical breakthroughs, 284–285
Medicare, 337, 341
Medication. *See also* Medicines
  quick reference chart, 303–320
Medicines, 94, 98, 105
  ACE inhibitors, 42, 94, 285, 299, 304–306,
    307
  adverse effects and, 22, 297
  alternative, xxiv–xxv, 281–295
  angina, 31
  Angiotensin II receptor blockers, 307–308
  anticoagulation, 299
  antiplatelets, 309
  aspirin, 34, 91, 93, 94, 169, 170, 171–172,
    191, 285, 298, 299, 309, 318
  atorvastatin, 229, 300
  Ayurvedic, 285–286, 287
  beta blockers, 31, 43, 94, 299
  birth control pills, 166
  blood cholesterol-lowering agents, 299
  bupropion, 219
  calcium channel blockers, 299, 310–313
  Chantix, 219
  chart for quick reference, 303–320
  Chinese, 287, 295
  cholesterol, 229–230, 299, 300
  cholestyramine, 229
  clofibrate, 229
  colesevelam, 229
  colestipol, 229
  complementary, 282
  digitalis, 299
  diuretics, 300
  ED, 155–159
  family impact and, 143–144
  fibrates, 229
  fluvastatin, 229, 300
  gemfibrozil, 229
  glycoprotein IIb/IIIa inhibitors, 313–314
  HBP, 299
  health care and keeping down costs of,
    334–335
  heart, 296–320
  heart attack and, 93–94

  heparin, 314–315
  hMaxi-K, 158
  integrative, xxv, 282
  living alone and compliance with exercise
    and, 330–331
  lovastatin, 229, 300
  low molecular weight heparin, 315
  meta-analysis of, 300
  nitrates, 299, 315–317
  not taking, 21–22
  oral anticoagulants, 317
  pravastatin, 230, 300
  resins, 229
  rosuvastatin calcium, 230
  salicylates, 318
  side effects and, xx, 5, 22, 297
  sildenafil, 155
  simvastatin, 230, 300
  smoking and, 218–219
  statins, 229–230
  tadalafil, 155
  TCM, 295
  things to know about heart, 300
  thrombolytic agents, 299, 319–320
  traveling with heart, 301–302
  using heart, 297–298
  vardenafil, 155
  varenicline, 219
  Viagra, 155
Meditation, 285
Mediterranean diet, 246–247, 359
Men
  cardiac symptoms in women v., 162–165
  common risk factors shared by women and,
    167–170
  ED statistics and, 155
  heart attack statistics and, 31, 33, 35
  heart attack symptoms and, 90
  heart disease and, 11, 185–186
Metoprolol, 94
Mevacor, 94
Mexican Americans, 12
  diabetes in, 18
  HBP in, 15
  obesity and, 234
MI. *See* Myocardial infarction
Micardis. *See* Telmisartan
Mind-body medicines, 288, 290
Minitran. *See* Nitroglycerin skin patches
Mitral valve prolapse (MVP), 48, 49
Mnemonics, 121

Moexipril (Univasc), 305
Monoket. *See* Isosorbide mononitrate
Monopril. *See* Fosinopril
Monounsaturated fats, 228
Mosca, Lori, 171
MRI. *See* Magnetic resonance imaging
MVP. *See* Mitral valve prolapse
Myocardial infarction (MI), xx, 4, 7, 31, 35, 106
  treatment, 33–34, 46 (*See also* Heart attack)
Myocardium, 38, 52–53

National Center for Health Statistics, 15
National Diabetes Education Program (NDEP), 20
National Heart, Lung, and Blood Institute, 34, 90, 94, 98, 228, 232
National Institute for Occupational Health and Safety (NIOSH), 114, 268
National Institute of Mental Health (NIMH), 131
National Institute on Drug Abuse (NIDA), 215
The National Center for Complementary and Alternative Medicine (NCCAM), 283, 285, 286, 288
Native Americans, 12
  diabetes in, 18
  heart disease statistics and, 190–191
  smoking and, 213
Native Hawaiians, 12
Naturopathy, 287, 294
Nausea, 22, 90
NCCAM. *See* The National Center for Complementary and Alternative Medicine
NDEP. *See* National Diabetes Education Program
Necrotic tissue, 32
Neiditch, Jean, 250
New England Journal of Medicine, 169
New Glucose Revolution (Brand-Miller, Foster-Powell, McMillan-Price), 360
The New Basics Cook (Rosso and Lukins), 358
Niacin, 230
Nicardipine (Cardene), 311–312
Nicardipine SR (Cardene SR), 312
Nicotine, 215, 216, 219, 221. *See also* Smoking
NIDA. *See* National Institute on Drug Abuse
Nifediac CC. *See* Nifedipine ER

Nifedipine, 94
Nifedipine ER (Adalat CC, Afeditab CR, Nifediac CC, Procardia XL), 312
NIMH. *See* National Institute of Mental Health
911, 32, 34, 37, 90, 91
NIOSH. *See* National Institute for Occupational Health and Safety
Nisoldipine (Sular), 312–313
Nitrates, 299
  isosorbide dinitrate, sublingual and chewable, 315–316
  isosorbide mononitrate, 316
  nitroglycerin ER, 316
  nitroglycerin skin patches, 316–317
  nitroglycerin spray, 317
Nitro-Bid Ointment. *See* Nitroglycerin ointment
Nitrodisc. *See* Nitroglycerin skin patches
Nitro-Dur. *See* Nitroglycerin skin patches
Nitroglycerin, 3, 30, 33, 91
Nitroglycerin ER (Nitroglyn), 316
Nitroglycerin ointment (Nitro-Bid Ointment, Nitrol), 316–317
Nitroglycerin skin patches (Deponit, Minitran, Nitro-Dur, Nitrodisc, Transderm-Nitro), 316–317
Nitroglycerin spray (Nitrolingual), 317
Nitroglyn. *See* Nitroglycerin ER
Nitrol. *See* Nitroglycerin ointment
Nitrolingual. *See* Nitroglycerin spray
Norvasc. *See* Amlodipine
Nuclear stress test, 5, 41

Obesity, 12, 196, 199. *See also* Weight loss
  apple or pear, 235
  BMI and, 232–234
  causes, 234–235
  children already at-risk for, 236–237
  contributing risk factors and, 13–15
  diabetes and, 18
  fats and, 232, 234, 235, 236
  HBP and, 14, 235
  overcoming, 237
  recognizing, 231–232
  results of, 235–236
  statistics, 14, 145, 231, 234, 236
  weight loss and, 15
Olmesartan (Benicar), 308
Oral anticoagulants, warfarin, 293, 317
Oral contraceptives, 214

Organ donation, 345–346
Ornish, Dean, 251, 249
Ornish diet, 251, 249
Osteopathy, 294–295
Oz, Mehmet C., 361

PA. *See* Physician assistant
Pain
  CAD and, 28
  chest, xix, 3, 26, 27, 29, 31, 33, 36, 48, 90,
    225
  surgery, recovery and, 123–124
Patent ductus arteriosus, 180
Patent foramen ovale (PFO), 44
Patients, types of, 201–202
PCI. *See* Percutaneous coronary intervention
Penicillin, 285
Percutaneous coronary intervention (PCI), 95
Pericarditis, 43–44
Perindopril (Aceon), 306
PFO. *See* Patent foramen ovale
Phlebotomist, 83
Physician assistant (PA), 73
The Pill Book (Chilnick), 3
Plaque, 28, 34, 94, 99
Plasma, 62
Platelets, 62, 83
Plavix, 98. *See also* Clopidogrel
Plendil. *See* Felodipine
Podleski, Greta, 357
Podleski, Janet, 357
Point-Of-Service plans (POS), 340
Polyunsaturated fats, 228
POS. *See* Point-Of-Service plans
PPOs. *See* Preferred Provider Organizations
Pravachol, 94
Pravastatin, 230, 300
Pre-eclampsia, 175
Preferred Provider Organizations (PPOs),
  339–340
Pregnancy
  amniotic fluid embolism and, 176
  blood clots and, 176
  congenital heart conditions and risks
    during, 176–177
  HBP and, 175
  heart disease and, 174–177
  heart murmurs and, 175
  non-heart problems and, 175–176
  pre-eclampsia and, 175
  smoking and, 221

stroke and, 175
  Type 2 diabetes and, 175
  varicose veins and, 176
Pre-hypertension, 16
*Prevention's Quick and Healthy Low-Fat
  Cooking* (Rogers), 358
Prinivil. *See* Lisinopril
Pritikin diet, 250
Pritikin, Nathan, 250
Procardia XL. *See* Nifedipine ER
Procrastination, 275
Programs
  diet and weight-loss, 246–251, 249–253
  exercise and FITT, 257–258, 260
  family impact and getting with, 139
  living alone and staying with cardio,
    329–330
  Make the Link!, 20
  NDEP, 20
  stress management, 275, 276, 270
Propranolol, 94
Protamine, 105
Pulmonary artery, 63
Pulse assessment, 125–127
Pure Comfort (Weight Watchers International
  Inc.), 359

Qi gong, 289, 295
Quinapril (Accupril), 306

Ramipril (Altace), 306
Rated Perceived Exertion Scale (RPE), 258
Recovery
  CABG, 106–127
  changing lifestyles and, 106–127, 202–210
  coronary artery bypass surgery and,
    106–127
  doctor's point of view, 200–202
  family impact and, 138–146
  getting control and, 195–210
  heart-attack, 106–127
  pulse assessment and, 125–127
  sex life and, 125
  surgery and emotions during, 124–125
  surgery, pain and, 123–124
  time, 145–146
Recumbent exercise bike, 264–265
Red blood cells, 61
Red flags
  diabetes, 5
  family history/high risk, 2, 3

HBP, 3
heart-disease, 1–8
MI, 4, 5
shortness of breath, 5
smoking and drinking, 2
Reiki, 289, 295
Relationships, personal, xxiv
with doctors, 70, 290
ReoPro. See Abciximab injection
Resentment, 129, 136–137
Resins, 229
Retavase. See Reteplase
Reteplase (Retavase), 319
RHD. See Rheumatic heart disease
Rheumatic fever, 44–45, 48, 101, 181–182,
186
Rheumatic heart disease (RHD), 44–45
Rimmerman, Curtis, M., xvii, 72, 107, 118,
199, 240, 361
Risk factors
African Americans and, 12
age and sex, 11
Asian Americans and, 12
contributing, 12–21
diabetes, 16–20
family history and ethnic background,
11–12
getting control and replacing, 198–200
HBP, 15–16
heart disease, 9–23
high blood cholesterol, 20–21
lack of knowledge about personal health,
22
major, 11–12
Mexican Americans and, 12
Native Americans and, 12
Native Hawaiians and, 12
obesity, 236–237
obesity and lack of exercise, 13–15
recognizing, 10–11
skipping meds, 21–22
smoking, 13, 214
stress, 22
top ten, 196
unofficial, 21–23
Rocky Mountain Spotted Fever, 182
Rogers, Gene, 358
Roizen, Michael F., 361
Rosen, Rochelle, 92
Rosso, Julee, 358
Rosuvastatin calcium, 230

RPE scale. See Rated Perceived Exertion
Scale (RPE)

Safety, living alone and, 331–332
Salicylates
aspirin, 318
aspirin gum, 318
Saturated fats, 228
Scarbrough, Mark, 354
Scars, 34, 40, 95, 108, 123, 124, 151, 328
SCD. See Sudden cardiac death
Schloss, Andrew, 355
Second opinions, getting, 76–80
Second-hand smoke, 13, 212–214
Self-esteem. See Low self-esteem
Septal defect, 180
Sex, 196, 199–200
ED meds and, 155–159
guidelines for resuming, 153–154
heart attacks and, 151–152
life, 125
returning to intimacy and, 149–159
where to start with, 150–151
Side effects, xx, 5, 22, 297
Sildenafil, 155. See also Viagra
Silent ischemia, 45
Simmons, Marie, 354
Simvastatin, 230, 300
60 Ways to Make Stress Work for You (Slaby),
274, 277
Slaby, Drew M., 274, 277
Sleep, 109–110, 118, 124, 132, 150, 152,
236, 275, 329
Smoking, xxiv, 2, 35, 45, 196, 199
addiction, 216–220
bans, 187–188
children, cigarettes and, 221–222
contributing risk factors and, 13, 168
damages sustained from, 188–189
death statistics, 188–189
difficulty quitting, 215
family impact and, 141–142
going cold turkey and, 219–220
HBP and, 15
heart-attack risk and, 13, 214
how to stop, 217–220
LDL and, 227
medicines and, 218–219
oral contraceptives and, 214
personal health enemy No. 1, 212
pregnancy and, 221

Smoking (*continued*)
  quitting, 28, 139, 211–222
  second-hand smoke and, 212–214
  START and, 218
  statistics, 188–189, 212, 213, 221–222
  support groups and, 218
  weight gain and, 220–221
  women and, 214, 225
Solomon, Harold, 22, 133
Sopko, George, 170
Sorbitrate. *See* Isosorbide dinitrate
South Beach diet, 251
Specialists. *See* Cardiologists
St. John's Wort, 291, 292
Standard of care, 70
START, 218
Statins, 229–230
Statistics
  African Americans, 190–191
  alternative medicines, 283, 288
  angina pectoris, 25
  Asian Americans, 190–191
  BMI, 234
  CAD, 25
  Caucasians, 190–191
  congenital heart disease, 178
  coronary artery bypass, 100
  CVD, 3
  death, 25, 46–47, 92, 160, 162, 185,
    188–189, 231
  depression, 132–133
  diabetes and heart-disease, 16–17, 18
  diets, 238
  diuretics, 15, 235
  ED, 155
  exercise, 261, 264
  HBP, 15, 235
  health care, 25, 33
  heart attack, 31, 116
  heart defects, 41
  heart disease, xix, 3, 9, 11, 16–17, 18, 25,
    185–186, 190, 191
  heart transplants, 344–345
  Hispanics, 190–191
  insurance, 338
  job stress, 116, 268
  living alone, 328
  men, 31, 33, 35, 155
  Native Americans, 190–191
  obesity, 14, 145, 231, 234, 236
  SCD, 46–47

  smoking, 188–189, 212, 213, 221–222
  stress, 269
  stroke, 25
  valvular disease, 47
  women, 25, 31, 33, 35, 125, 160, 162,
    185
Stem cells, 350–351
Stents, 43, 66, 71, 88, 104, 240, 298
  drug-eluting, 98
  heart attack, balloons and, 95–100
Stir It Up (Weight Watchers International
    Inc.), 359
Strep throat, 44–45
Streptase. *See* Streptokinas
Streptokinas (Streptase), 319–320
Stress, xxiii, 3–4, 6, 23, 169
  addicted to, 268–269
  biological basis for, 270–271
  cortisol and, 269, 271
  depression and, 268
  epinephrine and, 269
  Feng Shui and, 274
  fight-or-flight response and, 270, 271
  final word about, 277
  gaining control of, 275–276
  job, 116, 268
  making allies with, 274–275
  management programs, 275–276, 270
  managing, 273–272
  procrastination and, 275
  professional help with, 276–277
  risk factors, 22
  statistics, 116, 268, 269
  sympathetic nervous system and, 271
  tests, 5, 41, 85–87
  thallium test and, 86
  traveling and reducing, 325
  triggers, 272
  what's, 269–270
  women and, 269
  worldwide phenomenon of, 269
Stroke, 17, 22, 28
  mini, 44, 96
  pregnancy and, 175
  statistics, 25
Sudden cardiac death (SCD), statistics,
    46–47
Sular. *See* Nisoldipine
Superior vena cava, 64
Support teams
  diet programs and, 249–253

friends and family, 139–140, 203
smoking, 218
Surgeon General, U.S., 12
Sympathetic nervous system, 271
Symptoms
angina pectoris, 29
depression, 132
heart attack, 31–33, 89–92
heart disease, 26, 29, 31–33
heart failure, 41–42
specific cardiovascular risk, 165–167
Syndromes
Down's, 179
hypoplastic left heart, 181
Turner's, 179
WISE and, 163, 170
Woff-Parkinson-White, 53

Tachycardia, 37, 42
Tadalafil, 155
Tai chi, xxiv
Taztia XT. See Diltiazem
TCM. See Traditional Chinese Medicine
Telmisartan (Micardis), 308
Tenecteplase (TNKase), 320
Tests
blood, 83
heart disease, 41, 83, 85–87
nuclear stress, 5, 41
stress, 5, 41, 85–87
thallium stress, 86
Tetralogy of Fallot, 181
Teveten. See Eprosartan
Thallium stress test, 86
Therapeutic touch, 295
The 30-Minute Fitness Solution (Manson and
Amend), 361
Thrombolytic agents, 299
reteplase, 319
streptokinas, 319–320
tenecteplase, 320
urokinase, 320
Thrombus, 39
TIA. See Transient ischemic attack
Tiamate. See Diltiazem
Tiazac. See Diltiazem
Ticlid. See Ticlopidine
Ticlopidine (Ticlid), 309
Tirofiban (Aggrastat), 94, 314
TLC Diet (Therapeutic Lifestyle Changes),
228

TNKase. See Tenecteplase
Toxemia, 167
Traditional Chinese Medicine (TCM), 287,
295
Trandolapril (Mavik), 306
Trans fats, 228
Transderm-Nitro. See Nitroglycerin skin
patches
Transient ischemic attack (TIA), 44, 96,
99
Transplants. See Heart transplants
Transposition of great arteries, 181
Traveling
dining out and, 321–326
heart-healthy, 322
medicines and, 301–302
stress reduction and, 325
Treadmills, 263–264
Treatments
alternative medicines and ancient,
285–286
angina pectoris, 30–31
CAD, xxiii, xxiv, 28
cardiologists and plans for, 71–72
heart, 290–295
heart failure, 42–43
MI, 33–34, 46
where to seek, 341–343
Triglycerides, 20, 21, 225, 226, 227. See also
VLDL
Turner's syndrome, 179
Type 1 diabetes, 18–19. See also Diabetes
Type 2 diabetes, 2, 5, 17, 18, 19, 175. See
also Diabetes

Univasc. See Moexipril
Uremic pericarditis, 44
Urokinase (Abbokinase), 320

Valsartan (Diovan), 308
Valves. See Heart valves
Valvular disease
basic heart structure and, 47–50
statistics, 47
Van Rosendaal, Julie, 356
Vardenafil, 155
Varenicline, 219
Varicose veins, 176
Vascor. See Bepridil
Vasculitis, 182
Vasotec. See Enalapril

Veins, 63–64
  diagram, 102
  inferior vena cava, 64
  superior vena cava, 64
  varicose, 176
Verapamil (Calan, Isoptin), 94, 313
Verapamil, extended-release (Calan SR,
  Covera-HS, Isoptin SR, Verelan, Verelan
  PM), 313
Verelan. See Verapamil, extended-release
Verelan PM. See Verapamil, extended-release
Viagra, 155
Viral pericarditis, 43
Visceral fats, 234, 235, 236
Vision, blurred, 22
Vitamins, xxiv, 290, 291–292
VLDL (very low-density lipoproteins), 21
Vomiting, 22

Walking, 260–261
Waltzing, 287
Warfarin (Coumadin, Jantoven), 293, 317
The Wealthy Barber (Chilton), 357
WebMD, 364
Weight gain, 42, 196, 199, 227
  smoking and, 220–221
Weight loss, 15, 22
  changing diets, dieting and, 241–242
  cooking meals and, 243–246, 352–361
  diet programs and, 246–251, 249–253
  exercise and, 242
  gastric bypass surgery and, 253–254
  joining programs for, 249–253
  maintaining, 238–254
  other alternatives for, 246
  past history, lifestyle and, 239–240
  regaining health through, 240
  reinforcements and, 240–241
  requirements, 240–241
Weight Watchers, 248, 250, 249, 259, 359
Weight Watchers New Complete Cookbook,
  359, 360
Weil, Andrew, xxv, 281, 282, 283, 284, 286,
  361
Weinstein, Bruce, 354
White blood cells, 61, 83
WHO. See World Health Organization
Whole medical systems, 287
Willett, Walter C., 251
Williams Sonoma cookbooks, 354

WISE. See Women's Ischemia Syndrome
  Evaluation Study
Woff-Parkinson-White syndrome, 53
Women
  African-American, 125, 160
  birth control pills and, 166, 214
  breast cancer and, 25, 150, 161–162
  cardiac symptoms in men v., 162–165
  Caucasian, 25, 160, 167–170
  common risk factors shared by men and,
    167–170
  death statistics and, 25, 125, 160, 162, 185
  estrogen and, 163–165
  Go Red For, 161, 170, 171
  heart attack statistics and, 31, 33, 35
  heart attack symptoms in, 90
  heart disease and, xxiv, 11, 160–177
  heart murmurs in, 167
  obesity and, 234
  pregnancy and, 174–177
  reducing cardiovascular risk in, 170–173
  smoking and, 214, 225
  specific cardiovascular risk symptoms in,
    165–167
  statistics, 25, 31, 33, 35, 125, 160, 162,
    185
  stress and, 269
  treating heart disease in, 170
Women's Ischemia Syndrome Evaluation
  Study (WISE), 163, 170
  recommendations, 171
Work
  diets and, 116–117, 130
  heart attack and returning to, 114–118
World Health Organization (WHO), 186,
  187, 231

X-rays, 41, 84, 87, 285

Yoga, xxiv
You: The Owners Manual (Roizen and Oz),
  361
Your Heart: An Owner's Manual (American
  Heart Association), 361

Zestril. See Lisinopril
"Zipper," 123, 328. See also Scars
Zocor, 94
Zone diets, 249
Zorprin. See Aspirin